T0263228

Risk, Error and Uncertainty: Laboratory Quality Management in the Age of Metrology

Editors

JAMES O. WESTGARD
DAVID ARMBRUSTER
STEN A. WESTGARD

CLINICS IN LABORATORY MEDICINE

www.labmed.theclinics.com

March 2017 • Volume 37 • Number 1

ELSEVIER

1600 John F. Kennedy Boulevard ● Suite 1800 ● Philadelphia, Pennsylvania, 19103-2899

http://www.theclinics.com

CLINICS IN LABORATORY MEDICINE Volume 37, Number 1
March 2017 ISSN 0272-2712, ISBN-13: 978-0-323-47743-7

Editor: Stacy Eastman
Developmental Editor: Colleen Dietzler

© 2017 Elsevier Inc. All rights reserved.

This periodical and the individual contributions contained in it are protected under copyright by Elsevier, and the following terms and conditions apply to their use:

Photocopying
Single photocopies of single articles may be made for personal use as allowed by national copyright laws. Permission of the Publisher and payment of a fee is required for all other photocopying, including multiple or systematic copying, copying for advertising or promotional purposes, resale, and all forms of document delivery. Special rates are available for educational institutions that wish to make photocopies for non-profit educational classroom use. For information on how to seek permission visit www.elsevier.com/permissions or call: (+44) 1865 843830 (UK)/(+1) 215 239 3804 (USA).

Derivative Works
Subscribers may reproduce tables of contents or prepare lists of articles including abstracts for internal circulation within their institutions. Permission of the Publisher is required for resale or distribution outside the institution. Permission of the Publisher is required for all other derivative works, including compilations and translations (please consult www.elsevier.com/permissions).

Electronic Storage or Usage
Permission of the Publisher is required to store or use electronically anymaterial contained in this periodical, including any article or part of an article (please consult www.elsevier.com/permissions). Except as outlined above, no part of this publication may be reproduced, stored in a retrieval system or transmitted in any form or by any means, electronic, mechanical, photocopying, recording or otherwise, without prior written permission of the Publisher.

Notice
No responsibility is assumed by the Publisher for any injury and/or damage to persons or property as a matter of products liability, negligence or otherwise, or from any use or operation of any methods, products, instructions or ideas contained in the material herein. Because of rapid advances in the medical sciences, in particular, independent verification of diagnoses and drug dosages should be made.

Although all advertising material is expected to conform to ethical (medical) standards, inclusion in this publication does not constitute a guarantee or endorsement of the quality or value of such product or of the claims made of it by its manufacturer.

Reprints. For copies of 100 or more, of articles in this publication, please contact the Commercial Reprints Department, Elsevier Inc., 360 Park Avenue South, New York, New York 10010-1710. Tel. 212-633-3874, Fax: 212-633-3820, E-mail: reprints@elsevier.com.

Clinics in Laboratory Medicine (ISSN 0272-2712) is published quarterly by Elsevier Inc., 360 Park Avenue South, New York, NY 10010-1710. Months of issue are March, June, September, and December. Business and Editorial offices: 1600 John F. Kennedy Blvd., Suite 1800, Philadelphia, PA 19103-2899. Periodicals postage paid at NewYork, NY and additional mailing offices. Subscription prices are $258.00 per year (US individuals), $488.00 per year (US institutions), $100.00 per year (US students), $314.00 per year (Canadian individuals), $593.00 per year (Canadian institutions), $185.00 per year (Canadian students), $402.00 per year (international individuals), $593.00 per year (international institutions), $185.00 (international students). Foreign air speed delivery is included in all Clinics subscription prices. All prices are subject to change without notice. POSTMASTER: Send address changes to *Clinics in Laboratory Medicine*, Elsevier Health Sciences Division, Subscription Customer Service, 3251 Riverport Lane, Maryland Heights, MO 63043. **Customer Service: 1-800-654-2452 (US). From outside of the US and Canada, call 1-314-447-8871. Fax: 1-314-447-8029. E-mail: journalscustomerservice-usa@elsevier.com (for print support) or journalsonlinesupport-usa@elsevier.com (for online support).**

Clinics in Laboratory Medicine is covered in *EMBASE/Exerpta Medica, MEDLINE/PubMed (Index Medicus), Cinahl, Current Contents/Clinical Medicine, BIOSIS* and *ISI/BIOMED.*

Contributors

EDITORS

JAMES O. WESTGARD, PhD
Professor Emeritus, Department of Pathology and Laboratory Medicine, School of Medicine and Public Health, University of Wisconsin; Westgard QC, Inc, Madison, Wisconsin

DAVID ARMBRUSTER, PhD, DABCC, FACB
Director, Clinical Chemistry, Abbott Diagnostics, Abbott Park, Illinois

STEN A. WESTGARD, MS
Director, Client Services and Technology, Westgard QC, Inc, Madison, Wisconsin

AUTHORS

VIRTUDES ÁLVAREZ, MD
Spanish Society of Laboratory Medicine (SEQC), Commission of Analytical Quality, Barcelona, Padilla, Spain

ADA AITA, Biol Sci
Department of Laboratory Medicine, University Hospital of Padova, Padova, Italy

DAVID ARMBRUSTER, PhD, DABCC, FACB
Director, Clinical Chemistry, Abbott Diagnostics, Abbott Park, Illinois

CARMEN BIOSCA, PhD
Spanish Society of Laboratory Medicine (SEQC), Commission of Analytical Quality, Barcelona, Padilla, Spain

RAQUEL BLAZQUEZ, MD
Programa de Supervisión Externa de la Calidad y Comisión de Garantía de Calidad del Laboratorio Clínico, Spanish Association of Pharmaceutical Analists (AEFA), Madrid, Spain

BEATRIZ BONED, MD
Spanish Society of Laboratory Medicine (SEQC), Commission of Analytical Quality, Barcelona, Padilla, Spain

FERNANDO CAVA, MD
Spanish Society of Laboratory Medicine (SEQC), Commission of Analytical Quality, Barcelona, Padilla, Spain

NAVAPUN CHARURUKS, MD, FRCPath (Thailand)
Laboratory Department, Bumrungrad International Hospital, Bangkok, Thailand

ZORAIDA CORTE, PhD
Spanish Society of Laboratory Medicine (SEQC), Commission of Analytical Quality, Barcelona, Padilla, Spain

JORGE DÍAZ-GARZÓN, MD
Spanish Society of Laboratory Medicine (SEQC), Commission of Analytical Quality, Barcelona, Padilla, Spain

EMMA ENGLISH, PhD
Lecturer in Health Science, Faculty of Medicine and Health, School of Health Science, University of East Anglia, Norwich, United Kingdom

PILAR FERNÁNDEZ-CALLE, PhD
Spanish Society of Laboratory Medicine (SEQC), Commission of Analytical Quality, Barcelona, Padilla, Spain

PILAR FERNÁNDEZ-FERNÁNDEZ, MD
Spanish Society of Laboratory Medicine (SEQC), Commission of Analytical Quality, Barcelona, Padilla, Spain

JOSÉ VICENTE GARCÍA-LARIO, MD
Spanish Society of Laboratory Medicine (SEQC), Commission of Analytical Quality, Barcelona, Padilla, Spain

ELISABET GONZÁLEZ, MD
Spanish Society of Laboratory Medicine (SEQC), Commission of Analytical Quality, Barcelona, Padilla, Spain

HAROLD H. HARRISON, MD, PhD, FACB, FCAP
Director of Clinical Pathology, Geisinger Health System, Danville, Pennsylvania

GERALD A. HOELTGE, MD, FCAP
Checklist Commissioner, College of American Pathologists, Northfield, Illinois

JAMUNA JAIRAMAN, BSc, MPH
Senior Manager, Allied Health Support, Pathology Laboratory Department, Sunway Medical Centre, Selangor, Malaysia

JAY B. JONES, PhD, D(ABCC), FACB
Director (Ret.), Clinical Chemistry, Geisinger Regional Laboratories, Danville, Pennsylvania

JOSEP M. JOU, MD
Comité de Estandarización. Spanish Society of Hematology and Hemotherapy (SEHH), Madrid, Spain

ERNA LENTERS-WESTRA, PhD
HbA1c Researcher, European Reference Laboratory for Glycohemoglobin, Clinical Chemistry Department, Isala, Zwolle, The Netherlands

LEE SUAN LI, BSc
Senior Medical Laboratory Scientist, Pathology Laboratory Department, Sunway Medical Centre, Selangor, Malaysia

JOSEPH LITTEN, PhD
Corporate Technical and Development Manager, Laboratory, Valley Health, Winchester, Virginia

JOANA MINCHINELA, MD
Spanish Society of Laboratory Medicine (SEQC), Commission of Analytical Quality, Barcelona, Padilla, Spain

JORGE MORANCHO, MD
Programa de Supervisión Externa de la Calidad y Comisión de Garantía de Calidad del Laboratorio Clínico, Spanish Association of Pharmaceutical Analists (AEFA), Madrid, Spain

CARMEN PERICH, MD
Spanish Society of Laboratory Medicine (SEQC), Commission of Analytical Quality, Barcelona, Padilla, Spain

MARIO PLEBANI, MD
Department of Laboratory Medicine, University Hospital of Padova, Padova, Italy

ENRIQUE PRADA, MD
Comité de Calidad, Gestión, Seguridad y Evidencia. Spanish Association of Medical Biopathology-Laboratory Medicine (AEBM-LM), Madrid, Spain

FRANCISCO RAMÓN, MD
Comité de Programas Externos de la Calidad, Spanish Society of Clinical Chemistry and Laboratory Medicine (SEQC), Barcelona, Padilla, Spain

CARMEN RICÓS, PhD
Comité de Programas Externos de la Calidad, Spanish Society of Clinical Chemistry and Laboratory Medicine (SEQC), Barcelona, Padilla, Spain

ZARINAH SAKIMAN, BSc
Assistant Manager, Pathology Laboratory Department, Sunway Medical Centre, Selangor, Malaysia

ANGEL SALAS, MD
Comité de Programas Externos de la Calidad, Spanish Society of Clinical Chemistry and Laboratory Medicine (SEQC), Barcelona, Padilla, Spain

LAURA SCIACOVELLI, Biol Sci
Department of Laboratory Medicine, University Hospital of Padova, Padova, Italy

MARGARITA SIMÓN, MD
Spanish Society of Laboratory Medicine (SEQC), Commission of Analytical Quality, Barcelona, Padilla, Spain

ELVAR THEODORSSON, MD, PhD
Professor, Departments of Laboratory Medicine, Clinical and Experimental Medicine, Linköping University, Linköping, Sweden

JAMES O. WESTGARD, PhD
Professor Emeritus, Department of Pathology and Laboratory Medicine, School of Medicine and Public Health, University of Wisconsin; Westgard QC, Inc, Madison, Wisconsin

STEN A. WESTGARD, MS
Director, Client Services and Technology, Westgard QC, Inc, Madison, Wisconsin

Contents

> Biological variation gives valuable information about how the living organism regulates its constituents within and between subjects; this information on the behavior of body components allows us to derive consequences concerning reference populations and intervals. With a more pragmatic approach biological variation has three uses: setting the appropriate analytical performance specification for each analyte to limit the amount of error that laboratory could introduce in its measurements, to help distinguish health from disease, and to implement internal quality control with the automatic verification of results.

> This study uses three unique data sets to show the state of the art of hemoglobin A1c (HbA1c) analyzers in a range of settings and compares their performance against the international guidance set by the International Federation of Clinical Chemistry and Laboratory Medicine task force for HbA1c standardization. The data are used to show the effect of tightening those criteria, and the study serves as a guide to the practical implementation of the sigma-metrics approach in a range of clinical settings.

> Four external quality assurance programs combined their data to calculate the minimum acceptable quality specifications for laboratory testing. Other sources of quality specifications may be too stringent for the current market, or too lenient given the clinical demands on the test result, but these state-of-the-art goals may be practical and useful. Two main approaches were used: (1) defining the 95% percentile and comparing with other quality specifications, and (2) using an iterative approach to increase the quality specification until 90% of laboratories could achieve 75% of their results within the specification. 72 out of 82 analytes followed procedure 2.

> Six sigma concepts provide a quality management system (QMS) with many useful tools for managing quality in medical laboratories. This Six Sigma QMS is driven by the quality required for the intended use of a test. The most useful form for this quality requirement is the allowable total error. Calculation of a sigma-metric provides the best predictor of risk for an analytical examination process, as well as a design parameter for selecting the statistical quality control (SQC) procedure necessary to detect

medically important errors. Simple point estimates of sigma at medical decision concentrations are sufficient for laboratory applications.

Navapun Charuruks

Laboratory quality control has been developed for several decades to ensure patients' safety, from a statistical quality control focus on the analytical phase to total laboratory processes. The sigma concept provides a convenient way to quantify the number of errors in extra-analytical and analytical phases through the defect per million and sigma metric equation. Participation in a sigma verification program can be a convenient way to monitor analytical performance continuous quality improvement. Improvement of sigma-scale performance has been shown from our data. New tools and techniques for integration are needed.

David Armbruster

At the start of the twenty-first century, a dramatic change occurred in the clinical laboratory community. Concepts from Metrology, the science of measurement, began to be formally applied to clinical laboratory field methods, resulting in a new appreciation of metrological calibrator traceability. It is a change because clinical laboratories test complex patient samples, for example, whole blood, serum, plasma, urine, and so forth, using commercial assay systems, not reference methods, and patient samples are tested once, not in replicate. Analytical harmonization is necessary for optimal patient care but is challenging to achieve.

James O. Westgard

A new Clinical Laboratory Improvement Amendments option for risk-based quality-control (QC) plans became effective in January, 2016. Called an Individualized QC Plan, this option requires the laboratory to perform a risk assessment, develop a QC plan, and implement a QC program to monitor ongoing performance of the QC plan. Difficulties in performing a risk assessment may limit validity of an Individualized QC Plan. A better alternative is to develop a Total QC Plan including a right-sized statistical QC procedure to detect medically important errors. Westgard Sigma Rules provides a simple way to select the right control rules and the right number of control measurements.

Gerald A. Hoeltge

The Laboratory Accreditation Program of the College of American Pathologists (CAP) began in 2015 to allow accredited laboratories to devise their own strategies for quality control of laboratory testing. Participants now have the option to implement individualized quality control plans (IQCPs). Only nonwaived testing that features an internal control (built-in, electronic, or procedural) is eligible for IQCP accreditation. The accreditation checklists that detail the requirements have been peer-reviewed by content experts on CAP's scientific resource committees and by a panel of accreditation participants. Training and communication have been key to the successful introduction of the new IQCP requirements.

Sunway Medical Centre (SunMed) implemented Six Sigma, measurement uncertainty, and risk management after the CLSI EP23 Individualized Quality Control Plan approach. Despite the differences in all three approaches, each implementation was beneficial to the laboratory, and none was in conflict with another approach. A synthesis of these approaches, built on a solid foundation of quality control planning, can help build a strong quality management system for the entire laboratory.

Sigma metrics can be used to predict assay quality, allowing easy comparison of instrument quality and predicting which tests will require minimal quality control (QC) rules to monitor the performance of the method. A Six Sigma QC program can result in fewer controls and fewer QC failures for methods with a sigma metric of 5 or better. The higher the number of methods with a sigma metric of 5 or better, the lower the costs for reagents, supplies, and control material required to monitor the performance of the methods.

ISO 15189:2012 requires the use of quality indicators (QIs) to monitor and evaluate all steps of the total testing process, but several difficulties dissuade laboratories from effective and continuous use of QIs in routine practice. An International Federation of Clinical Chemistry and Laboratory Medicine working group addressed this problem and implemented a project to develop a model of QIs to be used in clinical laboratories worldwide to monitor and evaluate all steps of the total testing process, and decrease error rates and improve patient services in laboratory testing. All laboratories are invited, at no cost, to enroll in the project and contribute to harmonized management at the international level.

The authors developed a system-wide integrated network of instrumentation and Sigma-based quality control for fundamental chemistry, coagulation, and hematology analysis. The authors have based selection of Westgard rules for run management on a straightforward, Sigma-driven selection process. The network includes multiple hospitals and large regional clinic laboratories. Most hospitals have multiple instruments; overall there are at least four distinct instrument models active from each manufacturer. The authors have measured and monitored Sigma values in this network for more than five years, to verify and validate performance and to provide ongoing justification for rules selection and rules changes when necessary.

CLINICS IN LABORATORY MEDICINE

THE CLINICS ARE NOW AVAILABLE ONLINE!
Access your subscription at:
www.theclinics.com

Preface

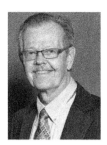
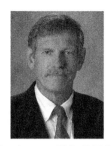
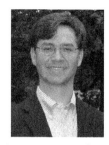

James O. Westgard, PhD   David Armbruster, PhD, DABCC, FACB   Sten A. Westgard, MS

Editors

"Look around, look around, how lucky we are to be alive right now…" This is the hopeful lyric that suffuses the smash hit musical, *Hamilton*. Despite its structure as a tragedy, where the eponymous hero dies in a duel with Aaron Burr, despite all the political infighting, jealousy, back-stabbing, and imperfections of that age, this tour de force is a testament to the optimism that embodies the American ideal.

While laboratory medicine lacks the music, choreography, and staging of a Broadway production, it is nevertheless a time for optimism in our field. True, we are equally beset by politics, jealousies, and vigorous debates, and we are still far from the ideals that laboratory medicine should achieve. But we are so lucky to be alive right now, and see so much progress, and work with so many individuals who are full of energy, generosity, and optimism.

Two years ago, when we first edited an issue of *Clinics in Laboratory Medicine*, the dawn of the Risk Management age was upon us. Laboratories were facing a new frontier: one built on new guidelines (Clinical and Laboratory Standards Institute [CLSI]'s EP23), new approaches (Risk Management), and new tools (Failure Modes and Effects Analysis). It seemed like a daunting task.

In the last 2 years, that challenge has only become more daunting and difficult.

When the Centers for Medicaid and Medicare Services released its guidelines for Individualized Quality Control Plans (IQCP), it became apparent the bar had been moved… but it was lowered, not raised. Instead of asking laboratories to embrace the procedures and power of the Risk Management tools used in industry, labs only have to perform a truncated, qualitative, subjective process for hazard analysis. So much for implementing the Right QC for patient care!

But that is not the only risk that emerged in the last 2 years.

In 2014, the European Federation of Clinical Chemistry and Laboratory Medicine (EFLM) convened a meeting to revisit the 1999 Stockholm Consensus on Quality Specifications. What had transpired to require a review of this consensus? Not much, as it happens. It appears the metrology wing of laboratory medicine wanted to reverse the course of laboratory quality management and prioritize Measurement Uncertainty (MU) as the universal measure of quality. This began as a distinctly European perspective, but was embraced by International Organization for Standardization accreditation

Clin Lab Med 37 (2017) xiii–xvii
http://dx.doi.org/10.1016/j.cll.2016.12.001
0272-2712/17/© 2016 Published by Elsevier Inc.

requirements, and therefore, it has been gaining prominence in the rest of the world. In the Clinical Laboratory Improvement Amendments part of the world, MU has not been adopted because it adds little practical value in laboratory quality management. However, related issues, such as goal setting models and requirements, will impact quality management practices worldwide.

In Milan, some major changes were proposed to the current status quo of quality management. (a) The "Ricos goals" (biological variability) that form the largest and most popularly adopted set of quality specifications and had been supported by numerous Spanish groups for the last 15 years would be absorbed into the EFLM/International Federation of Clinical Chemistry and Laboratory Medicine (IFCC) bureaucracy, to be administered with more control, more rigor, and more requirements. (b) The Stockholm consensus hierarchy of five different levels of quality specifications would be replaced by a slimmer three-level consensus, in which regulatory requirements, expert group recommendations, and "state-of-the-art" were lumped into an equivalent but lesser category. (c) Finally, but most crucially, a new set of "Task-Finishing Groups" was created to address more contentious topics, such as Total Analytic Error as a measure of analytical quality and Allowable Total Error (ATE or TEa as it is popularly known) as a quality goal. The committee's mission included questioning whether the Total Error (TE) approach should continue to exist or preferably be replaced by MU. While that was apparently considered to be a footnote in the meeting, it is truly a radical proposal, and risks compromising the quality management improvements that have been accomplished over the past 40 years.

Much of the debate following the Milan conference has been aired online and in print. Nearly a dozen papers devoted to "MU vs TE" have been printed, primarily in Clinical Chemistry and Laboratory Medicine, the flagship journal of the IFCC. The presidents of EFLM have voiced their opinions that the "uncertainty model" should take priority over the "total error model," with little concern for practical issues such as the daily management of analytical quality in routine clinical laboratories, which operate in stark contrast to highly specialized metrology reference laboratories.

It seems necessary, now more than ever, to present a counterpoint. This issue of Clinics in Laboratory Medicine explains the continuing value of the TE concept, the use of TE goals to determine quality on the Sigma scale, and the practical usefulness and application of the "total error toolbox" for routine quality management in a medical laboratory.

ABOUT OUR CONTRIBUTORS

It falls to me, Sten Westgard, the most junior of all the editors, to serve as the narrator and introduce our cast of characters. Each has a special role to play in this issue. Each has helped move the plot forward for quality improvement.

James O. Westgard, PhD, FACB is of course best known as the father figure of Quality Control, the originator of the eponymous "Westgard Rules" and a perennial paradigm pioneer. He brought no less than five revolutions to the laboratory medicine world, starting with the establishment of a series of Method Validation protocols, later officially codified by CLSI. Next, he introduced the concept of "Total Error" and "Total Allowable Error," a combination of the effects of imprecision and inaccuracy that was greeted as heresy at the time, but soon became the dominant paradigm for evaluating analytical error. It was only then that he completed the work that generated power function graphs and studied the different performance characteristics of various single and multirule QC procedures, one combination of which would eventually become known as the "Westgard Rules." Following that ground-breaking tool, he created the Critical-Error graph and the OPSpecs chart, tools that allowed laboratories for the first time to optimize their QC procedures based on the observed analytical performance. In 2001, he adapted the Six Sigma approach, so popular and successful in manufacturing and industry, to the medical analytical testing process, allowing laboratories to objectively benchmark their performance against a universal standard. This of course is only a brief summary of his books, chapters, papers, workshops, and webinars. A listing of the awards he has received during his career would require an additional article in the issue, so we summarize it by saying, he has been and continues to be thoroughly recognized for his achievements. All this he accomplished while holding just one job for more than 40 years—a distinguished professor at the University of Wisconsin in Madison, at the Medical Technology School and the Hospital and Clinics.

About myself, the less said the better; I am my father's son, a dutiful apprentice to the master for nearly 25 years. When I give lectures, I often explain that I am not following in my father's footsteps, but instead, simply trying to make his footsteps as big as possible. I cannot express how grateful I am, how lucky I feel, to be working with my father and making a difference in so many labs around the world. And, if the previous paragraph wasn't clear enough, I am very proud of my father.

Dave Armbruster, PhD, DABCC, FACB is our coeditor. We recruited him primarily to get a more objective opinion on many of these articles (hoping he would rein in some of our worst tendencies), but also because he has an excellent editor's eye. Dave serves on several scientific committees for key professional organizations, such as the Joint Committee for Traceability in Laboratory Medicine, which maintains a database of reference materials and methods that are the foundation for good laboratory medicine. His perspective as a representative of the in vitro diagnostic device industry is also crucial, because the goals of achieving comparability and traceability, so essential to an uncertainty of measurement approach, require industry to cooperate in establishing harmonization and standardization of assays.

Elvar Theodorsson, MD, PhD, Full Professor in the Department of Clinical and Experimental Medicine of Linkoping University, is a polymath of laboratory medicine, with hundreds of papers published. He has a strong interest in the philosophical approaches of the models of measurement uncertainty and TE. His contribution to this issue addresses the areas of overlap and contrast between these two models and proposes a future where both models can be utilized, rather than a future in which one model eliminates the other.

Carmen Ricos, PhD is one of the leading scientists who launched the compilation of data on biological variation. With colleagues from the Sociedad Española de Bioquímica Clínica y Patología Molecular (SEQC), she helped create the first database of desirable imprecision, inaccuracy, and allowable TE based on within-subject biological variation. This database is often popularly referred to as the "Ricos Goals." Currently, Dr Ricós and her colleagues are continuing this within one of the Task and Force groups derived from the Milan Conference, using a recently developed critical appraisal to classify papers for the final display of the revised data. Together with her colleagues, Virtudes Alvarez, Joana Minchinela, Pilar Fernández-Calle, Carmen Perich, Beatriz Boned, Elizabet González, Margarita Simón, Jorge Díaz-Garzón, José Vicente García-Lario, Fernando Cava, Pilar Fernández-Fernández, Zoraida Corte, and Carmen Biosca (active members of the SEQC-Analytical Quality Commission, some of them since 1982), she provides us with an article with key insights into the practical use of biological variation data in the laboratory as well as an article on the unique "state-of-the-art" goal approach on which the Spanish societies collaborated to generate for External Quality Assurance in Spain, which not only provides us with practical goals but also key information about which goals are practical to achieve for most laboratories.

Gerald A. Hoeltge, MD, FCAP is the checklist commissioner for the College of American Pathologists (CAP) Laboratory Accreditation Program. He provides us with the College's perspective in this issue. The CAP is the leading accreditation provider for full-service laboratories. Dr Hoeltge's narrative on IQCP and quality planning reflects the CAP's rigorous emphasis on laboratory quality. The CAP's implementation of IQCP is thus far the most detailed of all the regulators. It is setting the standard for IQCP implementation.

Erna Lenters-Westra, PhD is an HbA1c Research Coordinator at Isala Klinieken in the Netherlands. Her publications have, over the past decade, concentrated on benchmarking the performance of HbA1c assays. Along with her colleague, Emma English of the University of Nottingham, she participated in the IFCC Task Force on HbA1c standardization. Dr English is also part of the IFCC Committee on Education in the Use of Biomarkers in Diabetes. Together, they contribute an article that discusses the real-world application of TE goals as a way to not only evaluate the acceptability of methods but also drive the standardization, harmonization, and performance improvement of assays. HbA1c is one of the best success stories of standardization, harmonization, and performance improvement of assays, and their discussion reveals which parts of the success can be generalized to other assays and which parts of the success are unique to the nature of the HbA1c assay itself.

Navapun Charuruks, MD, a Diplomate of the Thai Board of Clinical Pathology, the Division Director of the Laboratory for Bumrungrad International Hospital in Bangkok, Thailand, is a tireless driver for laboratory improvement. For several years, she has been implementing Sigma-metrics to evaluate performance and optimize QC. But in her article, she demonstrates it is possible to apply Sigma-metrics not only to the analytical performance of laboratory assays but also to preanalytical and postanalytical processes as well. Thus, her article provides us with a Six Sigma perspective on the Total Testing Process and allows us, possibly for the first time, to make some true apples-to-apples comparisons among the error rates of the different testing phases.

Jamuna Jairaman, Senior Manager, Allied Health Support at Sunway Medical Centre in Selangor, Malaysia, has been implementing Sigma-metrics in her laboratory for nearly a decade. Together with colleagues, Zarinah Sakiman and Lee Suan Li, she contributes an article that compares the Sigma-metric approach to those other current contemporary approaches, MU and IQCP. The experience of Sunway Medical Centre in implementing all three approaches reveals some of the strengths and weaknesses of each technique.

Harold Harrison, MD, PhD is the Director of Clinical Pathology for Geisinger Medical Center in Danville, Pennsylvania. For more than five years, he has guided the implementation of Sigma-metrics across the entire Geisinger Health System, expanding its scope to cover not only chemistry but also hematology and coagulation assays. With years of data, he has enabled Geisinger Medical Laboratories to get a precise view of their long-term performance and comparability.

Joseph Litten, PhD, is the Technical and Development Manager of the Valley Health System in Virginia. A pioneer in the field of performance measurement, he began using Sigma-metrics to assess performance and compare vendors long before any other laboratory in the United States was doing so. His laboratory may have the longest continuously evaluated Sigma-metric performance data in the United States, more than six years of data. He has used that data to not only assess but also improve laboratory operations. His contribution to this issue discusses his monitoring of performance beyond the Sigma-metric and includes outliers, trouble-shooting, error types, and more.

Mario Plebani, MD is the Editor-in-Chief of *Clinical Chemistry and Laboratory Medicine* and perhaps the most-published laboratory professional in the world, with well over 1400 abstracts, books, and chapters to his name. He is a leading figure in the field of preanalytical and postanalytical error, having authored the groundbreaking studies on error rates in the laboratory. He has too many titles, committee chairmanships, and keynotes to mention here. Together with his colleague, Laura Sciacovelli, PhD, the Quality Manager at the Department of Laboratory Medicine of the University Hospital of Padova, Italy, they present an update of the project of the Working Group of the IFCC, "Laboratory errors and patient safety" and EFLM, "Performance specifications for the extra-analytical phases," to create a comprehensive set of quality indicators (QIs) that cover the preanalytical, postanalytical, and intra-analytical phases of the laboratory testing cycle. This represents decades of efforts to standardize QIs so that laboratories around the world can track their error rates in a comparable way.

It is with great pleasure that we, along with our colleagues, present this issue of *Clinics in Laboratory Medicine*, with the hope that we provide the reader with not only a stimulating discussion of about the debate on quality in the laboratory but also a meaningful series of real-world scenarios demonstrating that successful quality management can be accomplished at present with the tools at hand.

Look around, look around, there's plenty to be proud of in our labs right now. How lucky we are to have these colleagues, their examples, and practical tools to help us optimize and improve our performance.

James O. Westgard, PhD
Professor Emeritus
Department of Pathology and Laboratory Medicine
School of Medicine and Public Health
University of Wisconsin
Madison, WI 53705, USA

Westgard QC, Inc.
Madison, WI, USA

David Armbruster, PhD, DABCC, FACB
Clinical Chemistry, Abbott Diagnostics
Department 09AC, Building CP1-5
100 Abbott Park Road
Abbott Park, IL 60064, USA

Sten A. Westgard, MS
Client Services and Technology
Westgard QC, Inc.
7614 Gray Fox Trail
Madison, WI 53717, USA

E-mail addresses:
James@westgard.com (J.O. Westgard)
david.armbruster@abbott.com (D. Armbruster)
westgard@westgard.com (S.A. Westgard)

Measuring Analytical Quality

Total Analytical Error Versus Measurement Uncertainty

James O. Westgard, PhD[a,b,]*, Sten A. Westgard, MS[b]

KEYWORDS

- Total analytical error (TAE) • Allowable total error (ATE)
- Measurement uncertainty (MU) • Accuracy • Bias

KEY POINTS

- The accuracy of a laboratory test depends on both the trueness (bias) and imprecision (SD) of the examination procedure because only a single measurement is made to produce a reportable test result in a medical laboratory.
- Total analytical error (TAE) has been the common way of estimating a 95% limit of the error expected from the combined effects of random and systematic errors when a single measurement is reported as a test result.
- Trends in global practice (International Organization of Standards [ISO]15189) recommend the determination of measurement uncertainty (MU) to characterize the accuracy of medical laboratory tests and discourage the use of allowable total error (ATE).
- Bias is not included in an estimate of MU but rather should be eliminated, corrected, or ignored. If bias were truly eliminated, the TAE and MU models would reduce to a common form and provide consistent estimates of analytical quality.
- The concept of TAE and the definition of quality goals in the form of ATE are critical for a quantitative quality management system (QMS) that provides guidance on acceptability of methods, design of statistical quality control (SQC) procedures, development of risk-based quality control (QC) plans, and external assessment of comparability of results.

INTRODUCTION

Quality continues to be an issue in medical laboratories, both how good laboratory tests are today (precision, trueness or bias, accuracy, total analytical error, and MU) and how good they need to be (goals, allowable errors, and target specifications).

[a] Department of Pathology and Laboratory Medicine, School of Medicine and Public Health, University of Wisconsin, Madison, WI 53705, USA; [b] Westgard QC, Inc, Madison, WI 53717, USA
* Corresponding author. Department of Pathology and Laboratory Medicine, School of Medicine and Public Health, University of Wisconsin, Madison, WI 53705.
E-mail address: james@westgard.com

Clin Lab Med 37 (2017) 1–13
http://dx.doi.org/10.1016/j.cll.2016.09.001
0272-2712/17/© 2016 Elsevier Inc. All rights reserved.

labmed.theclinics.com

Quality is generally defined as conformance to requirements; thus, there is a need to compare the measured performance to a requirement for intended use. In analytical and metrological laboratories, the separate characteristics of precision (random error) and bias (systematic error) are evaluated when multiple measurements are made on each sample. In medical laboratories where only a single measurement is made on each sample, common practice is to estimate the combined effect of precision and accuracy, or TAE, to characterize an upper limit (often 95%) of the size of error expected in a medical test result. More recently, the ISO has recommended that MU be determined for all measurement procedures.

As shown in **Box 1**, accuracy is defined by ISO as the "closeness of agreement between a test result and the accepted reference values; note: The term *accuracy*, when applied to a set of test results, involves a combination of random components (imprecision) and a common systematic error or bias component (ISO 5725-1)." The estimation of TAE in medical laboratories conforms to this definition of accuracy because

---

Box 1
Definitions of important performance characteristics

Accuracy – closeness of agreement between a test result and the accepted reference value (ISO 5725–1); note: the term *accuracy*, when applied to a set of test results, involves a combination of random components (imprecision) and a common systematic error or bias component (ISO 5725-1).

Precision (measurement) – closeness of agreement between indications or measured quantity values obtained by replicate measurements on the same or similar objects under specified conditions (JCGM200:2012); note 1: measurement precision is usually expressed numerically by measures of imprecision, such as SD, variance, or CV under the specified conditions of measurement (JCGM 200:2012).

Trueness (measurement) – closeness of agreement between the average of an infinite number of replicate measured quantity values and a reference quantity value (JCGM 200:2012); note 1: trueness is expressed numerically using the observed bias.

Bias (of measurement) – difference between the expectation of the test result or measurement results and a true value (ISO 3534-2); note 1: bias is an estimate of the systematic measurement error (JCGM 200:2012).

Traceability – (metrological) property of a measurement results where the result can be related to a reference through a documented unbroken chain of calibrations, each contributing to the MU (JCGM 200:2012).

Uncertainty of measurement – parameter, associated with the result of a measurement, that characterizes the dispersion of the values that could reasonably be attributed to the measurand.

TAE – in the context of this guideline, TAE defines the interval that contains a specified proportion (usually 95% or 99%) of the distribution of analytical measurement differences between a measurement procedure operating in its stable in-control state and a comparative measurement procedure that is either a definitive reference method or one that is traceable to one. (Note: also called Total Error [TE])

ATE – an analytical quality requirement that sets a limit for both the imprecision (random error) and bias (systematic error) that are tolerable in a single measurement or single test result; note: also called total error allowable (TEa).

Total error – includes all random and systematic errors that can occur during the total testing process and also includes the combined effect of all precision and bias errors that can affect the accuracy of an analytical result; note: total error incorporates error sources from the preanalytical, analytical, and postanalytical phases of a measurement procedure.

only a single measurement is made to produce a test result; however, ISO does not officially recognize TAE and metrologists prefer MU.

The conflict between TAE and MU has received new attention after a recent conference by the European Federation of Clinical Chemistry and Laboratory Medicine on "Defining analytical performance goals 15 years after the Stockholm Conference on Quality Specifications in Laboratory Medicine." The proceedings were published in the journal, *Clinical Chemistry and Laboratory Medicine* in June 2015, and are available free on the journal's Web site.[1] In response, the authors published an opinion article that reviewed the use of different measures and models for managing analytical quality in medical laboratories and defended the use and practical applications of the total error model.[2] Both an opposing editorial[3] and opposing opinion[4] appeared in the same issue of that journal.

Given that this discussion is taking place in European conferences and documented in European journals, US laboratories may not be aware of the significance of the issue of TAE versus MU. US Clinical Laboratory Improvement Amendments (CLIA) regulations do not adhere to ISO guidelines for measurement traceability and uncertainty; thus, those characteristics need not be considered in validation of performance of laboratory methods in the United States. Instead, validation practices make use of the concept of TAE, the definition of ATE as acceptability criteria in proficiency testing (PT) surveys, and the application of sigma-metrics for characterizing quality, designing SQC procedures, and predicting risk. Risk-based thinking has been a recent trend in ISO guidelines and has also been adopted by Centers for Medicare & Medicaid Services in the new CLIA guidance for risk-based QC (called an individualized QC plan). The authors discuss "Quality Control in the Age of Risk Management" in a previous issue of *Clinics in Laboratory Medicine*.[5] Many of the articles in that issue rely on the concept of TAE and definition of quality goals in the form of ATE. Now the topic of TAE versus MU is even more critical for medical laboratory practice and US laboratories must be informed and become proactive in resolving this.

BACKGROUND

At the Antwerp Conference on Quality in the Spotlight in 1998, Dybkaer[6] recommended that MU should replace TAE based on the following arguments:

- The Guide to the Expression of Uncertainty in Measurement (GUM) approach to uncertainty is rapidly gaining acceptance by metrological institutes and industry and must be applied in ISO and European Committee for Standardization (Comité Européen de Normalisation [CEN]) standards. It should be used in accredited laboratory work, but chemists often find the implementation difficult...
- "Bias always impairs the comparability over space and time of the results for a given type of quantity and distorts the relationships between different types of quantity."
- "The necessary anchor for the trueness of a measurement procedure is obtained by strict metrological traceability of result, based on a calibration hierarchy."
- The upshot of these considerations is that defining a so-called ATE of result, with assessable biases of procedure and laboratory included, should be ceased. Instead, it is necessary to provide corrected results with a defined allowable maximum uncertainty at an agreed level of confidence.

Dybkaer[7] contributed a similar article to the proceedings of the Stockholm conference on quality specifications in 1999,[8] thus initiating the recommendation that MU replace TAE that became part of the Milan agenda. The Stockholm consensus has been the dominate guidance on "analytical quality specifications" for the past 15 years, defining specifications for allowable bias and allowable precision but also including ATE. It formalized a hierarchy of analytical goals and prioritized the use of studies that evaluate the effect of analytical performance on clinical outcome, biologic variability, published professional recommendations, regulatory and external quality assessment (EQA) performance goals, and state-of-the-art performance. The Milan recommendation is to reduce this to 3 models[1]:

Model 1. Based on the effect of analytical performance on clinical outcomes
Model 2. Based on components of biological variation
Model 3. Based on state of the art

An underlying issue is the analytical characteristics for which goals should be defined, for example, allowable bias, allowable precision, ATE, and/or MU (defined allowable maximum uncertainty). As part of the EFLM continuing efforts, a task and finish group (TFG) was initiated and charged with developing a proposal "for how to possibly combine performance specifications for bias and precision in a more scientifically sound way... This TFG is expected to... clarify when the use of TAE can still be useful... or when it should be replaced by the uncertainty estimated.[3] Thus, there is an ongoing effort to replace TAE with MU.

REALITY OF BIAS

The issue of bias is at the core of the arguments about TAE versus MU. The metrology perspective on errors is shown in **Fig. 1**,[9] where the types of errors are arranged to match different analytical concepts and related to appropriate measures. MU is shown as the measure of accuracy under the condition that bias has been eliminated or corrected or can be ignored (purpose of the dotted line (see **Fig. 1**) from bias to MU).

Dybkaer[6] outlined the following process to accomplish this: (1) define type of quantity; (2) select method of measurement for specificity; (3) describe practical measurement procedure; (4) define calibration hierarch for traceability; (5) devise SQC system to reveal any increases in bias; (6) define/validate correction procedures; and (7) participate in EQA. This approach depends on manufacturers to establish rigorous traceability chains for their examination procedures and to eliminate or correct identified error sources. Medical laboratories have a responsibility for establishing appropriate SQC procedures to detect changes in bias and for participating in PT/EQA surveys. The PT/EQA programs have a responsibility for monitoring comparability of

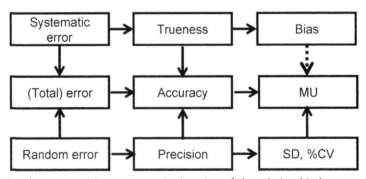

Fig. 1. Metrology perspective on errors. Explanation of the relationship between types of errors, analytical concepts, and measures from Hyltoft Peterson and colleagues.[9] Dotted line from bias to MU is indicates that if bias can be estimated, it should be eliminated.

results and assessing the biases of different analytical systems and methods. Manufacturers have the major responsibility for reducing bias because laboratories have limited capabilities to modify today's analytical devices and measurement procedures, plus there often are regulatory requirements that limit laboratories from making changes in approved analytical systems.

Unfortunately, biases still exist for laboratory tests, even those well standardized tests and certified analytical systems, such as hemogloblin A_{1c} (HbA_{1c}), as documented by evidence from method validation studies[10] and PT/EQA surveys.[11] For example, **Fig. 2** shows results from a 2016 College of American Pathologists survey for HbA_{1c} from 3237 laboratories with 24 different method subgroups for samples whose target value is 5.94% hemoglobin. Deviations of the points (method subgroups) on the Y axis represent the observed biases (as a percentage of the subgroup mean) whereas the values on the X axis represent the observed coefficients of variation (CVs). The solid line represents 2-sigma performance and the dashed line 3-sigma performance. Only 1 method subgroup achieves better than 3-sigma performance whereas 12 method subgroups provide worse than 2-sigma performance. Biases are the significant problem for 8 of those subgroups.

Such biases are understandable because of the physiochemical complexity of measurands, such as HbA_{1c}; the complex sample matrix; and the difficulty of establishing traceability.[12] The existence of bias is the reason TAE, rather than MU, is needed as a practical measure of accuracy in medical laboratories. Because bias

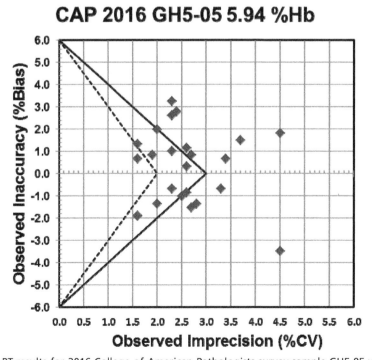

Fig. 2. PT results for 2016 College of American Pathologists survey sample GH5-05 with assigned reference value of 5.94% hemoglobin. Survey includes 3237 laboratories using 24 different methods. Observed subgroup biases are plotted on the Y axis as a percentage of the subgroup mean versus observed subgroup CVs on the X axis. Solid line, 2-sigma performance; dashed line, 3-sigma performance. (*Data from* NGSP.org. Accessed June 2, 2016.)

exists, it must be measured and managed. TAE provides a practical measure of accuracy that includes the effects of both imprecision and bias. ATE is the common form of quality requirement used in most PT/EQA surveys and is consistent with the industrial practice of defining *tolerance limits* that can be used for characterizing quality on the sigma scale. An error framework based on ATE/TEA provides a practical approach and practical tools for managing analytical quality. With specification of ATE, the performance of methods can be validated, quality determined on the sigma scale, appropriate SQC procedures selected, QC plans developed, and safety and quality monitored to identify needs for improvement.[13]

To provide a comprehensive QMS for medical devices and medical laboratories, there are important applications for both the error and uncertainty models. As shown in **Fig. 3**, TAE is the measure of accuracy when bias exists and MU is the measure of performance, either by top-down estimation of intermediate precision or the GUM bottom-up addition of components of uncertainty. MU is useful as a measure of the quality of the traceability chain and together with trueness provides a measure of the comparability results between methods.[2] Manufacturers should use the bottom-up GUM methodology to identify the contributions from individual error sources and hopefully eliminate or correct those errors. Laboratories can provide a top-down estimate of MU from SQC data collected under intermediate precision conditions to verify that the MU observed in production operations is consistent with a manufacturer's performance claims. PT/EQA programs should strive for commutable samples and assignment of target values based on reference methods, then characterize the trueness and MU of analytical systems and assess quality on the sigma scale.[11]

SOME SPECIFIC ISSUES AND ANSWERS

The latest discussions[2–4] highlight some of the ongoing issues that must be resolved to provide an improved and more comprehensive QMS.

Laboratory Versus Manufacturer Applications

Saying that medical laboratories should take care of TAE and IVD manufacturers of measurement uncertainty is a simplification that includes risk to separate responsibilities that should be conversely strongly integrated.[3]

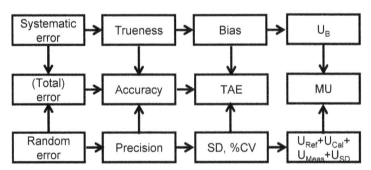

Fig. 3. Medical laboratory perspective on errors. Explanation of the relationship between types of errors, analytical concepts, and measures. In the presence of bias, TAE is the measure of accuracy. In the absence of bias, the uncertainty in the estimate of bias (U_B) is included in MU, along with other uncertainty components, which may be determined from a top-down estimate of imprecision or a bottom-up summations of all components of uncertainty.

Medical laboratories and in vitro diagnostics (IVD) manufacturers depend on each other to achieve quality in laboratory testing. Manufacturers develop examination procedures, validate their performance, and document those performance claims and instructions for use. Laboratories typically verify the manufacturers performance claims, then establish SQC procedures to verify the achievement of the intended quality in routine operation. Manufacturers use complex optimization methodologies during the development of new examination procedures and benefit from the application of the detailed bottom-up GUM methodology for estimation of MU, identification of sources of uncertainty, and reduction through improvements. Laboratories can verify the manufacturers' claims for MU by determination of precision under intermediate precision conditions. Such integration of responsibilities for validation of performance by manufacturers followed by verification in the laboratory is already common practice that can be extended to MU. Laboratories would be more accepting of MU if manufacturers documented their claims for MU, just as manufacturers do for other critical performance characteristics.

Metrology Versus Medical Laboratories

The two main issues favoring the measurement uncertainty paradigm are that most if not all other fields of metrology are using it and that it encourages estimation of the major components of uncertainty and favors actions for their minimization.[4]

There is a reason ISO developed a separate guidance document, 15189, to describe requirements for quality and competence in medical laboratories[12] versus existing guidance for analytical and standards laboratories (ISO/IEC 17025). Medical laboratories are almost unique in their practice of making a single measurement as an estimate of a test result. That single measurement is subject to both random and systematic errors, which is why the TAE concept is applicable as a measure of accuracy. In metrology laboratories, random error is typically minimized by replicate measurements and systematic error minimized by corrections. Corrections in medical laboratories could be hazardous to the health of patients; thus, that practice is often forbidden by regulations and accreditation standards.

Manufacturer Versus Laboratory Responsibility for Bias Correction

GUM states that all bias should be corrected when possible. This is one of the important contradictions within the TAE mode: why maintain the error (bias), when the value is known and can be used in the calculation of TAE?[4]

The idea that inclusion of bias in the estimate of accuracy somehow maintains the existence of bias is illogical. Bias does not exist because it is measured, but rather bias is measured because it exists. Use of MU does not lead or cause laboratories to eliminate bias. Laboratories actually have limited capabilities for eliminating bias, other than recalibrating methods and minimizing the number of changes in reagent lots, and so forth, whereas manufacturers have the capability of changing and redesigning all parts and components of the testing process. Applying corrections is both difficult and possibly hazardous, even when based on patient samples. Many analytical systems use proprietary measurement procedures that have different specificity and selectivity for complex measurands and complex matrices; therefore, bias is a fact of life in a medical laboratory and must be measured, monitored, and managed.

Practical Determination of Measurement Uncertainty

The error paradigm including TAE and ATE struggles when representing numerous and complex factors influencing measurement results and commonly resorts to the simplest models of reality, e.g., the common misconception amongst clinical chemists that the repeatability and reproducibility – as measures of short and long term imprecision – of a measurement result equals its overall measurement uncertainty.[4]

The TAE/ATE framework is a simple model that is easy to understand and has many practical tools to support applications (eg, method decision charts for judging acceptability of methods, sigma-metrics for characterizing quality on the sigma-scale, a sigma SQC selection tool, a chart of operating specifications for identifying appropriate control rules and numbers of control measurements, and a sigma quality assessment tool for monitoring long-term performance with trueness from PT/EQA surveys and intermediate imprecision from SQC data).[11] The simplicity of TAE/ATE is advantageous over the complexity of MU.

The apparent misconception among clinical chemists that MU can be estimated from precision data collected on control materials comes directly from ISO 15189,[14] section 5.5.1.4, note 2:

Measurement uncertainties may be calculated using quantity values obtained by the measurement of quality control materials under intermediate precision conditions that include as many routine changes as reasonable possible in the standard operation of a measurement procedure, e.g. changes of reagent and calibrator batches, different operators, schedule instrument maintenance.

Analytical Versus Preanalytical Factors

The [TAE/ATE] model is however only valid when imprecision and bias are the only variables involved… This model, e.g., does not cater for biological variation and other evident additional causes of variation. This is a serious drawback of this model going forwards as it needs to incorporate possibilities to deal with variation in additional factors. Biologic variation is not relevant when monitoring variation in control samples, but it certainly is when dealing with patient samples.[4]

MU, by definition, applies to only the analytical phase of the total testing process, according to ISO 15189. Biologic variation is not intended to be included as a measure of variation of the analytical testing process itself. See ISO 15189, section 5.5.1.4, note 1[14]:

The relevant uncertainty components are those associated with the actual measurement process, commencing with the presentation of the sample to the measurement procedure and ending with the output of the measured value.

Nonetheless, the TAE model can be expanded to encompass other variables, as illustrated by a clinical decision interval model that includes preanalytical biases and variation as well as within-subject biological variation, as documented in articles published more than 20 years ago.[15–17] This expanded model is particularly useful for assessing the effects of intraindividual biologic variability, number of patient tests on biologic variability, number of specimens on sampling variation, and preanalytical sampling bias as well as precision, bias, effect of number of sample replicates, and SQC performance characteristics. See **Fig. 4** for an example application for a cholesterol method with a decision interval of 20% (200–240 mg/dL) and within-subject biologic variability of 6.0%.

The real issue is a valid interest in characterizing diagnostic uncertainty to improve medical treatment. As discussed in a new report from the Institute of Medicine,[18]

…diagnostic error is underappreciated, even though the correct diagnosis is a critical aspect of health care. The data on diagnostic error are sparse, few reliable

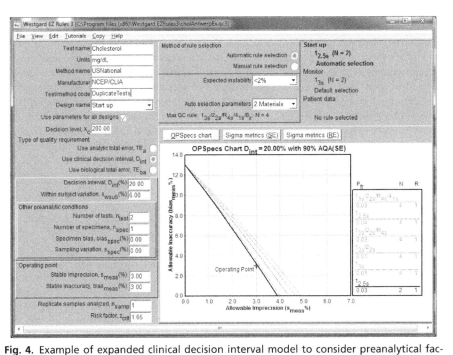

Fig. 4. Example of expanded clinical decision interval model to consider preanalytical factors, such as within-subject biologic variability, number of tests, number of specimens, specimen bias, and sampling variation as well as analytical factors, including imprecision, bias, number of replicate samples, and risk factor.

measures exist, and often the error is identified only in retrospect. Yet the best estimates indicate that all of us will likely experience a meaningful diagnostic error in our lifetime.

The capability to consider effects of preanalytical variability is especially important in optimizing the interpretation of laboratory test results. Both the MU model and the expanded TAE model (clinical decision interval) should be useful for this purpose.

Analytical Versus Clinical Goals for Intended Use

Usually we do not know whether ATE satisfies the intended quality for clinical use of the patient results despite the fact that "acceptance limits" in many proficiency testing/external quality assurance programs are expressed in the form of ATE.[4]

This criticism is not a limitation of the ATE concept, rather a difficulty in defining the goal for how good a measurement procedure should be. That is the purpose of goal-setting models and the reason why appropriate models are needed. MU suffers from the same problem, maybe even worse because advocates of MU are unable to agree on how to define targets for MU. In practice, ATE criteria may be adopted[19] because they are in the form of a 95% to 99.7% limit of error and can be compared with estimates of expanded MU with an appropriate coverage factor, for example, a coverage factor of 2 for a 95% estimate of MU and 3 for a 99.7% estimate.

DISCUSSION

Quality management practices in medical laboratories today favor the use of the error model over the uncertainty model. The TAE model is approximately 40 years old and is widely accepted because of its simplicity and its practicality for laboratory applications. The uncertainty model is approximately 20 years old and has not yet found widespread acceptance or practical use in medical laboratories, except when required for accreditation by ISO 15189.[14] The ISO 15189 requirement specifies that MU can be estimated by a simple top-down calculation of precision from QC data collected under intermediate precision conditions. Use of the detailed GUM bottom-up methodology is not practical in most service laboratories and is mainly applicable by manufacturers and academic medical laboratories in the planning, development, improvement, and validation of new analytical systems.

A major stumbling block in resolving the issues between the error model and the uncertainty model is the lack of acceptance of TAE in the official language and definitions of metrology.[20] Accuracy is defined as a primary characteristic of an examination procedure and is recognized to be a function of both random and systematic errors when a single measurement is reported as the test result. ISO, however, does not identify a practical measure of accuracy; instead it substitutes MU, along with the assumption that bias is to be eliminated and only random error included in the estimate of uncertainty. Bias continues to exist in the real world of medical laboratories; thus, the theory of metrology does not represent the reality of practice in a medical laboratory and the need for a measure of accuracy, such as TAE. Nonetheless, metrologists argue that TAE is not an acceptable concept because it is not defined in the International Vocabulary of Metrology (VIM).[20]

VIM does include a term, *maximum permissible measurement error*, that represents an "extreme value of measurement error, with respect to a known reference quantity value, permitted by specifications or regulations for a given measurement, measuring instrument, or measuring system". This term is consistent with the use of ATE goals for PT/EQA programs and implies there should be a related term, such as TAE, that represents the expected measurement error. Although VIM does define *measurement error* as a measured quantity minus a reference quantity value (2.16), that definition refers to an individual measurement minus a reference value and does not describe the range of measurement values that are expected for that measured quantity, which is characterized by TAE.

Even though VIM lacks a term for TAE, Farrance and colleagues[21] recently argued that GUM actually supports the concept of TAE in section F.2.4.5, which "specifically describes the procedure where a significant systematic effect may be taken into account by enlarging the uncertainty assigned to the result... This situation is directly comparable to the calculation of Total Error as described by Westgard and others, where the uncertainty includes both an imprecision and bias component..." Thus, terminology may actually be a bigger issue than the concept of TAE, which can be expressed an expanded uncertainty interval that includes bias. Magnusson and Ellison[22] have discussed this in greater detail in an article, "Treatment of Uncorrected Measurement Bias in Uncertainty Estimation for Chemical Measurements." One recommendation is to add the absolute value of the bias to 1.65 times the square root of the variance of measurements plus the uncertainty in the estimate of bias, which they say is similar to what is described in GUM section F 2.4.5. Thus there actually is support (in GUM and by some metrologists) for use of an expression like TAE for the case where bias is significant and cannot be readily corrected.

Other metrologists argue that combining trueness and precision in TAE leads to a loss of information about individual components and sources of errors and therefore TAE is not meaningful.[23] At the same time, they claim that the capability of combining all components of variance in one estimate of performance is an advantage of MU. Trueness and precision are generally estimated from separate experiments, for example, precision from a replication experiment during method validation and from routine SQC data under intermediate precision conditions and bias from comparison of results with a comparative method, certified reference materials, or survey results in PT/EQA programs. Thus, information about the trueness and precision components of TAE is available during the life cycle of an examination procedure and a transferable variance component for analytical performance can always be calculated from the estimate of precision.

TAE is criticized as an incomplete model, but there are also limitations with the uncertainty model. For example, although it is recommended that MU include the uncertainty in the estimate of bias (U_B), MU does not include the uncertainty in the estimates of the various SDs, which are likely to be much larger than U_B. MU does not include the uncertainties in the detection of unstable biases by SQC procedures, which are actually large. Furthermore, there must be uncertainties in the shape and width of type B components in the GUM bottom-up methodology. Note that type B components depend on scientific judgment, whereas type A components depend on experimental data. Different scientists would likely come up with different judgments on the shape and width of type B components as well as different estimates for type A components, depending on the experimental conditions. GUM, in fact, acknowledges these limitations[24]:

This 'uncertainty of the uncertainty'... can be surprisingly large; for n = 10, it is 24 percent... One may therefore conclude that Type A evaluations of standard uncertainty are not necessarily more reliable than Type B evaluations...

Ironically, the poor reliability of experimental determination of uncertainty when estimated from low numbers of measurements is a reason to accept the poor reliability of type B evaluations. Medical laboratories know better than to depend on only 10 replicates to estimate an SD. Furthermore, ISO 15189 specifically recommends control data collected under intermediate precision conditions, which implies a period of a few months and likely a minimum of 100 control measurements.[25] Therefore, estimation of type A components in medical laboratories is much more reliable than estimation of type B components. The point is that MU is not a perfect theoretic construct either but like TAE is still useful and necessary in a comprehensive QMS that considers manufacturers development of medical devices and laboratories operation of those devices to provide quality test results.

Goals for laboratory quality should be to provide comparability of results from method to method and laboratory to laboratory over time and space, as discussed previously by Dybkaer.[6] The conflict between theory and reality, however, limits both plans and achievements. In theory, traceability is the solution for achieving comparability of results, but the reality is that biases exist for the clinically complex measurands of interest in medical laboratories and today's many proprietary measurement procedures. Elimination or correction of those biases is not always possible, even with calibration based on comparative patient results; therefore, bias must still be measured and monitored and should not be ignored or assumed to be accommodated by long-term estimates of MU. A practical approach for managing biases in daily operations in medical laboratories involves the TAE/ATE error framework and related Six Sigma tools. Efforts to achieve comparability of results depend on manufacturers to use the GUM bottom-up methodology to identify error sources and eliminate their causes. PT/EQA programs should use the top-down methodology to characterize MU for different analytical systems across time and space, monitor trueness verses a reference method target value, and describe performance on the sigma scale to help laboratories select methods that provide accurate results.

REFERENCES

1. Sandberg S, Fraser CG, Horvath AR, et al. Defining analytical performance specifications: consensus statement for the 1st strategic conference of the European Federation of Clinical Chemistry and Laboratory Medicine. Clin Chem Lab Med 2015;53(6):829–953.
2. Westgard JO. Useful measures and models for analytical quality management in medical laboratories. Clin Chem Lab Med 2016;54:223–33.
3. Panteghini M, Sandberg S. Total error vs. measurement uncertainty: the match continues. Clin Chem Lab Med 2016;54:195–6.
4. Oosterhuis WP, Theodorsson E. Total error vs. measurement uncertainty: revolution or evolution. Clin Chem Lab Med 2016;54:235–9.
5. Westgard JO, Westgard SA. Quality control in the age of risk management. Clin Lab Med 2013;33:1.
6. Dybkaer R. From total allowable error via metrological traceability to uncertainty of measurement of the unbiased results. Accred Qual Assur 1999;4:401–5.
7. Dybkaer R. Setting quality specifications for the future with newer approaches to defining uncertainty in laboratory medicine. Scand J Clin Lab Invest 1999;59:579–84.
8. Hyltoft Peterson P, Fraser CG, Kallner A, et al. Strategies to set global analytical quality specifications in laboratory medicine. Scand J Clin Lab Invest 1999;59(No 7):475–585.
9. Theodorsson E, Magnusson B, Leito I. Bias in clinical chemistry. Bioanalysis 2014;6:2855–75.
10. Thienpont LM, Van Ufganghe K, Cabaleiro DR. Metrological traceability of calibration in the estimation and use of common medical decision-making criteria. Clin Chem Lab Med 2004;42:842–50.
11. Weykamp C, John G, Gillery P, et al. Investigation of 2 models to set and evaluate quality targets for HbA1c: bilogic variation and sigma metrics. Clin Chem 2015;61:752–9.
12. Westgard JO, Westgard SA. A graphical tool for assessing quality on the sigma-scale from proficiency testing and external quality assessment surveys. Clin Chem Lab Med 2015;53:1531–6.
13. Westgard JO, Westgard SA. Quality control review: implementing a scientifically based quality control system. Ann Clin Biochem 2016;53:32–50.
14. ISO 15189. Medical laboratories – requirements for quality and competence. Geneva (Switzerland): ISO; 2012.
15. Westgard JO, Hyltoft Petersen P, Wiebe DA. Laboratory process specifications for assuring quality in the U.S. National Cholesterol Education Program. Clin Chem 1991;37:656–61.
16. Westgard JO, Wiebe DA. Cholesterol operating specifications for assuring the quality required by CLIA proficiency testing. Clin Chem 1991;37:1938–44.
17. Westgard JO, Seehafer JJ, Barry PL. Allowable imprecision for laboratory tests based on clinical and analytical test outcome criteria. Clin Chem 1994;40:1909–14.

18. Balogh EP, Miller BT, Ball JR, editors. Board on health care services. Institute of medicine. improving diagnosis in health care. Washington, DC: The National academies Press; 2015.
19. White GH, Farrance I, AACB Uncertainty of Measurement Working Group. Uncertainty of measurement in quantitative medical testing: a laboratory implementation guide. Clin Biochem Rev 2004;25:S1–24.
20. JCGM 200;2012 International vocabulary of metrology – Basic and general concepts and associated terms (VIM), 3rd edition 2008 version with minor corrections. Available at: 222.bipm.org. Accessed February 1, 2016.
21. Farrance I, Badrick T, Sikaris KA. Uncertainty in measurement and total error – are they so incompatible? Clin Chem Lab Med 2016;54:1309–11.
22. Magnusson B, Ellison SLR. Treatment of uncorrected measurement bias in uncertainty estimation for chemical measurements. Anal Bioanal Chem 2008;390: 201–13.
23. Kallner A. Is the combination of trueness and precision in one expression meaningful? On the use of total error and uncertainty in clinical chemistry. Clin Chem Lab Med 2016;54:1291–7.
24. BIPM JCGM 100: 2008. GUM 1995 with minor corrections. Evaluation of measurement data – Guide to the expression of uncertainty in measurement. Available at: www.bipm.org/utils/common/documents/jcgm/JCGM_100_2008_E.pdf   Accessed February 22, 2016.
25. Westgard JO, Westgard SA. Basic quality management systems. Chapter 15. Measuring the uncertainty of measurements. Madison (WI): Westgard QC, Inc; 2014. p. 223–37.

Uncertainty in Measurement and Total Error

Tools for Coping with Diagnostic Uncertainty

Elvar Theodorsson, MD, PhD

KEYWORDS

- Law of propagation of uncertainty (LPU) • Uncertainty methods • Error methods
- Diagnostic uncertainty • Bayesian statistics • Frequentist statistics

KEY POINTS

- Error approaches are not likely to be replaced soon in laboratory medicine by uncertainty approaches because the latter are in their early phases of development and implementation.
- Uncertainty approaches are likely to gain increased ground as focus shifts from the property of the measurement system to the proper use of the measurement result in the diagnosis and monitoring of treatment effects, including all factors causing uncertainty.
- Revised versions of the Guide to the Expression of Uncertainty in Measurement and International Vocabulary of Metrology are likely to explicitly endorse both error and uncertainty approaches, including both frequentist and bayesian statistical methods, in chemical metrology.

INTRODUCTION

"Medicine is a science of uncertainty and an art of probability" claimed William Osler.[1,2] History, physical examination, imaging, electrocardiogram, and laboratory investigations are all fraught with uncertainties, frequently prompting further investigations, including laboratory methods, which usually reduce the diagnostic uncertainty. However, in extreme cases, numerous investigations may be expensive, painful, and lead nowhere; aptly coined the Ulysses syndrome.[3] Medical diagnosis must therefore rest on knowledge and skills in medicine combined with aptitude in the handling of uncertainties.

Department of Clinical Chemistry and Department of Clinical and Experimental Medicine, Linköping University, SE-581 85 Linköping, Sweden
E-mail address: elvar.theodorsson@liu.se

Clin Lab Med 37 (2017) 15–34
http://dx.doi.org/10.1016/j.cll.2016.09.002   labmed.theclinics.com
0272-2712/17/© 2016 The Author. Published by Elsevier Inc. This is an open access article under the CC BY-NC-ND license (http://creativecommons.org/licenses/by-nc-nd/4.0/).

Measurements have been the cornerstone of the quantitative sciences since antiquity. However, concepts, terms, units, and methods for expressing measurement results[4] and their uncertainties are still contested despite extensive and successful attempts at international consensus resulting in the International Vocabulary of Metrology (VIM) and Guide to the Expression of Uncertainty in Measurement (GUM) more than a decade ago.[5–11] The philosophy of measurement also continues to be a dynamic field of enquiry[12–15] rekindled since the early 2000s[16–19] when the Bureau International des Poids et Mesures (BIPM) began to engage in chemical measurements in addition to physical measurements.

According to Tal,[12] the following 5 theories dominate current philosophies of measurements:

1. Mathematical models of measurement view measurement as the mapping of qualitative empirical relations to relations among numbers.
2. Operationalist models view measurement as a set of operations that shape the meaning and/or regulate the use of a quantity terms.
3. Realist models view measurement as the estimation of mind-independent properties and/or relations.
4. Information models view measurement as the gathering and interpretation of information about a system.
5. Model theories view measurement as the coherent assignment of values to parameters in a theoretic/mathematical/statistical model of a process.

The realist models, represented in laboratory medicine by error methods[20] regard measurements as the estimation of "mind-independent properties"[12] of the measure and of the measurement system. Model theories, represented by measurement uncertainty methods[5] claim that other relevant and available information in addition to the measurement results themselves should be counted in as aid in the proper interpretation of the measurement results. Error methods currently dominate in laboratory medicine despite the introduction of measurement uncertainty methods in the early 2000s.[5,9]

Error methods focus on the practical measurement process and its results. Error is a property of a single measurement result in relation to a true value. Bias is estimated as the difference between the mean of replicate measurement results and of the true value. Repeatability, intermediate precision, and reproducibility imprecision are estimated as measures of random error. The combination of bias and imprecision (accuracy) expressed as total error (TE)[20,21] has gained prominence because it can be cost-effectively estimated by singleton measurements of control samples.

Error methods applied in laboratory medicine focus on the properties of measurement systems, and are also being developed for other measurement results in health care (**Fig. 1**).[22,23]

Uncertainty methods are also founded on the measurement results, but their primary focus is on their use for diagnosing and monitoring of treatment results. All factors influencing the interpretation of the measurement results are accounted for, including biological variation, preanalytical variation, analytical variation, and postanalytical variation (**Fig. 2**).

According to VIM,[9] measurement is a "process of experimentally obtaining one or more quantity values that can reasonably be attributed to a quantity."[9] Measurement thus consists both of estimating the mind-independent properties of the measurand obtained by the measurement system and the intellectual activity of interpreting the results of measurements in proper contexts.[5,15,24]

The harmonization of methods for describing measurement results and measurement uncertainties among all sciences, from physics, through environmental sciences, trade, and laboratory medicine, initiated by the highest authorities in international metrology (BIPM) constitutes an important development that is still ongoing; for example, in successive versions of GUM and VIM. The paradigm shift in chemistry and other measurement sciences encouraged by uncertainty methods has been, and is, questioned, including its value in practical health care.[25–27]

MEASUREMENT ERROR AND UNCERTAINTY

VIM[9] defines the crucial concepts and terms in metrology. The original version of GUM from 1993/1995 is still valid, but has been expanded by appendices.[28–30]

The error type TE (total error) in the terminology of VIM3[9] is the combination of random and systematic errors expressed on the nominal scale. In contrast, TE is the absolute value of the measured bias plus 2 standard deviations measured on the ratio scale in the terminology of Westgard[20,21] and others favoring error models in laboratory medicine.

Accuracy is also the combination of bias and random error, but measured on the ordinal scale according to VIM3.[9] Thus a measurement system is more or less accurate than another measurement system, but accuracy does not indicate how much more or less accurate (**Fig. 3**).

In the medical laboratory, patient samples are routinely measured once. The inherent error or measurement uncertainty is therefore only known indirectly from data obtained from repeated measurement of stabilized control samples or patient samples. It is therefore essential to perform repeated measurements of controls to estimate uncertainty in the analytical phase.

The GUM[5] states that measurement uncertainty "reflects the lack of exact knowledge of the value of the measurand." The distribution of results that describe measurement uncertainty should communicate the strength of a well-founded belief in where the true value of the measurand lies. The interval should include the true value of the measurand with a specified probability.[31,32]

Recent developments in the philosophy of measurement emphasize the relationship between the measurement and the theoretic models on which the use of measurement results are based.[12,14–19,33]

The 1993/1995 version of the GUM used both uncertainty and error approaches using bayesian and frequentist statistics, respectively.[30] Bayesian methods[34,35] quantify a state of knowledge or degree of belief, in contrast with frequentist methods, which regard probability as frequencies of occurrence. Bayesian methods assign probabilities to hypotheses, whereas frequentist methods test hypotheses without assigning them prior probabilities. Recent supplements to the GUM and the latest version of VIM (VIM3), published in 2008, went completely in the direction of the uncertainty approach and bayesian statistics. However, inconsistencies between the supplements and the main GUM text have been pointed out repeatedly.[28,36–38]

UNCERTAINTY METHODS

Uncertainty methods as developed by the BIPM (www.bipm.org)[5] have their roots in physical measurements.[11,39] The BIPM started to include chemistry in earnest as late as in the 1980s, which may explain why workers in chemistry and related sciences struggle when adapting to a long tradition established by physical metrology laboratories.[39,40]

In contrast with uncertainty methods, error methods require that a true value of a quantity is known because error is a property of a single measurement.[9,21] Uncertainty methods do not claim the absence of a true value,[9] but claim the absence of an exact knowledge about the true value.

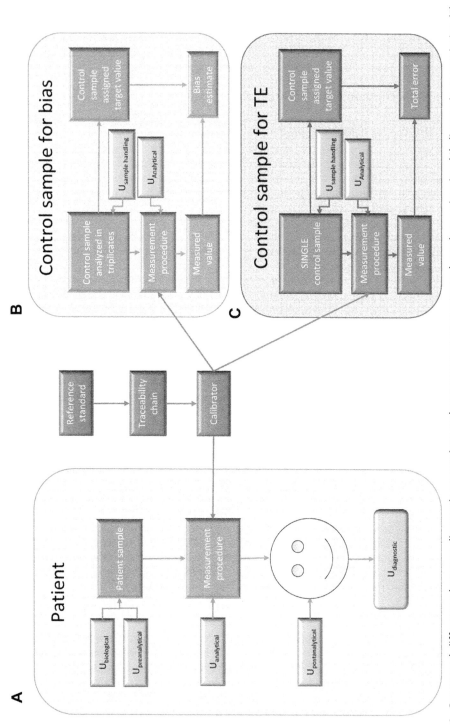

Fig. 1. Conceptual differences between diagnostic uncertainty and measurement error approaches when estimating (*A*) diagnostic uncertainties, (*B*) bias, and (*C*) TE in laboratory medicine. Diagnostic uncertainty approaches (*A*) provide estimates of diagnostic uncertainty; the combined uncertainty

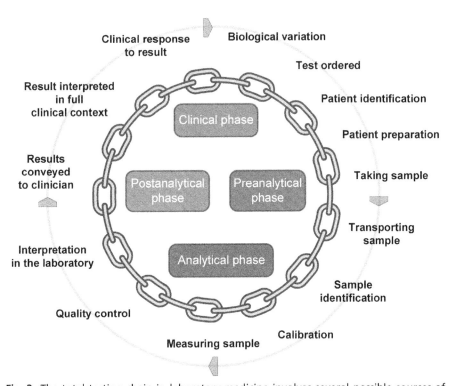

Fig. 2. The total testing chain in laboratory medicine involves several possible sources of uncertainty from the clinical decision to order a test through biological variation, the preanalytical, analytical, and postanalytical phases, to the value of the test result in the ongoing clinical decisions. Error methods focus primarily on the analytical phase (the properties of the measurement system), whereas uncertainty methods focus on counting all sources of uncertainties, including biological variation, preanalytical variation, analytical variation, and postanalytical variation, as an aid in diagnosis and in monitoring treatment effects.

of all causes of uncertainty in the total testing chain when using laboratory results for diagnosing patients, including biological variation and preanalytical, analytical, and postanalytical variations. Both the LPU favored by GUM and simple addition of variances according to the pythagorean theorem can be used to estimate diagnostic uncertainty. LPU methods have their major strength in their ability to deal with numerous and complex causes of uncertainty but their major weakness is their theoretic and practical complexity and lack of practical implementations in laboratory medicine.[81] Measurement error approaches (*B*, *C*) provide estimates of the uncertainty of the measurement methods; the analytical phase of the total testing chain. If the main purpose of the external quality control program is to determine bias and imprecision separately, approach (*B*) is preferred. External quality control programs aiming for estimation of TE use singleton measurements (*C*). They are supported by comprehensive theoretic models, acceptance by regulatory authorities, and widespread practical use in laboratory medicine. Biological, preanalytical, and postanalytical variations are not relevant when monitoring variation in control samples, but these variations are relevant when dealing with patient samples.[46]

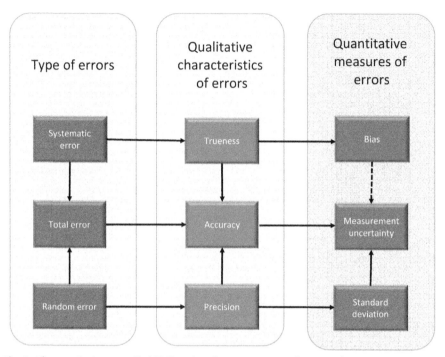

Fig. 3. The terminology used in VIM3 to describe components of error and measurement uncertainty.[91] Measurement error, or simply error, is a property of a single measurement: measured quantity value minus a reference quantity value.[9,21,92] The reference quantity value serves a surrogate true value" within the system (or model). A true value or reference value of the measurand in a particular patient sample cannot be known. Therefore, the true value of a single patient result cannot be known, and the confidence in a result must consequently be expressed in probabilistic terms based on frequentist statistics (confidence intervals) for error models and bayesian statistics (probability density) for uncertainty models.

Among the myths about measurement uncertainty methods is that they demand that bias be eliminated before uncertainty calculations and estimates can be made.[41] Uncertainty approaches claim that bias should be eliminated when identified. However, if bias cannot be eliminated, or when bias elimination risks increasing the overall measurement uncertainty, this can be handled as any other type B uncertainty.

Measurement uncertainty approaches in laboratory medicine face several challenges:

1. The level of knowledge in mathematics and advanced statistics in laboratory medicine is generally too low to fully understand and apply the law of propagation of uncertainty (LPU),[42] including measurement equations, covariance matrices, partial derivatives, Taylor expansions, and bayesian statistics necessary for the full implementation of uncertainty approaches.
2. Error/frequentist methods are implemented in all laboratories and generally are well understood. Their use when implementing International Standards Organization (ISO) standards is generally well accepted by accreditation authorities. There are limited incentives for the laboratories to leave error methods in favor of uncertainty methods with LPU.

3. The level of knowledge regarding biological, preanalytical, and postanalytical variation in laboratory medicine still lags far behind the knowledge of causes of analytical variation, and this diminishes the hope that the proper use of uncertainty methods will improve the clinical use of measurement methods.

Despite the obstacles, uncertainty methods have been properly implemented in laboratory medicine.[42–44]

ERROR METHODS

Although error methods are well developed and still dominate the quality assurance of measurement systems in laboratory medicine, a transition to the use of measurement uncertainty methods has already taken place in other fields of metrology. Differences between error and uncertainty methods need to be understood but should not be overemphasized.[41] The uncertainty approach represents an evolution of the error approach.

For a single measurement result, there is no way of knowing the separate contribution of bias and imprecision to the TE of that result. TE methods are favored and are particularly relevant when singleton samples are used for quality control. When TE methods are used,[21] bias and imprecision (multiplied by a z-factor) are added linearly, resulting in a value for the TE: TE = bias + zCVa. TE is used to estimate the limits of an interval around the true value where measured analytical results can be found with a certain probability, usually 95% probability.

Among the major challenges for the error approach are:

1. If a true value cannot be known, TE cannot be estimated.
2. Because bias is a scalar and the standard deviation represents variation, they seem incompatible. The various expressions of TE or maximum allowable deviation have in common the merger of quantities that are inherently incompatible; the bias has a sign, either positive or negative, whereas the standard deviation represents an interval (± 2 standard deviations) of quantity values.
3. There are several variants for how to calculate TE.[45]

It is hoped that the debate between proponents of uncertainty and error approaches in laboratory medicine will bring about increased understanding and development within both approaches in laboratory medicine.

Simple Addition of Variances Using the Pythagorean Theorem

Error methods use the pythagorean theorem to calculate total variance as the square root of the sum of the variances for all variance components making up the total uncertainty (**Fig. 4**). Just as the pythagorean theorem in trigonometry only applies to right triangles, only independent random variables can be added in this manner. Geometrically the random variables are represented as vectors whose lengths correspond with their standard deviations. When the variables are independent, their vectors are orthogonal. In this case the standard deviation of the sum or difference of the variables is just the hypotenuse of a right triangle. The pythagorean theorem is also not appropriate in the presence of significant bias/systematic error in any of the variance components.

Components of diagnostic variation in laboratory medicine are not necessarily orthogonal and not always corrected for bias. Error methods therefore struggle when representing numerous and complex factors influencing measurement results. They cater to the simplest models of reality, the simple addition of orthogonal variances.[46] Therefore, simple addition of variances are not always appropriate, calling for the more sophisticated methods for uncertainty calculation included in the LPU.

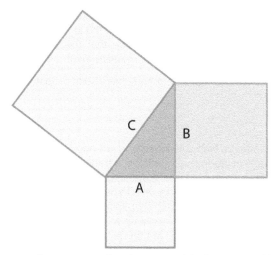

Fig. 4. The pythagorean theorem states that the square of the hypotenuse (the side opposite the right angle; marked C) is equal to the sum of the squares of the other 2 sides A and B. This means that the sum of the area of quadrant C is equal to the sum of the areas of the quadrants A and B.

The ISO 17025 and ISO 15189 standards require laboratories to estimate measurement uncertainty. However, methods for calculating measurement uncertainty are not prescribed in the standards so accreditation authorities accept both error and uncertainty approaches.[47] Top-down error methods for calculating measurement uncertainty from internal quality control samples are probably the most commonly used approaches for calculating measurement uncertainty in ISO-accredited medical laboratories.

The Law of Propagation of Uncertainty

GUM originally recommended primarily the LPU,[42] whereas GUM Supplement 1/JCGM 101 uses a Monte Carlo method.[43] Both methods are founded on forward uncertainty evaluation, which creates a mathematical input-output model (measurement equation), a description of the variation in the output caused by variations in the inputs. The uncertainty of the measurand is, if possible, expressed as a function of a set of influence quantities, including their covariances.[48]

LPU can accommodate nonorthogonality and bias using measurement models, covariance matrices, partial derivatives, and Taylor expansion[49–53] and are therefore theoretically preferable when calculating measurement uncertainty. The advantage of LPU is that all relevant uncertainty components are taken into account, both when they can be estimated directly by statistical methods (type A) and when estimated by other means (type B), including by educated estimation based on experience.

There is also a movement to apply bayesian statistics to the evaluation of measurement uncertainty,[35,36,54–57] in which a state of knowledge distribution about the quantity of interest is derived from (1) prior information about the quantity and other influence quantities; and (2) measured data, using probabilistic inversion or inverse uncertainty evaluation.[41,48]

Monte Carlo Simulation

Monte Carlo simulation is easier to understand than traditional LPU methods (**Fig. 5**). It requires information about the probability distributions of all factors influencing the

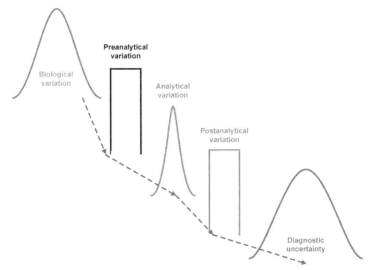

Fig. 5. Simplification of the principles of Monte Carlo techniques for estimating diagnostic uncertainty. The variance from the study used to estimate biological variation is used to model the contribution of the biological variation to the estimate of diagnostic uncertainty. Preanalytical variation is estimated from a quadratic probability function whose properties are estimated as type B uncertainty. Analytical variation is estimated as repeatability variance; all measurement results within the laboratory organization when measuring the same sample for a certain measurand using all measurement systems at different points in time. Postanalytical variation is estimated from a quadratic probability function whose properties are estimated as type B uncertainty. At least 100,000 repeated samples are simultaneously drawn from all probability functions in order to create the diagnostic uncertainty probability distribution.

variable of primary interest; in this case the diagnostic uncertainty of a measurand. The diagnostic uncertainty includes biological variation, preanalytical variation, analytical variation, and postanalytical variation. Biological variation and analytical variation may be expressed as coefficients of variation of a gaussian distribution and the preanalytical and postanalytical probability distributions may be expressed as rectangular distributions (either there is an error or not).

There are several software tools available for applying Monte Carlo methods,[58] including add-in modules for Microsoft Excel.[59]

Among other advantages of the Monte Carlo methods are that:

1. No mathematical function (output function) is needed to evaluate the diagnostic uncertainty
2. No assumptions about the input quantities is needed in addition to the assumption that they follow a gaussian distribution
3. There is no need to calculate partial derivatives
4. They are unaffected by partial derivatives that vanish when estimating input quantities

Resampling Methods

The wide availability of low-cost computing power in the 1980s drastically improved the options and cost of working with data, irrespective of theoretic distributions. A seminal work on resampling/bootstrap methods by Jones[60] in 1956 was followed by the influential works by Efron and colleagues,[61,62] which brought these methods into the mainstream of data analysis. There is a wealth of current and relevant literature on resampling methods.[63–66]

Resampling with replacement means that in the order of 100,000 to 1 million samples with replacement are then taken from the original sample and the statistics of interest are calculated from this pseudopopulation as an estimate of the corresponding parameters of the population (**Fig. 6**).

Resampling methods are free from the assumption that the observations are distributed according to a certain theoretic distribution, but importantly assume that the underlying population distribution is practically the same as that in a particular sample from the population. This assumption means that a sufficient number of observations is needed in the sample to make sure that it represents the population. In the order of 100,000 to 1 million resamples from the influencing distributions are preferable.

When a measured value is accompanied by its measurement uncertainty, the former becomes a result of measurement,[67] which is expressed by a coverage interval. In this kind of interval, 3 figures should be taken into account: the measured value and the lower and upper limits of that interval. This coverage interval is usually obtained after

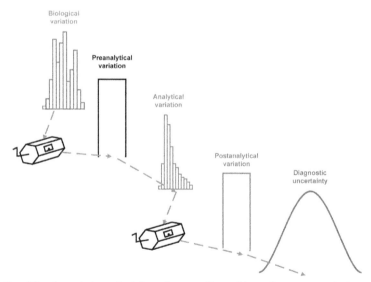

Fig. 6. Simplification of the principles of resampling with replacement techniques for resampling estimation of diagnostic uncertainty (here illustrated as gaussian distribution as example of any possible distribution). All original data from the study used to estimate biological variation are used for resampling (here illustrated as a tombola) the contribution of the biological variation to the estimate of diagnostic uncertainty. Preanalytical variation is estimated from a quadratic probability function whose properties are estimated as type B uncertainty. Analytical variation is estimated as reproducibility variation; all measurement results within the laboratory organization when measuring the same sample for a certain measurand using all measurement systems at different points in time. All data are used for resampling (here illustrated as a tombola) the contribution of the analytical variation to the estimate of diagnostic uncertainty. Postanalytical variation is estimated from a quadratic probability function whose properties are estimated as type B uncertainty.

adding and subtracting the expanded uncertainty to the measured value and the expanded uncertainty is the combined standard uncertainty multiplied by 2 in order to obtain a coverage interval of approximately 95%.[8]

The Kragten Method and Other Simplified Uncertainty Calculations

Kragten[68,69] published useful simplifications to these uncertainty calculations, which have been published in Nordtest guidelines[70,71] and implemented in freely available software for uncertainty calculations.[72]

THE BEST MAY BECOME AN ENEMY OF THE GOOD

The true purpose of laboratory results in medicine is to aid in making diagnoses and in the monitoring of treatment effects. Knowledge of the diagnostic properties of laboratory methods and efforts at minimizing the uncertainties involved are essential. Uncertainty estimates optimally include the probability densities of all causes of uncertainties in the total testing chain (**Fig. 2**), including preanalytical, postanalytical, biological, and analytical causes. This comprehensive approach is a prerequisite for proper quality specifications and a much more relevant goal than debating different statistical paradigms and formulas covering only a portion of the testing chain. Each laboratory should use the methods and tools for uncertainty calculations they are familiar with, being aware that they may not necessarily be optimal in all instances. Uncertainty calculations represent an important tool for quality management that no laboratory should miss because of conceived lack of mathematical skills.

Medical diagnosis is about making decisions under uncertainty rather than statistical inference. LPU and bayesian statistics are therefore, in theory, preferable to frequentist statistical methods in diagnostic medicine, including laboratory medicine. Because laboratory staff are usually better versed in frequentist statistics than in LPU and bayesian methods, simple addition of variances are commonly used. There is a risk that "Perfect becomes the enemy of good" (Pescetti 1603) in the choice between uncertainty and error methods. Error approaches, including frequentist statistics, are widely used for quality control in laboratory medicine.[20,22,73,74] Even after the advent of accreditation standards ISO 17025 and 15189 demanding uncertainty calculations, top-down variance component analysis used in error/frequentist statistics are commonly used for uncertainty estimation using internal quality control samples.[75,76] Error methods are well established in laboratory medicine and are likely to be used for singleton internal quality control procedures and for proficiency testing for the foreseeable future and for quality assurance purposes because of their familiarity and proven value.[15,24] The concept of measurement uncertainty should preferably be used for both frequentist and LPU/bayesian methods for estimating measurement uncertainty as long as the simplifications made (eg, in relation to LPU) are clearly expressed (eg, independence of causes of variation).

Error and uncertainty approaches should each be developed on its own merits as accepted but different philosophies and practical approaches to metrology.[14,15,24,77] Competition between them may prove to be more fruitful than attempting to reconcile them in a unified approach.[78–80] The approach that is applied in practice and contributes most substantially to improvements in medical care is likely to win.

DIAGNOSTIC UNCERTAINTY IN LABORATORY MEDICINE

Diagnostic uncertainty of a measurand in laboratory medicine is the combined uncertainty of all relevant sources of uncertainty when using the measurand for diagnostic purposes. These sources of uncertainty may be biological, preanalytical, analytical, and postanalytical variation. A measurand is the quantity intended to be measured.[9] The specification of a measurand requires knowledge of the kind of quantity; description of the state of the phenomenon, body, or substance carrying the quantity, including any relevant component; and the chemical entities involved.

Proficiency testing/external quality control schemes in laboratory medicine focus on the analytical phase and commonly use singleton-sample methods for quality control. This focus means that a control sample is measured only once before the result is reported. A mean of replicate measurements is therefore not available and thereby no separate estimate of imprecision. TE methods are particularly suitable for evaluating these results because they evaluate the combination of random error and bias (accuracy/TE). Singleton measurements are efficient for regulatory purposes because a minimum number of control samples (1) and measurements (1) are required. Diagram C in **Fig. 1** shows this. Only 2 uncertainty factors (factors causing variability in the results) are involved: (1) the uncertainty of the handling of the control sample, and (2) the analytical/measurement uncertainty. Because the uncertainty of handling a stabilized control material is minimal, the TE practically expresses the uncertainty of the measurement procedure. That uncertainty is commonly the primary focus of regulatory authorities and proficiency testing schemes based on TE are therefore is particularly useful in these contexts.

External quality control schemes can also be designed to enable participant laboratories to measure their bias. In this instance, shown in panel B of **Fig. 1**, the mean is calculated of at least 3 replicate measurements (for statistical reasons) of the control sample. External quality control programs for estimating bias do not focus on estimating imprecision, because the regular measurement of internal quality control samples is optimal for that purpose.

Measuring the concentration of a measurand in a stabilized control sample in internal quality control or in proficiency testing involves many fewer uncertainty factors than the factors encountered when preparing a patient for taking a sample, taking the sample, processing the sample, transporting the sample, analyzing the sample, and interpreting the results in a clinical context (see **Fig. 1**). The uncertainty factors involved when measuring a stabilized control sample are mainly the sample handling and the uncertainty of the measurement system. Therefore, the accuracy/combination of bias and imprecision/TE of the measurement result represent properties of the measurement system. The TE estimated from singleton measurements of control samples has been found to be appropriate for regulatory purposes and an extensive theoretic and practical framework has been developed around its use.[20,22]

Bias is commonly estimated by participation in proficiency testing schemes (external quality control programs), using certified reference materials or by comparisons with reference methods.[82,83] Comparisons commonly use stabilized samples that do not necessarily have all the properties of natural patient samples. Natural patient samples are commutable[75] by definition and in practice, whereas stabilized control materials may or may not be commutable. If the main purpose of a quality control system is to minimize the overall measurement uncertainty of all measurement systems and methods in an organization or geographic area, the use of fresh split patient samples is more efficient in finding clinically important bias and thereby for minimizing measurement uncertainty, especially when replicate measurements are used for minimizing random error. The purpose of laboratory medicine is to reduce uncertainty when physicians diagnose diseases and monitor treatment effects (diagnostic uncertainty). The TE of a measurement system estimated when measuring control samples is the main emphasis of many laboratories despite the TE only representing in the order of 20% of the diagnostic uncertainty related to laboratory medicine (see **Fig. 1**).[84]

The use of fresh split patient samples for quality control makes sense for several reasons: (1) the material has optimal matrix properties (is commutable), (2) the material is available without cost for all laboratories accepting routine patient samples, (3) there is general agreement that all measurement systems and reagents should optimally result in identical results when analyzing the same patient samples, and (4) the methods are optimal for identifying the measurement systems in the organization that contribute the largest part of the overall measurement uncertainty caused by bias (**Fig. 7**). Split sample methods are laborious in the absence of effective computerized systems, but convenient when properly implemented.[75,85]

Most laboratory organizations that introduce split sample methods prefer to continue their participation in external quality control schemes for the purpose of being able to compare their results nationally and transnationally.

ESTIMATED GLOMERULAR FILTRATION RATE: AN EXAMPLE OF A CLINICALLY IMPORTANT MEASURAND

The crucial differences between the concepts of measurand and analyte should be duly noted. The measurand estimated glomerular filtration rate (eGFR) is the quantity intended to be measured,[9] whereas the analyte creatinine or cystatin c is the substance of interest when measuring in plasma and urine the analytes whose concentrations are input in the equations used for that purpose. Clearance is used as a surrogate marker for glomerular filtration rate. Clearance is commonly estimated; for example, by EDTA (ethylenediamine tetraacetic acid) or iohexol clearance. The eGFR is a more indirect estimate of clearance: the volume of blood plasma completely cleared of creatinine/cystatin c per unit of time. There are several options when attempting to minimize the influence of the uncertainty of the creatinine concentrations on the eGFR estimate; for example, using enzymatic methods instead of Jaffe methods, or correcting for the influence of muscle mass by noting whether the subject is male or female, of African ancestry or not, and considering age (**Table 1**).

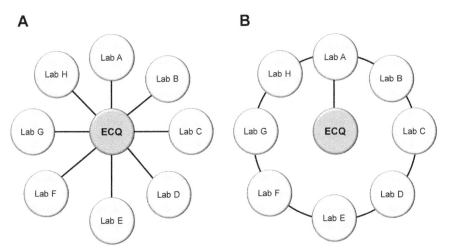

A   **B**

Fig. 7. Simplification of traditional external quality control (ECQ/proficiency testing) scheme (A) and control scheme (B) focused on minimizing bias within a conglomerate of laboratories (Lab) where laboratories B to H regularly send patient samples they have already analyzed to laboratory A, which participates in national or international ECQ.

Table 1
Estimates of factors, measurable or constants, in equations estimating clearance of concentrations of creatinine or cystatin c

Factors that Influence the Relation Between Creatinine Concentrations and Estimates of eGFR	Estimated by
Muscle mass	Male or female African ancestry or not
Age	Age
Body surface area	Calculated based on data on sex, height, and weight
Albumin concentrations in plasma	
Urea concentrations in plasma	
Ingestion of food containing creatinine	
Physical exercise	
Factors in various eGFR equations	Estimated in populations in which GFR has been measured by independent means; eg, using iohexol clearance

Other factors, including albumin or urea concentrations in plasma, are seldom factored into the calculation, because they play only a small part in improving the eGFR estimate of glomerular filtration. The substantial uncertainties involved when estimating the mathematical factors in the equations of eGFR are rarely displayed.[86] Various methods of calculating uncertainties have been used when estimating factors in equations or which measured quantities to include, but rarely according to harmonized methodology; for example, LPU. Despite eGFR being used to adjust the dosage of potent drugs to individuals, the diagnostic uncertainty in estimating eGFR as measure of glomerular filtration rate is seldom if ever reported with the results.[87]

Despite the theoretic advantages of advanced uncertainty estimates in laboratory medicine, it remains to be shown that reporting of eGFR together with proper uncertainty estimates will be successfully introduced and widely used in practice given the perceived lack of interest in uncertainty estimates in clinical medicine. It is probable that knowledge of data from full diagnostic evaluation[75] of medical tests[88–90] in practical health care will continue to be preferred to uncertainty estimates despite them being complementary.

The concept of true value, if used at all, is related to the measurement system used. However, the measurement system is only a part of the overall reality in laboratory medicine (see **Figs. 1–2**). The ultimate aim of measuring the concentration of a measurand in a patient is to improve the understanding of a possible disease condition or to monitor treatment effects. Fulfilling this aim is influenced by the uncertainties not only of the measurement system (measurement uncertainty) but of biological variation, preanalytical variation, and postanalytical variation. All these uncertainty components should be taken into account in a comprehensive model of reality that comprehensively reflects the diagnostic uncertainty of the measurement result. Predictive values are the diagnostic uncertainty, determined using a bayesian approach to combine the pretest probability with the performance specification (which is the same total uncertainty of testing process).

Statistics, philosophy of research, and metrology are fiercely debated sciences historically and at present. The present debate between error and uncertainty methods are, for example, reflections of the tensions between frequentists and bayesianists.[93] One or both of them may prevail in the long run or, perhaps, be challenged by new lines of thought,[12,33] including causal analysis.[94,95] In the words of Jordi Vallverdú,[93]

"Perhaps is time to admit that all our epistemological tools are provisional and fallible elements and that the path toward better knowledge is necessarily close to a critical thinking. Ontological disambiguation about causality and or statistics will not emanate by itself or due to any analytical process, instead of it, in an honest and critical activity of plenty of several failures and some successes. Let any one of you who is without priors be the first to throw a formula at the others." In the words of Luca Mari,[77] "'the error approach' and 'the uncertainty approach' are not only compatible but actually both required for an appropriate evaluation of measurement data: measurement errors are a component of the usually broader set of causes of measurement uncertainty."

SUMMARY

Error models, including TE models for quantifying the quality of measurement systems in laboratory medicine, are widely applied and have served laboratories well since their introduction in the 1970s. Developments in other fields of international metrology have introduced generalized and even more comprehensive methods (LPU) for quantifying the combination of several uncertainties, not only of the measurement systems but the combined effects of all the parts of the total testing chain (preanalytical, analytical, postanalytical, and clinical) when used for diagnosing and for monitoring treatment results. LPU and bayesian calculations have yet to fully show their practical added value in the laboratory and in clinical medicine. Such developments depend on the sophistication of the end user of the measurement results in practical health care. However, uncertainty concepts are increasingly used in all fields of human endeavor, including commerce, engineering, and environmental sciences, and are taught in general curricula, including medicine, so their practical value is likely to be increasingly appreciated. LPU approaches are likely to gain increased acceptance in laboratory medicine as focus shifts from the property of the measurement system to the proper use of the measurement result in the diagnosis and monitoring of treatment effects, including all factors causing uncertainty. Revised versions of the GUM[5] and VIM[9] are likely to explicitly endorse both error and uncertainty approaches, including both frequentist and bayesian statistical methods.[14,15,96–100]

REFERENCES

1. Osler W. The historical development and relative value of laboratory and clinical methods in diagnosis. The evolution of the idea of experiment in medicine. Transactions of the Congress of American Physicians and Surgeons 1907;7:1–8.
2. Bean RB, Bean WB. Sir William Osler: aphorisms from his bedside teachings and writings. New York: H Schuman; 1950.
3. Rang M. The Ulysses syndrome. CMAJ 1972;106:122–3.
4. Marciano JB. Whatever happened to the metric system? How America kept its feet. 1st edition. New York: Bloomsbury; 2014.
5. JCGM. Evaluation of measurement data — Guide to the expression of uncertainty in measurement. Paris: Joint Committee for Guides in Metrology; 2008. JCGM 100:2008, GUM 1995 with minor corrections. Available at: http://www.bipm.org/utils/common/documents/jcgm/JCGM_100_2008_E.pdf. Accessed February 15, 2016.
6. Barwick V, Prichard E. Terminology in analytical measurement - introduction to VIM 3. Brussels: Eurachem; 2011. Available at: https://www.eurachem.org/index.php/publications/guides/terminology-in-analytical-measurement. Accessed February 15, 2016.

7. De Bievre P. The 2007 International Vocabulary of Metrology (VIM), JCGM 200:2008 [ISO/IEC Guide 99]: meeting the need for intercontinentally understood concepts and their associated intercontinentally agreed terms. Clin Biochem 2009; 42(4–5):246–8.

8. Dybkaer R. ISO terminological analysis of the VIM3 concepts 'quantity' and 'kind-of-quantity'. Metrologia 2010;47:127–34.

9. JCGM. International vocabulary of metrology — Basic and general concepts and associated terms (VIM 3). 3rd edition. 2012. Available at: http://www.bipm.org/utils/common/documents/jcgm/JCGM_200_2008.pdf. Accessed February 15, 2016.

10. Zender R. Whims on VIM. J Int Fed Clin Chem 1992;4:115–6.

11. Page CH, Vigoureux PE. The International Bureau of Weights and Measures 1875-1975. Paris: National Bureau of Standards; 1975. Vol NBS Special Publication 420.

12. Tal E. Measurement in Science. In: Zalta EN, editor. Stanford Encyclopedia of Philosophy; 2015. Available at: http://plato.stanford.edu/entries/measurement-science/#Bib. Accessed February 16, 2016.

13. Boumans M, Hon G, Petersen AC. Error and uncertainty in scientific practice. London: Pickering & Chatto; 2014.

14. Mari L, Giordani A. Modeling measurement: error and uncertainty. In: Boumans M, Hon G, Petersen A, editors. Error and uncertainty in scientific practice. London: Pickering & Chatto; 2014. p. 79–96.

15. Giordani A, Mari L. Measurement, models, and uncertainty. IEEE T Instrum Meas 2012;61(8):2144–52.

16. Psillos S. Scientific realism: how science tracks truth. London: Routledge; 1999.

17. Giere RN. Explaining science: a cognitive approach. Chicago: University of Chicago Press; 1988.

18. Giere RN. Cognitive models of science. Minneapolis: University of Minnesota Press; 1992.

19. Giere RN. Scientific perspectivism. Chicago: University of Chicago Press; 2006.

20. Westgard JO. Useful measures and models for analytical quality management in medical laboratories. Clin Chem Lab Med 2016;54(2):223–33.

21. Westgard JO, Carey RN, Wold S. Criteria for judging precision and accuracy in method development and evaluation. Clin Chem 1974;20(7):825–33.

22. Westgard JO, Westgard SA. Quality control review: implementing a scientifically based quality control system. Ann Clin Biochem 2016;53(Pt 1):32–50.

23. Petersen PH. Performance criteria based on true and false classification and clinical outcomes. Influence of analytical performance on diagnostic outcome using a single clinical component. Clin Chem Lab Med 2015;53(6):849–55.

24. Mari L, Carbone P, Petri D. Measurement fundamentals: a pragmatic view. IEEE T Instrum Meas 2012;61(8):2107–15.

25. Robinson R. Critical review of uncertainty guidance documents final report. Teddington, UK: NPL; 2004.

26. Aarons GA. Transformational and transactional leadership: association with attitudes toward evidence-based practice. Psychiatr Serv 2006;57(8):1162–9.

27. Goldschmidt H, Libeer JC, De Bievre P, et al. How far can the concepts of traceability and GUM/VIM can be applied to measurement results in laboratory medicine - Antwerp conference consensus statements on the applicability of the concepts metrological traceability, measurement uncertainty, and VIM in laboratory medicine. Accred Qual Assur 2004;9(3):125–7.

28. Kyriazis GA. Contributions to the revision of the 'Guide to the expression of uncertainty in measurement'. Journal Physics: Conference Series 2015;575:1.

29. Evaluation of measurement data — Supplement 1 to the "Guide to the expression of uncertainty in measurement" — Propagation of distributions using a Monte Carlo method. 2006. Available at: http://www.bipm.org/utils/common/documents/jcgm/JCGM_101_2008_E.pdf. Accessed February 13, 2016.

30. Kacker R, Jones AW. On use of Bayesian statistics to make the guide to the expression of uncertainty in measurement consistent. Metrologia 2003;40:235–48.

31. Tyler Estler W. Measurement as inference: fundamental ideas. CIRP Ann Manufacturing Technology 1999;48(2):611–31.

32. Possolo A. Five examples of assessment and expression of measurement uncertainty. Appl Stoch Model Bus 2013;29(1):1–18.

33. Tal E. Old and new problems in philosophy of measurements. Philos Compass 2013;8(12):1159–73.

34. Bayes T. An essay towards solving a problem in the Doctrine of Chances. Phil Trans 1763;53:370–418.

35. Weise K, Woger W. A Bayesian theory of measurement uncertainty. Meas Sci Technol 1993;4(1):1–11.

36. Lira I. The GUM revision: the Bayesian view toward the expression of measurement uncertainty. Eur J Phys 2016;37(2):1–16.

37. Bich W. How to revise the GUM? Accred Qual Assur 2008;13(4–5):271–5.

38. Michel R. Measuring, estimating, and deciding under uncertainty. Appl Radiat Isot 2016;109:6–11.

39. Williams A. What can we learn from traceability in physical measurements? Accred Qual Assur 2000;5(10–11):414–7.

40. Williams A. Traceability and uncertainty - a comparison of their application in chemical and physical measurement. Accred Qual Assur 2001;6(2):73–5.

41. Bich W. Error, uncertainty and probability. P Int Sch Phys 2013;185:47–73.

42. Farrance I, Frenkel R. Uncertainty of measurement: a review of the rules for calculating uncertainty components through functional relationships. Clin Biochem Rev 2012;33(2):49–75.

43. Farrance I, Frenkel R. Uncertainty in measurement: a review of Monte Carlo simulation using Microsoft Excel for the calculation of uncertainties through functional relationships, including uncertainties in empirically derived constants. Clin Biochem Rev 2014;35(1):37–61.

44. White GH, Farrance I, AACB Uncertainty of Measurement Working Group. Uncertainty of measurement in quantitative medical testing: a laboratory implementation guide. Clin Biochem Rev 2004;25(4):S1–24.

45. Oosterhuis WP. Gross overestimation of total allowable error based on biological variation. Clin Chem 2011;57(9):1334–6.

46. Oosterhuis WP, Theodorsson E. Total error vs. measurement uncertainty: revolution or evolution? Clin Chem Lab Med 2016;54(2):235–9.

47. Farrance I, Badrick T, Sikaris KA. Uncertainty in measurement and total error - are they so incompatible? Clin Chem Lab Med 2016;54(8):1309–11.

48. Forbes AB, Sousa JA. The GUM, Bayesian inference and the observation and measurement equations. Measurement 2011;44(8):1422–35.

49. Taylor JR. An introduction to error analysis. The study of uncertainties in physical measurements. 2nd edition. Sausalito (CA): University Science Books; 1997.

50. Salicone S. Measurement uncertainty: an approach via the mathematical theory of evidence. New York: Springer; 2007.

51. Bandemer H. Mathematics of uncertainty: ideas, methods, application problems. Berlin: Springer; 2006.

52. Dieck RH. Measurement uncertainty: methods and applications. 4th edition. Research Triangle Park (NC): ISA; 2007.
53. Lindley DV. Understanding uncertainty. Hoboken (NJ): Wiley; 2006.
54. Weise K, Wöger W. Comparison of two measurement results using the Bayesian theory of measurement uncertainty. Meas Sci Technol 1994;5:879–82.
55. Attivissimo F, Giaquinto N, Savino M. A Bayesian paradox and its impact on the GUM approach to uncertainty. Measurement 2012;45(9):2194–202.
56. Elster C. Bayesian uncertainty analysis compared with the application of the GUM and its supplements. Metrologia 2014;51(4):S159–66.
57. Willink TJ, White R. Disentangling classical and bayesian approaches to uncertainty analysis. Available at: http://www.bipm.org/cc/CCT/Allowed/26/Disentangling_uncertainty_v14.pdf. Accessed February 2, 2016.
58. Foundation TR. The R Project for statistical computing. 2016. Available at: https://www.r-project.org/. Accessed February 2, 2016.
59. Wikipedia. Comparison of risk analysis Microsoft Excel add-ins. 2016. Available at: https://en.wikipedia.org/wiki/Comparison_of_risk_analysis_Microsoft_Excel_add-ins. Accessed February 2, 2016.
60. Jones HL. Investigating the properties of a sample mean by employing random subsample means. JASA 1956;51:54–83.
61. Efron B, Tibshirani R. Statistical-data analysis in the computer-age. Science 1991;253(5018):390–5.
62. Efron B, Tibshirani R. An introduction to the bootstrap. New York: Chapman & Hall; 1993.
63. Good PI. Resampling methods: a practical guide to data analysis. 3rd edition. Boston: Birkhäuser; 2006.
64. Efron B. A 250-year argument: belief, behavior, and the bootstrap. B Am Math Soc 2013;50(1):129–46.
65. Andersson MK, Karlsson S. Bootstrapping error component models. Stockholm (Sweden): Stockholm School of Economics; 1999.
66. Shao J, Tu D. The jackknife and bootstrap. New York: Springer-Verlag; 1995.
67. De Bievre P. Meeting the need for intercontinentally understood concepts and intercontinentally agreed terms for Metrology in Chemistry (at the occasion of the 2007 edition of the VIM) - "To prevent war, be very precise in your speaking" [Kongfutze 551-479 BC]. Accred Qual Assur 2007;12(8):439–42.
68. Kragten J. Calculating standard deviations and confidence-intervals with a universally applicable spreadsheet technique. Analyst 1994;119(10):2161–5.
69. Kragten J. A standard scheme for calculating numerically standard deviations and confidence-intervals. Chemometr Intell Lab Syst 1995;28(1):89–97.
70. Magnusson B, Näykki T, Hovind H, et al. Handbook for calculation of measurement uncertainty in environmental laboratories. Oslo, Norway: Nordtest; 2012.
71. Hovind H, Magnusson B, Krysell M, et al. The TROLL book. Internal quality control - handbook for chemical laboratories. Oslo (Norway): Nordtest; 2011. Available at: http://nordtest.info/index.php/7-technical-reports/22-trollboken-a-new-edition.html. Accessed February 2, 2016.
72. Virtanen A, Näykki T, Varkonyi E. MUkit - Measurement uncertainty kit. 2012. Available at: http://www.syke.fi/en-US/Services/Calibration_services_and_contract_laboratory/MUkit__Measurement_Uncertainty_Kit. Accessed February 13, 2016.
73. Westgard JO, Groth T, Aronsson T, et al. Combined Shewhart-Cusum control chart for improved quality control in clinical chemistry. Clin Chem 1977;23(10):1881–7.

74. Westgard JO, Groth T, Aronsson T, et al. Performance characteristics of rules for internal quality control: probabilities for false rejection and error detection. Clin Chem 1977;23(10):1857–67.

75. Theodorsson E. Validation and verification of measurement methods in clinical chemistry. Bioanalysis 2012;4(3):305–20.

76. Theodorsson E, Magnusson B, Leito I. Bias in clinical chemistry. Bioanalysis 2014;6(21):2855–75.

77. Mari L. The 'error approach' and the 'uncertainty approach': are they incompatible? Leiden (Netherlands): Lorentz Center; 2011.

78. Rozet E, Marini RD, Ziemons E, et al. Total error and uncertainty: friends or foes? Trends Anal Chem 2011;30(5):797–806.

79. Hubert P, Marini RD, Rozet E, et al. Estimation of uncertainty from the total error strategy: application to internal and normative methods. Acta Clin Belg 2010;65: 100–4.

80. Panteghini M. Application of traceability concepts to analytical quality control may reconcile total error with uncertainty of measurement. Clin Chem Lab Med 2010;48(1):7–10.

81. Badrick T, Hawkins RC, Wilson SR, et al. Uncertainty of measurement: what it is and what it should be. Clin Biochem Rev 2005;26(4):155–8 [author reply: 159–60].

82. Büttner J. Reference methods in clinical chemistry. Objectives, trends, problems. Eur J Clin Chem Clin Biochem 1991;29:221–2.

83. Thienpont LM. Quality specifications for reference methods. Scand J Clin Lab Invest 1999;59(7):535–8.

84. Bonini P, Plebani M, Ceriotti F, et al. Errors in laboratory medicine. Clin Chem 2002;48(5):691–8.

85. Norheim S. Computer support simplifying uncertainty estimation using patient samples. Linkoping (Sweden): Institute of Technology; Linkoping University; 2008. Available at: http://liu.diva-portal.org/smash/record.jsf?pid=diva2:417298.

86. Grubb A, Horio M, Hansson LO, et al. Generation of a new cystatin C-based estimating equation for glomerular filtration rate by use of 7 assays standardized to the international calibrator. Clin Chem 2014;60(7):974–86.

87. Kallner A. Estimated GFR. Comparison of five algorithms: implications for drug dosing. J Clin Pathol 2014;67(7):609–13.

88. Pepe MS. The statistical evaluation of medical tests for classification and prediction. Oxford (United Kingdom): Oxford University Press; 2004.

89. Galen RS, Gambino SR. Beyond normality: the predictive value and efficiency of medical diagnoses. New York: John Wiley and Sons; 1975.

90. Zhou XH, Obuchowski NA, McClish DK. Statistical methods in diagnostic medicine. New York: Wiley-Interscience; 2002.

91. Menditto A, Patriarca M, Magnusson B. Understanding the meaning of accuracy, trueness and precision. Accred Qual Assur 2007;12:45–7.

92. Ehrlich C, Dybkaer R. Uncertainty of error: the error dilemma. OIML Bull 2012; LIII(2):12–7.

93. Vallverdú J. Bayesian versus frequentists. A philosophical debate on statistical reasoning. Heidelberg (Germany): Springer; 2016.

94. Pearl J. Causality: models, reasoning, and inference. 2nd edition. Cambridge (United Kingdom): Cambridge University Press; 2009.

95. Pearl J. Causal inference in statistics: an overview. Stat Surv 2009;3:96–146.

96. Bich W. Revision of the 'Guide to the Expression of Uncertainty in Measurement'. Why and how. Metrologia 2014;51(4):S155–8.

97. Bich W, Cox MG, Dybkaer R, et al. Revision of the 'Guide to the Expression of Uncertainty in Measurement'. Metrologia 2012;49(6):702–5.

98. Bich W. From errors to probability density functions. Evolution of the concept of measurement uncertainty. IEEE T Instrum Meas 2012;61(8):2153–9.

99. Ehrlich C. Terminological aspects of the Guide to the Expression of Uncertainty in Measurement (GUM). Metrologia 2014;51(4):S145–54.

100. Ehrlich C, Dybkaer R, Wöger W. Evolution of philosophy and description of measurement (preliminary rationale for VIM3). Accred Qual Assur 2007;12:201–18.

Rhetoric Versus Reality? Laboratory Surveys Show Actual Practice Differs Considerably from Proposed Models and Mandated Calculations

Sten A. Westgard, MS

KEYWORDS

- Measurement uncertainty • Individualized quality control plans • Allowable total error
- Total error • Performance specifications

KEY POINTS

- There is a large difference between the scientific debate about goals, measurement uncertainty, and analytical goals and the reality of how laboratories routinely operate.
- Online surveys of laboratory professionals in the United States and around the world were conducted in 2014, 2015, and 2016.
- Most laboratories that implement measurement uncertainty do so only because of regulatory mandate by ISO (International Organization for Standardization) 15189. They do not have a practical use for the calculation.
- Most US laboratories that implement individualized quality control (QC) plans (IQCPs) did so only to fulfill the US regulatory mandates. The IQCPs did not substantively change their QC practices. In particular, most laboratories made no change to their QC frequency after completing their IQCPs.
- Most laboratories use allowable total error to set their analytical goals, along with other goals from a variety of resources. Only a small percentage of laboratories set their goals using target measurement uncertainty.

Although the scientific literature is full of publications proposing new models for errors and new statistics to calculate, the real world of laboratory practice is different. The academic debates often seem to take place in a separate reality, arguing over what is the perfect, pure expression, while ignoring the economic and work-flow pressures that drive the current practice of laboratory medicine.

Client Services and Technology, Westgard QC, Inc., 7614 Gray Fox Trail, Madison, WI 53717, USA
E-mail address: westgard@westgard.com

Clin Lab Med 37 (2017) 35–45
http://dx.doi.org/10.1016/j.cll.2016.09.004   labmed.theclinics.com
0272-2712/17/© 2016 Elsevier Inc. All rights reserved.

Over the past 3 years (2014–2016), the authors have conducted 3 online surveys on analytical goals,[1] measurement uncertainty,[2] and individualized QC plans (IQCPs)[3] that attempted to capture the real-world practices of laboratories all over the world. The findings of these surveys are different than what is recommended or condemned in the literature. The contrast between reality and theory is stark. When the 3 surveys are summarized, a very different picture of laboratory practice is revealed than what the literature describes, debates, or recommends.

That the scientific literature should differ so considerably from reality is to be expected, particularly for new models that are being introduced. Novel approaches are by definition previously unknown. However, in the measurement uncertainty (MU) and total error (TE) debate, both approaches have been around for decades, and most laboratories are already applying one if not both of these models. The difference between the scientific literature and reality therefore should not be large, but it is.

For IQCPs,[4] this is a new approach, in which US laboratories are in effect "guinea pigs" in a kind of regulatory experiment. After an unsuccessful attempt in the early 2000s to justify reduced quality control (QC) frequency through the equivalent QC (EQC) protocols,[5,6] the Centers for Medicare and Medicaid Services asked the Clinical Laboratory Standards Institute to develop an alternative justification for running QC only once a month or once a week. Although the motivation espoused for this regulatory initiative was that the advanced engineering of modern instrumentation no longer requires the traditional regulatory default minimum of daily QC (ie, running controls once every 24 hours), the more honest reason for this approach was the proliferation of point-of-care (POC) devices that are not designed for practical daily QC. For institutions using POC devices for which operators are not well versed in QC, with devices that are not well designed to mimic operations with daily QC, and in situations in which the number of devices and operators can run into the hundreds, the traditional QC approach was daunting and a reduced application of QC was desirable.

There is always a need for scientific debate that is separate from market realities; a discussion that envisions the future ideal state of the marketplace and that shows the optimal possibilities and urges both the diagnostic industry and laboratories to innovate and improve to make those possibilities into practical realities. However, if the discussion is so lofty as to be unrealistic, the debate has little relevance to industry or laboratory. It is a tragic waste of scientific focus if research concentrates on issues that have no practical impact on laboratories and the diagnostic industry. In addition, if there is an ideal state that laboratories and industry need to achieve but is currently beyond their reach, then, at least in the interim, a model is needed that is practical and achievable.

MATERIALS AND METHODS

In late 2014 through 2016, Westgard QC sent out invitations to online surveys on MU, analytical goal setting, and IQCPs. The survey requests were sent to more than 24,000 laboratory professionals who had voluntarily joined the electronic newsletter list of westgard.com and nearly 15,000 LinkedIn connections who had voluntarily connected with one of the authors. Surveys were conducted on the SurveyMonkey site and consisted of a variety of single-choice, multiple-choice, and free-form comments. Results were downloaded from the site and saved as Microsoft Excel files. Survey results were initially posted on Westgard Web.

LIMITATIONS

The surveys were subject to several biases common to voluntary polling. Although the authors sent out survey requests to more than 24,000 laboratory professionals and

15,000 LinkedIn connections in 2016, both of those are opt-in, self-selecting groups; the type of laboratory professional who chooses to subscribe to a Westgard newsletter may have already expressed a preference and thus results will be affected by self-selection bias. It is also possible that the authors did not search widely enough to address the entire global laboratory marketplace. Furthermore, with the IQCP survey, the voluntary respondents might represent a biased portion of IQCP users: those motivated by their experience to share their results. There may be a silent majority that is satisfied with their IQCP experience but not as highly motivated as the vocal few who were disgruntled. There may also be more laboratories that enjoy their MU calculations and use them widely in their practice but did not feel the imperative to share those views, and that would prefer to abolish allowable TE (TEa) goals and replace them with some other model, but simply did not want to participate in our survey to express that opinion. Also, given our strong views on the subject, the authors are subject to confirmation bias, wherein we ask the questions in a way to solicit the answers we want to receive. All of these biases are well known to survey research and not unique to this particular set of surveys.

As with any survey of this sort, it cannot be concluded that this is the true picture of laboratory sentiment or practice. It is one picture, but it may be the only one that the public gets to see. Although business groups and the vendors conduct countless surveys, they rarely share them with the general public, but instead exploit them for their own economic interests.

What is surprising is that for all the scientific journals and trade press that serve the laboratory market, survey results of this type are rarely available.

THE REAL STATE OF ANALYTICAL GOAL SETTING

At the end of 2014 and early 2015, Westgard Web conducted a survey, announcing it in an electronic newsletter, which reached more than 20,000 laboratory professionals.[1] Similar announcements were made via Twitter, LinkedIn, and various electronic mailing lists that are dedicated to the medical laboratory profession. The authors received more than 450 responses from more than 80 countries.

The most common type of analytical goal used by nearly 2 out of 3 laboratories is the TEa. Target MU was only used by 15% of the responding laboratories (**Fig. 1**).

Even more striking is that, when laboratories were asked how they want goals to improve, less than 6% of laboratories responded that they wanted to eliminate TEa. There are a lot of items that these laboratories would like to happen, such as harmonization of the external quality assessment (EQA) and proficiency testing (PT) goals, or the development of more evidence-based goals. However, the form of those goals is not really in question. Most laboratories accept and prefer TEa (**Fig. 2**).

THE REAL STATE OF MEASUREMENT UNCERTAINTY

In 2015, Westgard Web conducted a global survey of analytical goal setting. This survey obtained more than 550 responses from more than 85 countries, which is the largest response we have had to date. The results were significantly different within the United States, where MU is almost unknown as a concept and rarely implemented save by a handful of laboratories. Thus the authors broke out the responses for non-US or rest of world into 1 set of results, and then the US responses were collected in another set of results.

Outside the United States, nearly 2 out of 3 respondents calculate MU, but only 7.5% of those laboratories include MU in their test reports. Because most of these

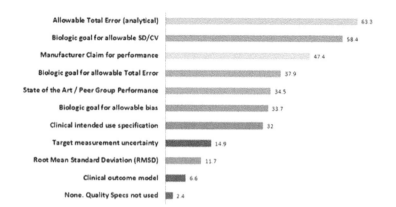

Fig. 1. Type of analytical goals used within the laboratory. Multiple choices allowed. Specs, specifications. CV, coefficient of variation; SD, standard deviation.

laboratories are not communicating MU, we asked whether they were using it internally. The most common response was that MU is not being used at all (**Fig. 3**).

Even if most laboratories do not routinely report or use MU, there is the possibility that clinicians could request MU, to help them interpret the uncertainty around a particular laboratory result. However, that is an even more rare event. Most laboratories report that MU has never been requested by a clinician (**Fig. 4**).

Probing further, we asked whether clinicians have ever changed their diagnoses or decisions based on the MU reported with the test result. Less than 10% of laboratories report that this happened even once a year, with more than 84% of respondents reporting that MU has never had a clinical impact or, if it has had any impact, they do not know about it (**Fig. 5**).

Within the United States, it is different: more than 73% of laboratories reported that they do not calculate MU, and another 13% do not know about the concept. Most of these laboratories do not calculate MU because they are not required by their regulations to do so.

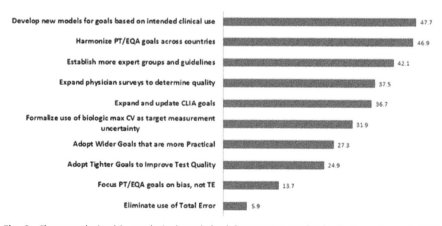

Fig. 2. Changes desired in analytical goals by laboratories. Multiple choices allowed. CLIA, Clinical Laboratory Improvement Amendments; CV, maximum allowed coefficient of variation.

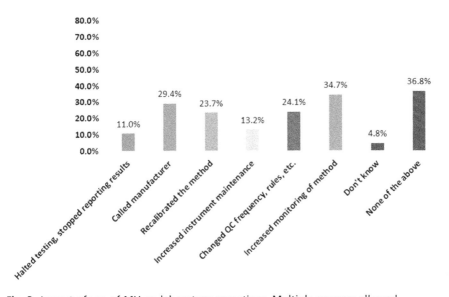

Fig. 3. Impact of use of MU on laboratory operations. Multiple answers allowed.

This sharp division in the calculation of MU has not produced wildly different treatments or choices in laboratories, calling into question the utility of MU. If a laboratory can be operated perfectly well with or without MU, why is MU needed? In economic terms, there is a natural experiment with the United States and the rest of the world, but no studies exist that report the rest of the globe achieving any superior patient outcomes because of the use of MU.

THE REAL STATE OF INDIVIDUALIZED QUALITY CONTROL PLAN IMPLEMENTATION

In early 2016, after a 2-year educational period, IQCPs became a matter of law in US laboratories. The previous EQC protocols became illegal. For many laboratories, despite 2 years of advanced notice, the details of IQCP implementation remained vague, and it was also a mystery how IQCPs were going to be interpreted by inspectors.

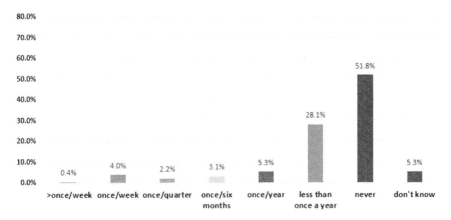

Fig. 4. How often is MU requested by clinicians. One answer allowed.

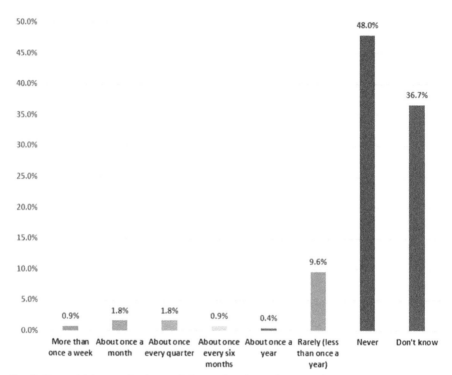

Fig. 5. Non-US laboratories (n=229): how often have clinicians changed their diagnosis or decisions based on measurement uncertainty?

After 6 months of implementation, the authors initiated a survey of laboratories that had implemented IQCPs. Of the surveys we conducted, this one had the smallest response rate: 210 respondents from within the United States and around the world. Our own theory of this reduced response could be termed IQCP fatigue: that most laboratories were tired of researching, developing, and implementing these policies, and thus did not want to share their experiences.

Within the United States, most respondents were from core laboratories with volumes of more than 1000 tests per day. Most laboratories had implemented just a few (between 1 and 5) IQCPs and the plurality were implemented only for 1 site. There was a dichotomy in the personnel tasked with IQCP implementation: nearly 1 in 5 laboratories only devoted 1 staff member to the IQCP implementation, whereas more than a quarter of laboratories had 5 people or more dedicated to the task (**Fig. 6**).

That is a big difference in resources and it reflects a divergence from the recommended practice of risk assessment. Guidelines like EP23 (trademarked)[7] and other official risk management standards are clear that this should be a multidisciplinary project; it requires multiple people from different parts of the testing cycle in order to gain an accurate picture of all the possible failure modes. However, 1 in 5 laboratories are cutting corners on risk assessment, and only 1 in 5 laboratories are addressing the resource requirements appropriately.

When it comes to the time required to develop IQCPs, there is a similar split in effort: nearly 1 in 4 laboratories spent more than 15 hours developing their IQCPs, whereas slightly more than 1 in 4 laboratories spent between 1 and 4 hours developing their IQCPs. Although it is possible that some laboratories have far fewer hazards and risks,

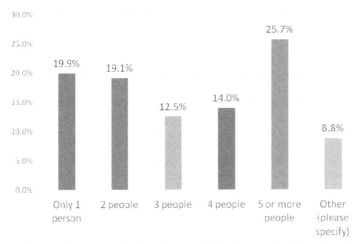

Fig. 6. Number of staff persons dedicated to IQCP development and implementation. One answer allowed.

it is also possible that some laboratories are simply not spending the appropriate amount of time to develop their IQCPs, the danger being that they develop inadequate risk controls (**Fig. 7**).

More than 60% of US respondents reported that their IQCPs had 20 or fewer failure modes or hazards addressed. In a recent online example, the authors compared an IQCP developed by a single laboratory[8] for a chemistry POC device with an IQCP for the same device developed by an expert group. The single laboratory identified 30 sources of error for the POC device, whereas the expert group identified 97.[9]

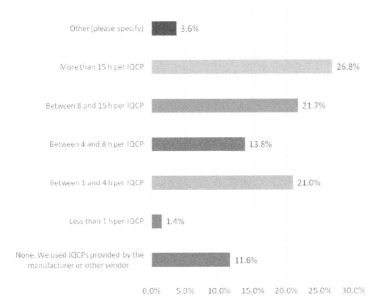

Fig. 7. Number of hours required to develop IQCPs. One answer allowed.

This analysis was performed on one of the most prevalent POC devices on the market, but both the independent laboratory and the expert group not only disagreed about how many sources of error there were, they were both finding more error sources than the typical laboratory reported in our survey. It could be concluded that most US laboratories have fewer sources of error than the 2 examples, or that most US laboratories are not fully aware of all their risks, despite their IQCP efforts. This conclusion would lend credence to the argument that failure mode effects analysis, which is a strong influence on EP23 (trademarked) and IQCP, does not generate reproducible or reliable results.[10–12]

Despite all this effort (5 staff members conducting 15 hours of work per IQCP, with about 5 IQCPs per laboratory, is 375 hours of staff time), the IQCP results in the United States have not prompted major changes to previous practices. More than 68% of US respondents reported discovering no unacceptable risks as a result of their IQCP development, and nearly 80% of laboratories reported that their current control mechanisms were adequate to control both known and newly discovered risks. That is, all those hours of effort produced no modifications in the laboratory operation.

Furthermore, most laboratory practices did not change as a result of their IQCP implementation. Most laboratories remained on once-a-month QC, which was the old option 1 of the EQC regulations that were replaced by IQCP. In other words, same QC frequency, different regulation (**Fig. 8**).

The most cynical conclusion about IQCP implementation is that it was a paperwork exercise, designed to justify an already-reduced QC frequency by giving it the appearance of a scientific process. However, there is nothing scientific about once-a-month QC; no equation or calculation can be found that will tell clinicians to base their QC on a lunar cycle. This conclusion may seem too jaded, but the comments that many users shared about their IQCP experience were much harsher.[13]

The laboratories implementing IQCPs outside the United States seem to be far more satisfied with the process.[14] It is a curious development to see that laboratories outside the United States are implementing IQCPs, because it is only mandatory within the United States. However, because accreditation agencies like the College of American Pathologists (CAP) are deemed providers of US laboratories, they are required to implement all Clinical Laboratory Improvement Amendments (CLIA) regulations. Thus, despite any objections to the regulations they might have expressed,

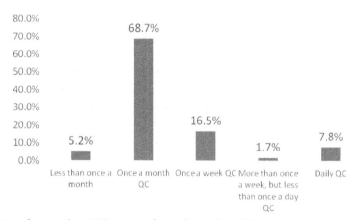

Fig. 8. How frequently is QC being performed now that IQCPs have been implemented. One answer allowed.

CAP and other US accreditation providers have their own implementation of the IQCP regulations. In addition, when laboratories outside the United States apply for CAP certification, they are then exposed to the IQCP regulations. Even though the IQCP regulations are only mandatory within the United States, and only then when the laboratory opts out of the default minimum QC frequency of once a day, foreign laboratories have been swept up in the IQCP fervor. Fewer responses were garnered in the IQCP survey from foreign laboratories, but those who did respond were more positive about their experience than the US laboratories. When the IQCP process is adopted voluntarily by a laboratory it may be more palatable than when it is an imposed mandate.

More than 70% of global respondents reported that they identified fewer than 10 failure modes or hazards in their IQCP process, suggesting either that the United States is far more error-prone, or that these laboratories are conducting a less rigorous risk assessment. Also in contrast the US findings, most of the foreign laboratories found unacceptable risks after their IQCP implementation. As a result of this, 44% of global laboratories with IQCP implementations increased their QC frequency, whereas slightly less than a third of laboratories reduced their QC frequency; this is almost the opposite outcome of what has been observed in the United States, where IQCP has been a justification to reduce QC frequency. The outcome of the IQCP process outside the United States is very different from what happened inside the United States: 76% of laboratories are still running daily QC, and very few laboratories have reduced to once-a-month QC (**Fig. 9**).

Again, this speaks to the variability (or individuality) of the IQCP process. It is possible that significantly different outcomes will be generated by laboratories that implement the technique.

The final result of IQCP implementation remains to be seen. Risk management has been used with various degrees of success in other industries, with notable failures on Wall Street in recent memory, but broad acceptance across the world. If the current IQCP evolves into a more rigorous risk assessment protocol, with more reproducible, reliable measurements of risk and application of control mechanisms, there is no reason for it not to produce better quality, better laboratories, and better patient

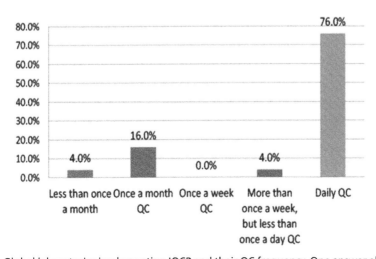

Fig. 9. Global laboratories implementing IQCP and their QC frequency. One answer allowed.

care. If it remains a mere paperwork exercise, a type of QC theater instead of a real risk management implementation, the authors suspect that it will experience the same fate as the EQC protocols: eventual abandonment as a regulation.

DISCUSSION

In the scientific literature, because of the ISO 15189[15] mandate, MU is supreme. In reality, it is a calculation that even compliant laboratories find virtually useless. In the marketing of IQCP, it was promised that this approach would help laboratories choose the right QC and right-size their QC, when in practice it has been mostly used to justify exactly the same QC and same QC frequency. In the scientific literature, there are continuing attacks on the TEa approach, despite its near-universal adoption and acceptance by laboratories around the globe.

It may be that the arguments in the scientific literature are so vigorous because the reality is so challenging. MU cannot make inroads into practical laboratory use until the existence of other approaches is eliminated. Therefore, MU proponents are also the most vociferous critics of TEa. Similarly, IQCP has been forced on laboratories rather than offered as an option, and the chief supporters of the approach have been quick to criticize the perceived shortcomings of all other approaches, such as the traditional statistical QC approach, as a method of making IQCP look better. Because reality is not amenable to the MU and IQCP approaches, their only path to broader implementation in laboratories is through compulsion and mandate. The survey results strongly suggest that if laboratories were given free choice tomorrow, they would eliminate their calculations of MU, they would cease developing IQCPs, and they would return to traditional QC techniques and approaches that include TEa.

To take the perspective of a marketplace of ideas, the current debate is one in which real laboratories choose TEa and the traditional statistical QC approach. That may reflect more laziness and a reluctance to change the status quo than an informed choice, but the mandates of MU and IQCP have not generated an enthusiastic following. Laboratories are performing these calculations and implementing these requirements only when forced, and they are not embracing them.

For more than 40 years, TE has provided an imperfect but useful model of how to approach errors and adapt QC to detect those errors. MU-IQCP may promise improvements, but the fact that they must be forced on laboratories in order to be implemented shows that they have little traction in the marketplace. They are ideas that do not thrive because they represent approaches that are not practical or useful in the real world.

SUMMARY

There is a common saying about academic debates, that the arguments are so large because the differences are so small. In this case, the differences are significant, but the reason the debate is so loud is because the reality is so unforgiving. Despite all the articles published on the superiority of MU and IQCP, or the imperfections of TEa, laboratories still use the TEa instead of MU and IQCP, and prefer the TEa approach to the forced implementations of MU and IQCP. When laboratories are given a voice, such as through these surveys, they speak volumes.

REFERENCES

1. Analytical global goal survey results. 2015. Available at: https://www.westgard. com/global-goal-results.htm. Accessed October 26, 2016.

2. Measurement uncertainty survey results. 2015. Available at: https://www.westgard.com/mu-global-survey.htm. Accessed August 22, 2016.
3. IQCP survey results 2016. 2016. Available at: https://www.westgard.com/iqcp-user-survey.htm. Accessed August 22, 2016.
4. IQCP homepage. Available at: https://www.cms.gov/regulations-and-guidance/legislation/CLIA/Individualized_Quality_Control_Plan_IQCP.html. Accessed August 22, 2016.
5. Equivocal QC. Coming soon to a laboratory near you. 2007. Available at: https://www.westgard.com/essay119.htm. Accessed August 22, 2016.
6. Laessig RH, Ehrymeyer SS. CLIA 2003's new concept: equivalent quality control. MLO Med Lab Obs 2005;37:32–4. Available at: http://www.mlo-online.com/articles/200501/0105labmgmt_quality.pdf. Accessed August 22, 2016.
7. EP23–A. Available at: http://shop.clsi.org/method-evaluation-documents/EP23.html. Accessed August 22, 2016.
8. IQCP for a POC device. 2016. Available at: https://www.westgard.com/iqcp-poc-chemistry.htm. Accessed August 18, 2016.
9. An outside review of an IQCP for POC. 2016. Available at: http://www.westgard.com/iqcp-poc-review.htm. Accessed August 18, 2016.
10. Shebl NA, Franklin BD, Barber N. Failure mode and effects analysis outputs: are they valid? BMC Health Serv Res 2012;12:150.
11. Franklin BD, Shebl NA, Barber N. Failure mode and effects analysis: too little for too much? BMJ Qual Saf 2012;21:607–11.
12. Shebl NA, Franklin BD, Barber N. Is failure mode and effect analysis reliable? J Patient Saf 2009;5:86–94.
13. 2016 IQCP users survey – the comments section2016. . Available at: https://www.westgard.com/iqcp-user-survey-comments.htm. Accessed August 18, 2016.
14. 2016 IQCP users survey global results. 2016. Available at: https://www.westgard.com/iqcp-user-survey-global.htm. Accessed August 18, 2016.
15. ISO 15189:2012. Available at: http://www.iso.org/iso/catalogue_detail?csnumber=56115. Accessed August 22, 2016.

Biologic Variation Approach to Daily Laboratory

Carmen Ricós, PhD*, Virtudes Álvarez, MD, Joana Minchinela, MD,
Pilar Fernández-Calle, PhD, Carmen Perich, MD,
Beatriz Boned, MD, Elisabet González, MD, Margarita Simón, MD,
Jorge Díaz-Garzón, MD, José Vicente García-Lario, MD,
Fernando Cava, MD, Pilar Fernández-Fernández, MD,
Zoraida Corte, PhD, Carmen Biosca, PhD

KEYWORDS

- Biological variation • Error limits • Quality control • Reference change value

KEY POINTS

- Biologic variation is an unavoidable result of the continuous changes inherent in a living organism and has been studied within subject and between subjects.
- Biologic variation can be used to set the analytical performance specifications for total allowable error, imprecision, and bias (trueness).
- Biologic variation can also be used to assess the significance of changes in serial patient results through a reference change value.
- Biologic variation can be used to determine rules to help autoverification of patient results.
- Recent conferences and studies have made important observations about the validity and usefulness of today's biologic variation estimates. An international effort is working toward improving these estimates.

INTRODUCTION

Laboratory medicine is the science that gives information on the patient health status on the basis of measurements of biological fluids. It is well-known that concentration of analytes in these fluids are not the always exactly at the same concentration owing to the simple fact of being a living, constantly changing organism; this is what in general is named biological variation (BV). Characterization and understanding of BV enables a valid assessment of the significance of a laboratory result.

There are many sources of BV that have been very well-described,[1] with random variation around a central value the focus of this article. There are 2 components of

Spanish Society of Laboratory Medicine (SEQC), Commission of Analytical Quality, Spain
* Corresponding author.
E-mail address: cperich.bcn.ics@gencat.cat

random BV: within-subject BV and between-subject BV. Within-subject BV is the random variation around the homeostatic setting point[1] or the random variation that assures an equilibrium state of the human body (data not published[2]). Between-subject BV is the variation among the central points of different individuals. Both terms are usually expressed in terms of percentage coefficient of variation (intraindividual coefficient of variation [CVı] and intragroup coefficient of variation, respectively).[3]

The way to estimate the components of BV was thoroughly described by Fraser and Harris[4] and data on BV have been compiled in a BV database since 1999 (Ricós-Stockholm conference).[5] This database has been updated every 2 years by the Analytical Committee of the Spanish Society of Clinical Chemistry and Molecular Pathology (SEQC) and has been regularly published at the Westgard website.[6]

More recently, some weaknesses of this database have been described, such as the lack of published studies available for an important number of analytes, discrepancies among the papers that have been compiled, and so on[7,8]; these points were discussed at the European Federation of Clinical Chemistry and Laboratory Medicine Milan Strategic Conference where a Task and Finish group was created with the aim to improve the current database and transform it to a more comprehensive and granulated one as well as reliable as reference data. All the information compiled may be available and will no longer merely the list of quality specifications, but also supporting data such as confidence intervals, and so on.[2,9]

USES OF BIOLOGICAL VARIATION

The currently available data on BV are important information for the medical laboratory that may be used for different applications. These are (1) setting analytical quality specifications, also named performance quality specifications, which are mainly used within the laboratory, (2) assessing the significance of changes in serial results from an individual, reference change value (RCV) that can be used both intralaboratory (delta-check) and can be shown to the clinicians in the laboratory report to inform them about significant changes in patient health status (RCV), and (3) autoverification of results.

Analytical Quality Specifications

Since the Aspen conference in 1977,[10] it has been an accepted standard that the analytical coefficient of variation should be maintained below one-half of the within-subject CV, so that the amount of variability added to the true variability of the result is only about 10%.[11] Further, Gowans stated that when bias is limited below one-quarter of the within-subject plus between-subject coefficients of variation, only a limited percentage of results should be falsely considered outside the upper and lower limits of the population-based reference interval.[12] Accordingly, Ricós and colleagues[13] suggested a limit for total allowable error (TAE) for a single measurement based on the combination of both criteria. The formulae that summarize these statements are:

$$CV_A \leq 0.5 * CV_I$$

$$Bias \leq 0.25 * (CV_I^2 + CV_G^2)^{1/2}$$

$$TAE \leq 1.65 * 0.5 * CV_I + 0.25 * (CV_I^2 + CV_G^2)^{1/2}$$

Although the formula for TAE has been debated[14] and some alternatives have been proposed, no revised formula has been generally accepted to date. From the first

Strategic Conference of Milan TFG ("Task Finishing Group") has been created to review and debate this concept.

In addition, Fraser and colleagues[15] suggested also minimum and optimum levels of quality based on fractions different that 0.5 for imprecision and 0.25 for bias, which may be used in the case of testing analytes with very narrow or very wide CV_I according to the current methodological technology.

Nevertheless, the current list of quality specifications from the SEQC group, based on the estimates of CV_I and intragroup coefficient of variation, uses these standard formulae and establishes 3 classes of limits (desirable, minimum, and optimum) so that each laboratory can select the best alternative for its own performance capability. Analytical quality specifications are applied for 2 basic activities of the medical laboratory: internal quality control procedures and evaluation of laboratory performance.

Internal quality control procedure

According to the Westgard's internal quality control protocol, for each analyte and analytical procedure, the laboratory has to estimate its stable performance (in terms of CV_A) and has to define the corresponding quality specification. Briefly, a simple ratio between both terms (6 sigma concept) gives an idea on how restrictive or how relaxed the control rules must be for proper error detection.[16] If any bias exists it should be subtracted from the TAE before calculating the mentioned ratio.[17]

The most important issue is to use the appropriate control rule for each analyte and procedure (even for each control level) instead of using a uniform control rule on all tests in the laboratory (ie, 1:2s). **Table 1** shows an example of a number of analytes tested on a single instrument of a laboratory with different sigma values for the various analytes. The quality specification (desirable) for each analyte is derived from BV; as the TAE narrows, the sigma-metric lowers and more rules and controls are required.

Evaluation of laboratory performance

At a regular interval, the laboratory should review its performance to establish priorities for making improvements and to apply resources when necessary. A simple way to do this is to elaborate monthly figures with CV_A and bias for each analyte and procedure. **Fig. 1** shows an example of serum albumin internal quality control results (at concentration within population based reference values) compared with desirable specifications derived from BV for a 1-year time study.

Problems and solutions applied in daily routine may also be recorded so that requirements for accreditation according to ISO 15189 standard are satisfied.

Laboratory performance is also evaluated and monitoring by participating in external quality assurance (EQA) programs. The recommendations for analytical

Table 1
Control rules for a single instrument used in a stat laboratory

Analyte	Level	Goal	TAE	B_A	CV_A	σ	Rule	N	$P_{de\,(\%)}$	$P_{fr\,(\%)}$
Ferritin	3	BV_{des}	16.9	0.0	1.39	12.2	1:5s	2	90	0
IgG	3	BV_{des}	7.99	0.0	2.37	3.37	1:3s/s:2s.R:4s/3:1s/12x	6	90	8.93
IgA	3	BV_{des}	13.5	0.0	2.39	5.64	1:3.5s	2	90	0.08
IgM	3	BV_{des}	16.8	0.0	2.08	5.46	1:3s	2	90	0.56
Rheumatoid factor	3	BV_{des}	13.5	0.0	2.13	6.32	1:4s	2	90	0.01

Abbreviations: B_A, analytical bias; BV_{des}, desirable biological variation; CV_A, analytical coefficient of variation; P_{de}, probability for detection of error; P_{fr}, probability for false rejection; TAE, total allowable error.

ALBUMIN
(Normal control)

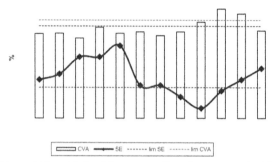

Fig. 1. Monthly CV_A and bias obtained for serum albumin compared with desirable quality specifications. CV_A, analytical coefficient of variation; lim CVA, limit for analytical coefficient of variation; lim SE, limit for systematic error; SE, systematic error.

performance specifications among EQA are not harmonized. Some of them use statistical approaches (United Kingdom National External Quality Assessment Service), others apply state of the art goals aligned with legislated limits of performance (Rilibak, Clinical Laboratory Improvement Amendments), whereas still others recommend biologically derived specifications (Royal College of Pathologists of Australasia).

The most widely used EQA in Spain is organized by the Spanish Society of Clinical Chemistry and Laboratory Medicine (SEQC), which uses acceptability limits for total error derived from BV. **Fig. 2** shows a report of serum calcium from a laboratory using

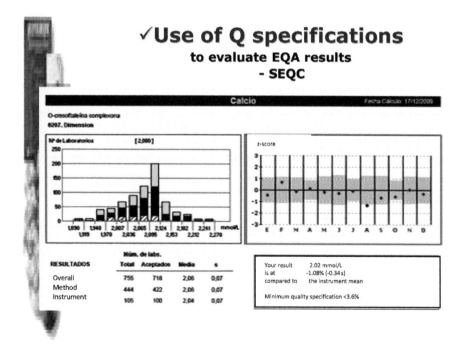

Fig. 2. External quality assurance (EQA) report for serum calcium.

the ortho-cresolftalein method in a Siemens dimension instrument as an example. The left part of the figure shows the frequency histogram of all results and description of total number of results, accepted number of results (after exclusion of outliers), and mean values and standard deviation(s) for overall group and instrument grouped values. The right part shows the deviation of results compared with the instrument mean, expressed both in z-score and as a percentage deviation for the last 12 months; also, the minimum specification for total error is shown. Using this report, the laboratory can evaluate its performance (judged as acceptable in the example) for the entire EQA cycle.

Another application of quality specifications is to evaluate performance of all laboratories participating in an EQAS program. **Fig. 3** shows the percentage of results reported to the SEQC-EQA for the basic biochemistry program of 1-year period satisfying the TAE derived from BV (2015).[18] The majority of analytes have 80% or more results within the acceptable limits for total error. The exceptions are acid phosphatase with a high dispersion of results in our setting, sodium and chloride with a very narrow within-subject BV, as well as creatinine with a lot of laboratories using the Jaffé kinetic method, which is nonspecific at levels of creatinine that are less than the upper limit of reference interval, with great impact on the pediatric population.

Reference Change Value

Interpretation of serial results of an analyte in a patient is an important challenge for health care today. Calculation of the individuality index ratio between the within-subject and the between-subject variation gives key information on whether a result from a patient should be compared with the population-based reference interval (the classical procedure) or with previous results from only the same patient and analyte. When the within-subject variability is narrower than the between-subject variability, comparison with previous patient results is much more sensitive to detect changes on health status than comparing with the reference population value.

According to the SEQC database[19] the majority of analytes have high individuality (individuality index <0.6), indicating that a significant change versus the previous result

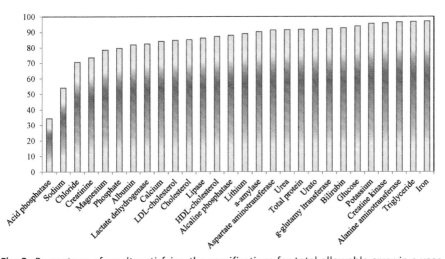

Fig. 3. Percentage of results satisfying the specifications for total allowable error in a year revision. Analytes are shown in ascending order according to the percentage of accomplishment. HDL, high-density lipoprotein; LDL, low-density lipoprotein.

is more important than comparison with the population-based reference value. Laboratories should use this calculation when monitoring patients and incorporate the resulting information into their reports; otherwise, a useful tool for medical decision making could remain hidden.

The formula used to calculate the RCV was proposed by Harris[20]: $RCV = 2^{1/2}Z$ $(CV_A^2 + CV_I^2)^{1/2}$. The Z score determines the level of significance of the change being 1.65 or 2.32 as 95% or 99% of probability for a change for unidirectional changes (1 tailed) and 1.96 or 2.528 for bidirectional changes (2 tailed). Despite 2-tailed Z scores being the most commonly used, the more stringent 1-tailed RCV seems to be more appropriate when a significant increase or decrease is the only change to be considered, as Cooper and colleagues[21] recommended. Fraser published similar advice using an example the assessment of serial observations of cardiac troponins to recognize an acute cardiac event.[22]

When monitoring pathologic status, it is of upmost importance to know the CV_I value in the concrete pathology. That is, we must not only know BV in healthy patients, but the particular variation of analytes in patients with disease. It has been demonstrated that CV_I for a number of analytes, which are the key determinant in some organ-related pathologies, is greater than the CV_I estimated in healthy subjects.[23] This is summarized in **Table 2**.

The use of RCV derived from healthy individuals for monitoring pathologies could lead to an increased risk of false-positive results with the consequent impact on clinical decision making. It is very important to check the distribution of results, because if a skewed distribution is presented, the formula to estimate RCV is different than the formula shown above.

The classical formula to estimate RCV assumes a Gaussian distribution for both CV_A and CV_I; however, it has been observed that a significant number of clinically relevant quantities have a skewed distribution. In these cases, the RCV should be calculated using a lognormal approach that was first described in equations formulated by Fokkema and colleagues.[24] In this approach the total CV_I of non–log-transformed data is used to estimate the σ parameter of the lognormal distribution:

$$\sigma = [Ln\ (CV_I^2 + 1)]^{1/2}$$

The asymmetrical limits for the upward value for the lognormal RCV (RCV_{pos}) and for the downward value (RCV_{neg}) are determined as follows:

$$RCV_{pos} = [exp\ (1.96 \times 2^{1/2} \times \sigma) - 1] \times 100$$

$$RCV_{neg} = -\ [exp\ (1.96 \times 2^{1/2} \times \sigma) - 1] \times 100$$

In a recent review, Roraas and colleagues[25] recommend the use of the logarithmic method for calculating the RCV regardless of the distribution of data because in statistical terms patient results will always have a certain asymmetry.

Autoverification of Patient Results

Authoverification is a control application within the laboratory aimed at detecting errors that may have been missed by the traditional controls. The formula is: Δ Check $< 2^{1/2} * Z\ (CV_A^2 + CV_I^2)^{1/2}$ and Z in this case is recommended to be $Z = 1.96$ (very significant change). **Fig. 4** shows the diagnostic detection outcome in a primary care laboratory (outpatients). Taking into account that autoverification output is a compromise between sensitivity and specificity to detect errors in requests and results. There is a

Table 2
Analytes with CV$_I$ in pathologies different than in healthy

Analyte	Patients Pathology CV$_I$	Type of Pathology	Mean	Units	Healthy Subjects CV$_I$
α-Amylase	12.4	IDDM	0.50	AE/L	9.5
α-Fetoprotein	38.0	Hepatic diseases	3.97	mg/L	12.0
Alanine aminotransferase	12.6	Chronic liver, IDDM	2.04	μmol/s.L	24.3
Albumin	5.5	Myocardial infarction, IDDM	38.1	g/L	3.1
Albumin concentration. first morning	61.0	Diabetes	14.4	mg/L	36.0
Alkaline phosphatase	12.4	Paget	586	U/L	6.4
CA 125	46.2	Ovarian neoplasia on complete remission	8.77	U/L	29.2
CA 15.3	14.0	Breast cancer patients	16.2	U/mL rev	6.2
CA 19.9	24.5	Ovarian neoplasia on complete remission	8.8	U/L	16.0
CA 19.9	24.5	Lung neoplasia on complete remission	1.3	U/L	16.0
Calcium	4.8	Myocardial infarction	2.25	mmol/L	1.9
CEA	26.9	Breast cancer (operated)	1.6	ng/mL	12.7
CEA	27.0	Breast cancer	ND	ND	12.7
CEA	44.9	Colorectal neoplasia on complete remission	1.99	mg/L	12.7
CEA	23.6	Lung cancer on complete remission	1.77	mg/L	12.7
Creatine kinase	43.3	Inpatients	75.2	U/L	22.8
Creatinine	6.1	IDDM/inpatients	190	μmol/L	4.3
Creatinine	12.3	Renal recipients/myocardial infarction	85	μmol/L	4.3
C-Telopeptide type I collagen	12.4	Paget	5976	pmol/L	9.6
γ-Glutamyl transferase	4.7	Chronic liver disease	6.8	μmol/s.L	13.4

Abbreviations: CEA, carcinoembryonic antigen; CV$_I$, intraindividual coefficient of variation; IDDM, insulin-dependent diabetes mellitus; ND, not done.

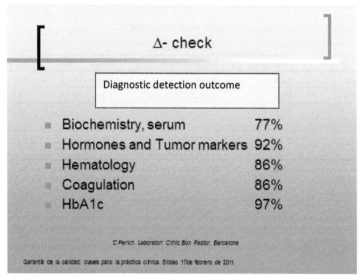

Fig. 4. Delta check diagnostic detection outcome in a primary care laboratory. HbA1c, hemoglobin A1c.

wide dispersion among the output described by different authors: Auxter-Parham[26] found that 70% of detection in oupatients and 10% in hospitalized patients, Dunikoski[27] describes 80% output for biochemistry and coagulation tests, in a hospital laboratory, and Fraser and associates[28] obtained an outcome of 60% in hospitalized patients.

SUMMARY

BV gives valuable information about how the living organism regulates its constituents both within and between subjects; this information on the behavior of body components allows us to derive consequences concerning reference population and reference intervals.

With a more pragmatic approach, BV has a 3 uses: setting the appropriate analytical performance specification for each analyte to limit the amount of error that laboratory could introduce in its measurements, to help to distinguish health from disease (a significant change in a measure and for a particular individual, establishing such a kind of parallelism with current trends of personalized medicine), and, last, to implement internal quality control with the automatic verification of results.

REFERENCES

1. Fraser CG. The nature of biological variation. In: Biological variation: from principles to practice. Washington, DC: AACC Press; 2001. p. 1–28.
2. Panteghini M, Sandberg S. Defining analytical performance specifications 15 years after the Stockholm conference. Clin Chem Lab Med 2015;53:829–32.
3. Simundic AM, Bartlett AW, Fraser CG. Biological variation: a still evolved facet of laboratory medicine. Ann Clin Biochem 2015;52:189–90.
4. Fraser CG, Harris EK. Generation and application of data on biological variation in clinical chemistry. Crit Rev Clin Lab Sci 1989;27:409–37.

5. Ricós C, Ávarez V, Cava F, et al. Current databases on biological variation: pros, cons and progress. In: Hyltoft Petersen P, Fraser CG, Kallner A, et al. Strategies to set global quality specifications in laboratory medicine. Scand J Clin Lab Invest 1999;59(7):491–500.

6. Minchinela J, Ricós C, Perich C, et al. Biological variation database and quality specifications for imprecision bias and total error (desirable and minimum). The 2014 update. Available at: http://www.westgard.com/biodatabase-2014-update.htm. Accessed September 15, 2016.

7. Aarsand A, Roraas T, Sverre S. Biological variation- reliable data is essential. Clin Chem. Lab Med 2015;53:153–4.

8. Carobene A. Reliability of a biological variation data available in an online database: need for improvement. Clin Chem Lab Med 2015;53:801–7.

9. Bartlett WA, Braga F, Carobene A, et al. A checklist for critical appraisal of studies on biological variation. Clin Chem Lab Med 2015;53:879–85.

10. Elevitch FR, editor. 1976 aspen conference on analytical goals in clinical chemistry. Skokie (IL): College of American Pathologists; 1977.

11. Fraser CG. Quality specifications. In: Biological variation: from principles to practice. Washington, DC: AACC Press; 2001. p. 29–66.

12. Gowans EMS, Hyltoft Petersen P, Blaabjerg O, et al. Analytical goals for the acceptance of reference intervals for laboratories throughout a geographical area. Scand J Clin Lab Invest 1988;48:757–64.

13. Ricós C, Baadenhuijsen H, Libeer JC, et al. Currently used criteria for evaluating performance in EQA in European countries and a proposal for harmonization. Eur J Clin Chem Clin Biochem 1996;34:159–65. Also in: Uldall A. Compendium on advanced external quality assurance in clinical biochemistry. DEKS. Herlev University Hospital. Denmark 2000.

14. Oosterhuis WP, Sandberg S. Proposal for the modification of the conventional model for establishing performance specifications. Clin Chem Lab Med 2015;53:925–37.

15. Fraser CG, Hyltoft Petersen P, Libeer JC, et al. Proposals for setting generally applicable quality goals solely based on biology. Ann Clin Biochem 1997;34:8–12.

16. Westgard JO. Six sigma basics. In: Six sigma quality design and control. Madison (WI): Westgard QC Inc; 2006. p. 69–91.

17. Westgard JO. Charts of Operational Process Spacificatins ("OPSpects charts") for assessing the accuracy, precision and quality control needed to satisfy proficiency testing performance criteria. Clin Chem 1992;38:1226–33.

18. Ramón F, Alsina MJ, Álvarez V, et al. XXXVI Programa de Garantía Externa de la Calidad de Bioquímica suero de la SEQC. 2015. Available at: http://www.contcal.org/qcweb/Documents/90%20Avaluacio%20anual/80%20 Programas%202015/40.Suero.pdf. Accessed October 5, 2016.

19. Ricós C, Álvarez V, Perich C, et al. Rationale for using data on biological variation. Clin Chem Lab Med 2015;53:863–70.

20. Harris EK. Statistical aspects of reference values in clinical pathology. Prog Clin Pathol 1981;8:45–66.

21. Cooper G, DeJonge N, Ehrmeyer S, et al. Collective opinion paper on findings of the 2010 convocation of experts on laboratory quality. Clin Chem Lab Med 2011;49:793–802.

22. Fraser CG. Improved monitoring of differences in serial laboratory results. Clin Chem 2011;57:1635–7.

23. Ricós C, Iglesias N, García-Lario JV, et al. Within-subject biological variation in disease: collate data and clinical consequences. Ann Clin Biochem 2007;44: 343–52.

24. Fokkema MR, Herrmann Z, Muskiet FA, et al. Reference change values for brain natriuretic peptides revisited. Clin Chem 2006;52:1602–3.

25. Roraas T, Stove B, Hyltoft Petersen P, et al. Biological variation: the effect of different distributions on estimated within-person variation and reference change values. Clin Chem 2016;62:725–36.

26. Auxter-Parham S. Taking autoverification to the next level: new tools make it easier to increase efficiency. Clin Lab News 2003;29:11.

27. Dunikoski LK. The advantages of autoverification. Adv form Med Lab Professionals 2003;15:25.

28. Fraser CG, Stevenson HP, Kennedy IMG. Biological variation data are necessary prerequisites for objective autoverification of clinical laboratory data. Accred Qual Assur 2002;7:455–60.

Understanding the Use of Sigma Metrics in Hemoglobin A1c Analysis

Erna Lenters-Westra, PhD[a,b,*], Emma English, PhD[c]

KEYWORDS

• HbA1c • Diabetes • Sigma metrics • Analytical performance criteria

KEY POINTS

• Performance of hemoglobin A1c (HbA1c) analyzers is, on the whole, very good, with many attaining the international guidance target of sigma greater than 2 at a total allowable error (TAE) of 10%. In addition, many analyzers perform well in excess of these targets, as individual analyzers or in networks of analyzers across a wide geographic area.

• In strict evaluation conditions, point-of-care test devices can perform as well as routine laboratory analyzers and may in future be considered suitable for use in the diagnosis of diabetes.

• Using direct calibration traceable to the primary reference measurement procedure, the authors have shown that there is the capacity to improve performance of analyzers in routine clinical practice.

• Although few analyzers currently meet tighter targets of a 10% TAE and 4 sigma and a 6% TAE at 2 sigma, the outcomes for pass or fail are comparable for the 2 criteria.

• Precision has a greater impact on the calculated sigma than bias does, in the current data set. There are many ways in which to calculate bias and imprecision and the method used to establish these values must be detailed in any evaluation or study.

INTRODUCTION

Global standardization of hemoglobin A1c (HbA1c) methods, in particular through the International Federation of Clinical Chemistry and Laboratory Medicine (IFCC) primary reference method, has been the forerunner to a marked improvement in the analytical performance of many HbA1c assays. The IFCC primary reference method has been proved to be stable in many intercomparison studies with designated comparison

Disclosure Statement: The authors have nothing to disclose.
[a] Clinical Chemistry Department, Isala, Dr. Van Heesweg 2, Zwolle 8025 AB, The Netherlands; [b] European Reference Laboratory for Glycohemoglobin, Isala, Dr. Van Heesweg 2, Zwolle 8025 AB, The Netherlands; [c] Faculty of Medicine and Health, School of Health Science, University of East Anglia, Norwich Research Park, Norwich NR4 7TJ, UK
* Corresponding author. Dr. Van Heesweg 2, Zwolle 8025 AB, The Netherlands.
E-mail address: w.b.lenters@isala.nl

Clin Lab Med 37 (2017) 57–71
http://dx.doi.org/10.1016/j.cll.2016.09.006
0272-2712/17/© 2016 Elsevier Inc. All rights reserved.

methods (the National Glycohemoglobin Standardization Program [NGSP] and the Japanese Diabetes Society [JDS]/Japanese Society of Clinical Chemistry [JSCC] method) and is recognized in a 2010 consensus statement as the only valid anchor for the standardization of HbA1c.[1,2] The development of this reference method enabled the World Health Organization (WHO) and American Diabetes Association to advocate the use of HbA1c for the diagnosis of type 2 diabetes.[3] WHO guidance stipulates that "stringent quality assurance tests are in place and assays are standardized to criteria aligned to the international reference values."[4] In addition to standardization, it is imperative that tests used for the diagnosis of diabetes meet strict analytical performance criteria for bias and imprecision because both have the potential to affect reported values. Suboptimal analytical performance may cause misclassification of patients' result, and thus give rise to either inappropriate positive diagnoses or missed diagnoses.

In 2015 the IFCC Task Force on Implementation of HbA1c Standardization published an investigation of 2 different models to set and evaluate quality targets for HbA1c.[5] The biological variation model and the sigma-metrics model were investigated. The IFCC task force advocates the use of the sigma-metric model as the model of choice because the within biological variation of HbA1c is very small and analytical performance criteria derived from biological variation of HbA1c are too strict even for the best performing HbA1c methods currently on the market.[6] The task force set out guidance for the application of the sigma-metrics model for HbA1c in all countries with the purpose of engaging international stakeholders in diabetes to further the development of analytical quality at a global level.

In the laboratory, sigma metrics is a quality management strategy that provides a universal benchmark for process performances. Sigma metrics places analytical characteristics (bias and imprecision) in the form of total allowable error (TAE) within a framework of clinical requirements. Sigma metrics allows users to define the TAE they wish to achieve and how often results can acceptably be outside of this target value. The higher the sigma value, the fewer times a system is allowed to fall short of the required target. A sigma of 2 implies a 5% risk to fail the TAE; that is, it is acceptable for 5% of results to not meet the TAE value that has been preset. TAE for HbA1c has been set by the IFCC Task Force on Implementation of HbA1c Standardization as a default of 5 mmol/mol (0.46% DCCT) at an HbA1c level of 50 mmol/mol (6.7% DCCT), which corresponds with a relative TAE of 10% ([5/50] × 100%) in SI (International System) units (6.9% DCCT units; [0.46/6.7] × 100%).[7]

The aim of this study was to explore the ways in which sigma metrics are applied in clinical laboratory testing using the criteria set by the IFCC task force. Three approaches were used as exemplars of the range of different uses of the sigma-metrics approach. These were:

1. Data from an external quality assurance (EQA) program of 134 individual laboratories in the Netherlands using a variety HbA1c methods, showing how sigma is used in real-life routine settings.[7]
2. Data from a recent evaluation of the performance of 7 HbA1c POC (POC) instruments to calculate sigma, which show how sigma metrics can be used to evaluate new or existing instruments at a laboratory level.[8]
3. Data from the IFCC monitoring program from 6 certified secondary reference measurement procedures (SRMPs) to the IFCC reference method procedure (RMP) to calculate sigma, showing how well methods perform at higher order levels.[9]

In addition, changing the TAE of 10% to 6% in SI units was investigated to indicate the potential impact of tightening the criteria in the future.

METHODS
Part 1

Data from the recent (March 2016) Stichting Kwaliteitsbewaking Medische Laboratoria (SKML) External Quality Assurance Services (EQAS) in the Netherlands were used to assess the individual laboratory performance of various HbA1c methods using sigma metrics.[7] In the SKML EQA program 4 fresh whole-blood ethylenediamine tetraacetic acid (EDTA) samples are distributed to individual laboratories 6 times per year. The samples should be analyzed within 48 hours of receipt and the results are submitted to the Web site of SKML. The results of the latest survey were used to calculate sigma. The target values of the distributed samples were assigned with the following 6 IFCC-certified SRMPs based at 2 European reference laboratories, with values determined on 2 individual days in duplicate[10]:

European Reference Laboratory for Glycohemoglobin, location Isala, Zwolle, The Netherlands:

- Roche Tina-quant Gen.2 HbA1c on Integra 800, immunoassay (Roche TQ Isala)
- Premier Hb9210 Isala, boronate affinity high-pressure liquid chromatography (HPLC) (Trinity Biotech);
- Tosoh G8 Isala, cation-exchange HPLC (Tosoh Bioscience)

European Reference Laboratory for Glycohemoglobin, location Queen Beatrix Hospital, Winterswijk, The Netherlands:

- Sebia Capillarys 2 Flex Piercing, capillary electrophoresis (Sebia Capillarys SKB)
- Premier Hb9210 SKB, boronate affinity HPLC (Trinity Biotech)
- Menarini HA8180 SKB, cation-exchange HPLC (Menarini Diagnostics)

The 6 SRMPs were all calibrated with IFCC secondary reference material and showed excellent performance in the 2015 IFCC monitoring program.

The mean of the 4 samples minus the mean of the target value set by the 6 SRMPs was used to calculate bias. The within-laboratory standard deviation (SD) was calculated from the residual SD regression line through the laboratory results versus the target values and was used to calculate the coefficient of variation (CV).[11] Sigma was calculated with the formula: $\sigma = (TAE - B)/CV$ where B is bias compared with a reference method and CV is imprecision of the method (all values expressed as percentages). The TAE used was 5 mmol/mol (0.46% DCCT) at an HbA1c level of 50 mmol/mol (6.7% DCCT), which corresponds with a relative TAE of 10% [(5/50) × 100%] in SI units [6.9% DCCT units; (0.46/6.7) × 100%].[5]

Part 2

Data from an evaluation study of 7 HbA1c POC instruments performed in our laboratory in 2014[8] and the latest results of an evaluation of the Quo-Test method after the manufacturer claimed to have adjusted the calibration are included. The CLSI EP-5 and EP-9 protocols were used to establish precision and accuracy (bias) for the POC testing (POCT) instruments. The CLSI EP-9 protocol was performed twice, with 2 different reagent lots, and the bias was determined as the difference between the POC instrument values and the mean of the first 3 SRMPs detailed earlier. The sigma value was calculated 3 different ways using the CV, of a sample with an HbA1c value of approximately 48 mmol/mol (6.5% DCCT), established in the EP-5 protocol, and the CVs calculated from the duplicates in the EP-9 protocol using 2 different lots. The bias was calculated at 48 mmol/mol using Deming regression analysis compared with the mean of the first 3 SRMPs.

Part 3

The design of the IFCC monitoring program is based on 24 interconnected EDTA whole-blood samples. The samples are sent annually to IFCC-certified reference laboratories and subsequently stored at or below −70°C. One sample is then analyzed every fortnight, and the results are to be submitted to the Web site of HbA1c/IFCC.[9] The 24 samples are 12 blinded samples in duplicate. From these duplicates the CV is calculated. Values of samples were assigned by the whole IFCC network (18 approved IFCC primary reference laboratories) each performing the IFCC primary reference method.[10] Data from the 2015 monitoring program were used to calculate the performance of 6 IFCC SRMPs mentioned earlier.

In addition, data were reanalyzed to investigate the impact of changing targets from a TAE of 10% to a TAE 6% to elucidate the likely impact of tightening the performance criteria. The pass and fail rate calculated with a TAE of 10% and 4 sigma was compared with the pass and fail rate with a TAE of 6% and a 2 sigma.

STATISTICS

Calculations were performed using Microsoft Excel 2010 (Microsoft Corporation). Statistical analyses were performed using Analyse-It (Analyse-It Software) and EP Evaluator Release 9 (Data Innovations LLC).[12]

For the duplicates in the EP-9 protocol and in the IFCC monitoring program, CV was calculated with the following formula:

$$CV_a = \frac{\sqrt{\frac{\sum (\Delta)^2}{n}}}{\bar{x}\sqrt{2}} \times 100\%$$

where CV_a is the analytical CV, Δ is the difference between duplicates, n is the number of duplicates, and $\bar{x}$ is the mean of the duplicates.

RESULTS
Part 1

Of the 134 laboratories that participated in the SKML-EQAS in the Netherlands, 90.3% of the methods used in these laboratories met the criteria of having σ greater than 2, and 74.6% met standards for σ greater than 4 with a TAE of 10%. With a TAE of 6%, 70.1% met the criteria for σ greater than 2 and 41.0% for σ greater than 4 (**Fig. 1A, B, Table 1**). As an example, the Menarini HA8180 in one laboratory had a calculated sigma of 32.7 because of a CV of 0.30% and a bias of 0.2%. Using the formula σ = (TAE − B)/CV resulted in a calculated sigma value of 32.7 [(10−0.2)/0.30 = 32.7]. A very high sigma is generated with a low CV, generally less than 1%. The opposite effect is also possible. A bias greater than the TAE of 10% results in a negative sigma value. In practice a sigma of 32.7 is essentially equal to a sigma of 6 because world-class performance is world-class performance no matter how high the calculated sigma. A negative sigma indicates that the method fails to meet the set criteria more often than it achieves these set criteria. **Table 1** details the range of sigma values that were calculated for each method, representing the distribution of the performance of that particular method between laboratories. However, this is better shown in **Fig. 1A**. Most of the methods cluster around a certain sigma, except for the Roche method group, which shows the widest range of sigma values among users.

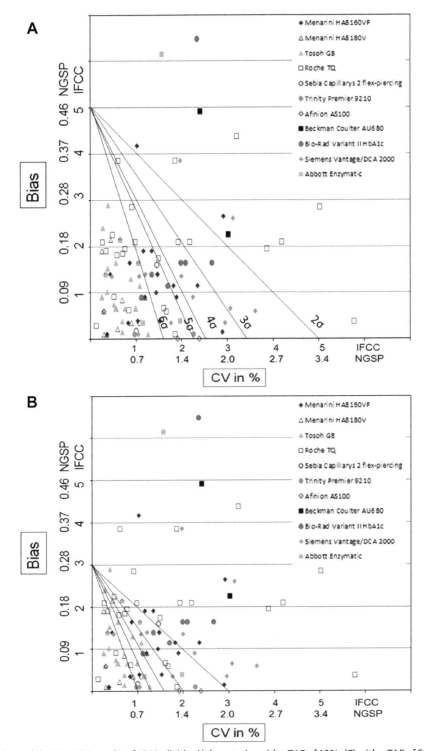

Fig. 1. (*A*) SKML EQA results of 134 individual laboratories with a TAE of 10%, (*B*) with a TAE of 6%, and (*C*) with a TAE of 10% and 4 sigma (*unbroken line*) and TAE of 6% and 2 sigma (*dashed line*).

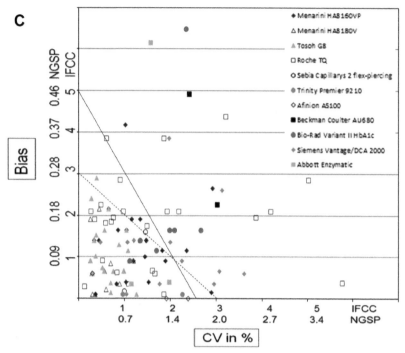

Fig. 1. (*continued*).

Fig. 1C compares the distribution of performance when using the alternative criteria of either a TAE of 10% and 4 sigma or a TAE of 6% and 2 sigma. Fewer individual laboratories would meet the criteria if the TAE was reduced than if the sigma target was increased.

Part 2

Table 2 shows the results of the sigma calculations using data from a previous POCT evaluation study. All POCT methods, except the first evaluations of the Quo-Lab and the Quo-Test, had a sigma greater than 2 (TAE 10%) and this was independent of which CV was used (EP-5 or CV from duplicates in EP-9 lot number A or B). Only the B-analyst had a sigma greater than 4 with TAE of 10% and sigma greater than 2 with a TAE of 6%. **Fig. 2**A and **Table 2** show that a method can pass the criteria of having a sigma greater than 2 with TAE of 10% even if the bias is 5.7% and 6% (Inno-vaStar) because of a very low CV (1.9%, 1.4%, and 0.9%). Taking a TAE of 6% and 2 sigma as the criteria, this method would have failed (**Fig. 2**B), as would the DCA Vantage and, potentially, the Afinion analyzers. **Fig. 2**C shows that the pass and fail rate for the POCT methods when using criteria of TAE of 10% and 4 sigma was almost equal to a TAE of 6% and 2 sigma.

Part 3

Table 3 shows the current criteria of the IFCC monitoring program. The 6 SRMPs evaluated showed excellent performance in 2015 concerning deviation from IFCC target, reproducibility, and linearity. High sigma values were observed at HbA1c values of 30, 60, and 90 mmol/mol, which are the levels at which deviation from IFCC target values

Table 1
Sigma calculated for various hemoglobin A1c methods in Stichting Kwaliteitsbewaking Medische Laboratoria external quality assurance with total allowable error of 10% and 6%

Method	N	Mean σ, (Range σ), TAE 10%	Laboratories with σ >2 (%)	Laboratories with σ >4 (%)	Mean σ, (Range σ), TAE 6%	Laboratories with σ >2 (%)
Menarini HA 8160 VP	21	7.9 (1.8–27.2)	95.2	80.9	3.7 (−2.2–16.1)	76.2
Menarini HA 8180 V	14	17.3 (6.9–32.7)	100	100	8.9 (3.5–19.4)	100
Tosoh G8	35	12.2 (0.5–32.7)	97.5	97.5	5.5 (−5.5–16.7)	91.4
Roche TQ WB/Hem Gen 2 and 3	25	9.9 (0.4–72.9)	80.0	68	5.6 (−1.6–41.9)	56
Sebia Capillarys 2 Flex Piercing	2	7.2 (4.7–9.7)	100	100	3.8 (2.0–5.7)	100
Trinity Premier 9210	2	7.3 (4.3–10.2)	100	100	4.3 (2.6–6.0)	100
Afinion AS100	3	12.4 (3.1–30.3)	100	33.3	6.6 (1.0–16.5)	66.7
Beckman Coulter AU680/P/ACE MDQ	2	2.3 (2.1–2.5)	100	0.0	0.8 (0.5–1.2)	0.0
Bio-Rad Variant II HbA1c/Turbo A1c	8	3.6 (−1.2–7.4)	87.5	37.5	1.3 (−2.9–3.8)	37.5
Siemens Vantage/DCA 2000	12	5.1 (1.6–15.6)	91.7	41.7	2.4 (−0.8–7.0)	41.7
Abbott Architect Enzymatic test	3	6.4 (4.6–8.1)	100	66.7	3.6 (2.6–4.6)	100

Table 2

Sigma calculated using the results of an evaluation of 7 hemoglobin A1c point-of-care testing instruments. The coefficient of variation from EP-5 (Evaluation Protocol), coefficient of variation calculated from the duplicates in EP-9 and bias at 48 mmol/mol compared with 3 secondary reference measurement procedures were used for the calculation of sigma

	σ at 48 mmol/mol TAE = 10%, CV (%) from EP-5 Lot A	σ at 48 mmol/mol TAE = 6%, CV (%) from EP-5 Lot A	σ at 48 mmol/mol TAE 10%, CV (%) from duplicates EP-9 Lot A	σ at 48 mmol/mol TAE 6%, CV (%) from duplicates EP-9 Lot A	σ at 48 mmol/mol TAE 10%, CV (%) from duplicates EP-9 Lot B	σ at 48 mmol/mol TAE 6%, CV (%) from duplicates EP-9 Lot B
Afinion	4.3	2.4	3.0	1.7	3.2	1.8
DCA Vantage	2.6	1.3	2.5	1.3	3.1	1.8
Cobas B101	3.3	1.8	4.8	2.7	6.1	3.4
InnovaStar	2.3	0.2	3.1	0.2	4.4	<0
B-analyst	6.1	3.6	5.8	3.4	5.1	3.3
Quo-Lab	1.0	0.3	1.6	<0	1.6	<0
Quo-Test	1.5	0.0	1.5	0.0	1.6	<0
Quo-Test[a]	2.3	1.1	4.1	1.9	6.4	3.1

σ = (TAE − B)/CV.

[a] After manufacturer recalibration.

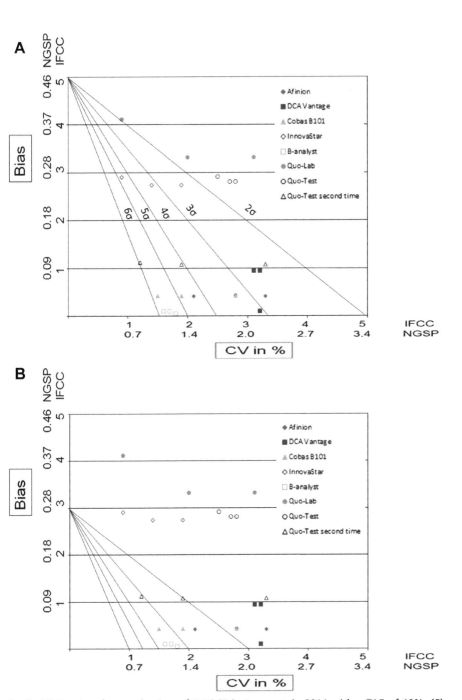

Fig. 2. (*A*) Results of an evaluation of 7 POCT instruments in 2014 with a TAE of 10%, (*B*) with a TAE of 6%, and (*C*) with a TAE of 10% and 4 sigma (*unbroken line*) and TAE of 6% and 2 sigma (*dashed line*).

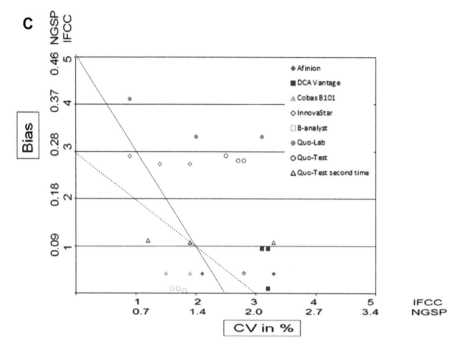

Fig. 2. (*continued*).

are detailed on the annual monitoring certificate (**Table 4**). Again it can be seen from **Table 4** that a CV less than 1.0% leads to sigma values greater than 6 (Tosoh G8 and Menarini HA8180). **Fig. 3**A shows the results of the 6 SRMPs using the bias at 60 mmol/mol and a TAE of 10%, and **Fig. 3**B shows the same results but with a TAE of 6%. All SRMPs had a sigma greater than 4 with a TAE of 10% and a sigma greater than 2 with a TAE of 6% (**Fig. 3**C).

DISCUSSION
The Global Context

This study used data from 3 different clinical settings in order to highlight the current state of the art of HbA1c analyzers that are in routine use around the world. The TAE of 10% (5 mmol/mol at an HbA1c value of 50 mmol/mol) was set as a default by the IFCC task force and these goals should serve as a starting point for discussion with

Table 3
Current criteria International Federation of Clinical Chemistry and Laboratory Medicine monitoring program

Issue	Deviation from IFCC Target (mmol/mol)	Reproducibility (%)	Linearity
Excellent	0.0–1.9	<2	>0.9950
Good	2.0–3.9	2.00–3.49	0.9901–0.9950
Acceptable	4.0–6.9	3.50–4.99	0.9851–0.9900
Poor	7.0–9.9	5.00–6.99	0.9801–0.9850
Unacceptable	>9.9	>6.99	<0.9801

Table 4
Sigma calculated for 6 International Federation of Clinical Chemistry and Laboratory Medicine secondary reference measurement procedures derived from the International Federation of Clinical Chemistry and Laboratory Medicine monitoring program of 2015

SRMP	CV (%)	HbA1c Value (mmol/mol)	Absolute Bias (mmol/mol)	Relative Bias (%)	Sigma TAE 10%	Sigma TAE 6%
Roche TQ	1.47	30	0.5	1.7	5.6	2.9
		60	0.2	0.3	6.7	3.9
		90	1.0	1.1	6.1	3.3
Premier HA9210	1.34	30	0.1	0.3	7.2	4.3
		60	0.1	0.2	7.3	4.3
		90	0.1	0.1	7.4	4.4
Tosoh G8	0.67	30	0.5	1.7	12.3	6.4
		60	0.2	0.3	14.4	8.5
		90	0.2	0.2	14.6	8.7
Sebia	1.36	30	0.4	1.3	6.4	3.5
		60	0.6	1.0	6.6	3.7
		90	0.8	0.9	6.7	3.8
Premier	1.61	30	0.1	0.3	6.0	3.5
		60	0.3	0.5	5.9	3.4
		90	0.6	0.7	5.8	3.3
Menarini	0.85	30	0.1	0.3	11.4	6.7
		60	0.2	0.3	11.4	6.7
		90	0.5	0.6	11.1	6.4

international stakeholders in diabetes. This cut point was chosen because it is based on the difference in HbA1c results in 2 consecutive HbA1c tests that clinicians use as a guide to change therapy and is therefore a clinical decision limit.[5] Previous guidance focused on the imprecision of methods with instruments expected to perform at a within-laboratory CV of less than 3% for SI units and less than 2% for percentage (NGSP) units. The sigma metrics approach allows for both bias and imprecision to be taken into account when assessing analytical performance, generating a more comprehensive view of performance.

Performance Within and Between Countries

Results from part 1 of this study clearly show that most individual laboratories (90%) are meeting these targets of a sigma value of greater than 2 at a TAE of less than 10%. Two method groups (Roche and Bio-Rad) performed less well, with a wide range of sigma values calculated for the within-method group. A reason for this large distribution might be that in this EQA program the Roche method was taken as 1 group (whole-blood application and hemolysate application, Generation 2 and Generation 3 reagent, using different instruments [Cobas Integra 800, Cobas c8000, Hitachi]), giving considerable heterogeneity to the group. In addition, all methods factors, such as the technical/analytical skills required to perform the analysis and maintenance of instruments and so forth, can have an impact on performance and thus on sigma values. In general, the smaller the distribution (range) of sigma values the more robust and reproducible that particular method is likely to be at that sigma level.

It is difficult to draw conclusions for some method groups because of small user numbers, but increasing the sigma cut point to greater than 4 sigma leads to a reduction in the number of laboratories meeting that target (80%). This number decreases further to 75% with a TAE of 6% and sigma of greater than 2.

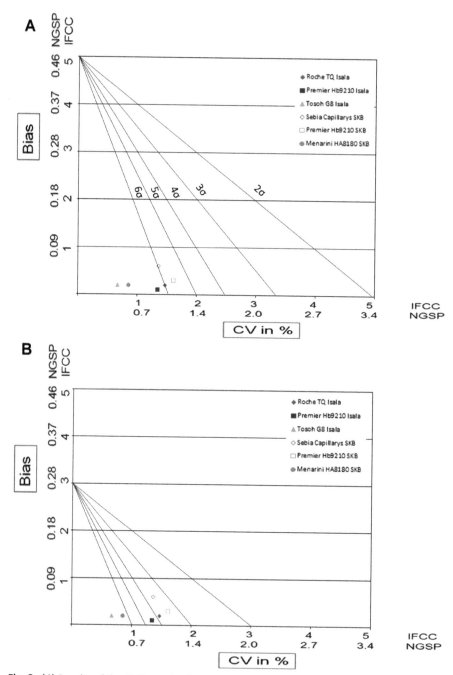

Fig. 3. (A) Results of the IFCC monitoring program of 6 SRMPs with a TAE of 10%, (B) with a TAE of 6%, and (C) with a TAE of 10% and 4 sigma (*unbroken line*) and TAE of 6% and 2 sigma (*dashed line*).

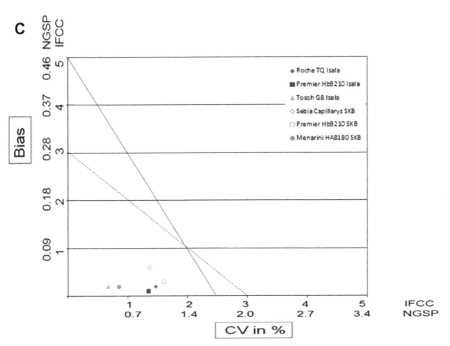

Fig. 3. (*continued*).

Individual laboratories or networks of laboratories in any country can use the results of their EQA data to calculate their bias and imprecision and use this model to assess the performance of their own analyzers. The minimum expected standard is a sigma value of 2 or greater at a TAE of 10%.

How Do Point-of-Care Devices Compare?

Part 2 data show that, under strict evaluation conditions, most POCT devices perform to the same limits that are expected of laboratory analyzers. Only the Quo-Lab and Quo-Test did not reach these targets; however, the Quo-Test did meet the targets after a manufacturer recalibration. This finding is significant because the question as to whether or not POC devices can be used for the diagnosis of diabetes is regularly raised. These findings indicate that most methods could be used in this setting; however, the performance shown here may not reflect the performance of these devices in the clinical setting, with multiple users and multiple lot numbers, and further evidence is required before advocating the use of POCT devices for the diagnosis of diabetes. When the criteria are tightened to 4 sigma at a TAE of 10%, only 1 analyzer showed a consistent ability to meet that target, and with a reduced TAE of 6% and 2 sigma only 2 instruments met the targets, indicating that a TAE of 10% at 2 sigma is the current state of the art of these analyzers.

Establishing the Limit of Performance of Routine Analyzers

Part 3 data show how well routine laboratory analyzers can perform when directly calibrated to the IFCC RMP. Each of the 6 SRMPs performed exceptionally well, meeting both the sigma greater than 2 and sigma greater than 4 targets at a TAE of 10%; in addition, all also met the sigma greater than 2 at a TAE of 6% target. This finding shows that routine analyzers have the capacity to meet these stringent performance targets and the aim should be to increase performance to these levels in the clinical setting.

Future Aims

Overall, the performance of most laboratory and POC analyzers for HbA1c is very good. Although not all analyzers are currently meeting the proposed target of greater than 2 sigma at a TAE of 10%, some analyzers are already performing far in excess of this target, clearly indicating the capacity for excellent performance in routine clinical settings. Manufacturers and users of all instruments should strive to further improve the quality and consistency of the results they produce, to ensure that 100% of methods meet the basic quality targets. Once this has been achieved, then the criteria can be further tightened, and this will allow HbA1c analysis to become the benchmark for performance of all laboratory testing. Note that the IFCC task force also advocated the use of analyzers that perform to the level of 4 sigma with a TAE of 10% when used for clinical trials; this is achievable with a range of current analyzers, but not all, and care should be taken when selecting and the instrument to be used for collecting trial data.

Should the Performance Guidelines Be Changed?

This study also evaluated the impact of tightening the performance criteria to greater than 4 sigma at 10% TAE or greater than 2 sigma at 6% TAE. Both targets produced similar findings, with slightly fewer methods attaining the latter target. Although increasing the sigma level will still allow some methods to pass with a considerable bias, it could be used to give clinicians the confidence to know that the result they have is true, within a specific range, and it is unlikely that the value is ever likely to be outside of that range. However, decreasing the TAE means that the range of values around the true value will be much smaller, with the caveat that up to 5% of results will not be in that range. This option leaves some uncertainty because clinicians would not know which results were outside of the expected range; however, for a situation in which minimum deviation from the true value is required, this would be the preferred choice.

The primary focus for the immediate future should be to ensure that all analyzers perform to the minimum standards set by the IFCC task force and this performance should be considered when deciding on which analyzer to choose. Once this goal is achieved, further tightening of the criteria can be discussed.

ACKNOWLEDGMENTS

This article could not have been written without the results of the Dutch SKML. The authors thank the SKML for sharing these results with us.

REFERENCES

1. Weykamp C, John WG, Mosca A, et al. The IFCC reference measurement system for HbA1c: a 6-year progress report. Clin Chem 2008;54(2):240–8.
2. Hoelzel W, Weykamp C, Jeppsson JO, et al. IFCC reference system for measurement of hemoglobin A1c in human blood and the national standardization schemes in the United States, Japan, and Sweden: a method-comparison study. Clin Chem 2004;50(1):166–74.
3. International Expert Committee. International Expert Committee report on the role of the A1C assay in the diagnosis of diabetes. Diabetes Care 2009;32(7): 1327–34.

4. 2011 WHO Guidelines. Use of glycated haemoglobin (HbA1c) in the diagnosis of diabetes. Available at: www.who.int/diabetes/publications/report-hba1c_2011. pdf. Accessed November 14, 2016.

5. Weykamp C, John G, Gillery P, et al. Investigation of 2 models to set and evaluate quality targets for Hb A1c: biological variation and sigma-metrics. Clin Chem 2015;61(5):752–9.

6. Lenters-Westra E, Roraas T, Schindhelm RK, et al. Biological variation of hemoglobin A1c: consequences for diagnosing diabetes mellitus. Clin Chem 2014; 60(12):1570–2.

7. SKML. Available at: http://www.skml.nl/en/home. Accessed October 1, 2016.

8. Lenters-Westra E, Slingerland RJ. Three of 7 hemoglobin A1c point-of-care instruments do not meet generally accepted analytical performance criteria. Clin Chem 2014;60(8):1062–72.

9. International Federation of Clinical Chemistry and Laboratory Medicine. Available at: http://www.ifcchba1c.net/node/1. Accessed October 1, 2016.

10. International Federation of Clinical Chemistry and Laboratory Medicine. IFCC HbA1c network. Available at: http://www.ifcchba1c.net/network/approved? page=1. Accessed October 1, 2016.

11. SKML. Scoring and reporting system. Available at: http://www.skml.nl/en/home/ schemes/reportings/inputs/great-britain-frgi. Accessed October 1, 2016.

12. Data Innovations. EP Evaluator. Available at: https://www.datainnovations.com/ products/ep-evaluator. Accessed October 1, 2016.

State-of-the-art Approach to Goal Setting

Angel Salas, MD[a],*, Carmen Ricós, PhD[a], Enrique Prada, MD[b],
Francisco Ramón, MD[a], Jorge Morancho, MD[c], Josep M. Jou, MD[d],
Raquel Blazquez, MD[c]

KEYWORDS

- Quality assurance • Laboratory testing • Analytes • Quality specification

KEY POINTS

- A consensus of 4 external quality assurance programs combined their data to calculate the minimum acceptable quality specifications for laboratory testing.
- Where other sources of quality specifications may be too stringent for the current market, or may be too lenient given the clinical demands on the test result, these state-of-the-art goals may be practical and useful.
- More than 4 million test results from more than 4000 laboratories covering 82 different analytes were examined.
- Two main approaches were used: (1) defining the 95% percentile and comparing with other quality specifications, and (2) using an iterative approach to increase the quality specification until 90% of laboratories could achieve 75% of their results within the specification.
- Seventy-two out of 82 analytes followed procedure 2.

INTRODUCTION

Spanish clinical laboratories are involved regularly in external quality assurance programs (EQAPs), also known as proficiency testing. This participation is mandatory for clinical laboratories in most autonomic regions of Spain, although there is not a requirement for reaching a predetermined quality specification for each analyte.

Conflict of Interest: The authors have no conflicts of interest regarding the publication of this article.
[a] Comité de Programas Externos de la Calidad, Spanish Society of Clinical Chemistry and Laboratory Medicine (SEQC), Barcelona, Padilla 323-325 BCN 08025, Spain; [b] Comité de Calidad, Gestión, Seguridad y Evidencia, Spanish Association of Medical Biopathology-Laboratory Medicine (AEBM-LM), Madrid, Condado de Treviño 2, portal 2, local 1, Madrid 28033, Spain; [c] Programa de Supervisión Externa de la Calidad y Comisión de Garantía de Calidad del Laboratorio Clínico, Spanish Association of Pharmaceutical Analists (AEFA), Madrid, Modesto Lafuente 3, Madrid 28010, Spain; [d] Comité de Estandarización, Spanish Society of Hematology and Hemotherapy (SEHH), Madrid, Fortuny 51, local 5, Madrid 28010, Spain
* Corresponding author.
E-mail address: asalasrooms@gmail.com

The EQAP organizations that cover most of the hospital and primary care laboratories, private institutions, and public institutions working all over the country are 4 scientific societies, covering various laboratory disciplines: the Spanish Association of Pharmaceutical Analysts, Spanish Association of Medical Biopathology–Laboratory Medicine; Spanish Society of Laboratory Medicine, and Spanish Society of Hematology and Hemotherapy.

Although these organizations are competitors, they decided to work together on defining common quality specifications, based on scientific evidence. The aim of this study was to establish common specifications that are considered the minimum level of quality that each laboratory has to reach, to ensure harmonized analytical services. An additional purpose was to avoid the possibility of a legal imposition concerning quality specifications from the administration, defined without any scientific basis.

For this reason, a committee of experts from the 4 scientific societies was created in 2007, with the aim of agreeing on common analytical minimum quality specifications for total error, which have to be achieved by laboratories enrolled in any of the 4 EQAPs.[1]

The basis for the rationale was to use results from the 4 EQAPs, according to lowest level defined in the hierarchical model of Stockholm,[2] transferred to an ISO (International Organization for Standardization) technical report,[3] and further confirmed in the Milan strategic conference,[4] which are based on the current state of the art from the EQAP results.[5]

These 4 EQAP organizations have performances that make it feasible to agree on the level of quality required of participant laboratories:

- Working from the ISO/IEC (International Electrotechnical Commission) 17043:2010 standard.[6]
- Following recommendations of the IFCC/Education and Management Division/ Committee of Analytical Quality.[7]
- Using confidentiality as an essential ethic criterion.
- Being nonprofit organizations, independent of commercial interests.
- Having great experience in the field (the scientific societies began to organize programs around 1980).
- Using blind stabilized control material, with the overall or peer-group mean of participant results as a consensus value for comparison, after exclusion of outliers.
- Distributing 12 (biochemistry) and 24 (hematology) control materials per year, and asking for monthly results.
- Covering a wide range of concentration values for each analyte, including critical values for medical decisions.

The 4 programs are certified according to the ISO 9001 standard[8] and are in the process of accreditation, according to the ISO 17043 standard.[6]

MATERIAL AND METHODS

The materials used in this study were all results obtained from 2005 to 2010, 6 cycles of EQAP programs of the 4 societies, being the results of 2005 and 2006 and the basis of a preliminary study[1,9]; in total, 6 cycles of EQAP programs of the 4 societies were considered. All these data were compiled in a database, called Datum, which includes the 82 analytes included in at least 2 programs of the 4 societies (25 basic biochemistry, 15 hormones and tumor markers, 22 hematology and coagulation, 3 immunology, 12 urine, and 5 therapeutic drugs tests).

The overall number of results compiled in the Datum was 4,883,798, divided into:

- 619,430 from the basic biochemistry programs of 2005 and 2006[1]
- 1,262,623 from the basic hematology and special biochemistry programs of 2005 and 2006[9]
- 2,468,365 from the basic and special biochemistry and basic hematology programs during the 2007 to 2010 cycles[10]
- 266,690 from urine biochemistry and special hematology programs during the 2007 to 2010 cycles[11]

The number of laboratories involved was 4,104, distributed throughout the Spanish territory.

The variables of the Datum were laboratory code, annual cycle, monthly period, analyte, result reported by the laboratory, and value for comparison. This value was the overall mean or the peer-group (method and instrument) mean, depending on the analyte.

The method used for each analyte studied had 3 steps:

1. Basic calculations (procedure A)
   a. Percentage difference of each result versus the target (in absolute value)
   b. Plotting distribution of the differences
   c. Eliminating 5% of the higher differences
   d. Defining the 95th percentile as the candidate minimum quality specification (cMQS)
   e. Rounding this specification up to whole values
2. Comparison with other values
   a. The cMQS was compared with specifications that are mandatory in 2 countries, such as Richtlinie in Germany[12] and Clinical Laboratory Improvement Amendments (CLIA) in the United States.[13] When the cMQS result was equal to or higher than the lower limit of at least 1 of these mandatory specifications, cMQS was accepted as definitive (procedure A)
   b. Moreover, for data obtained from 2007 to 2010, the cMQSs were also compared with the preliminary study (2005–2006); in case of discrepancies, the (2005–2006) values were disregarded.
3. Procedure B
   If the cMQS result was lower than the German (Richtlinie) or US (CLIA) specifications and, in the opinion of the Expert Committee, would be not plausible to be used in our country, a complementary calculation procedure was added (procedure B; **Figs. 1** and **2**). This iterative procedure consisted of increasing the cMQS value by 0.01% (probe error value) and counting the amount of laboratories obtaining 75% of their results within this probe error value. The process finished when 90% of laboratories had 75% of results within the probe error value. This value was considered to be the minimum quality specification (MQS) agreed by the Expert Committee.

Figs. 1 and **2** summarize our working algorithm.

RESULTS

The analytes studied, the mandatory specifications in the United States and Germany as well as their highest values (when there are more than 1), our provisional specifications, the pathway used to arrive at our final decision, the process chosen, and the final specifications defined are shown in **Table 1**.

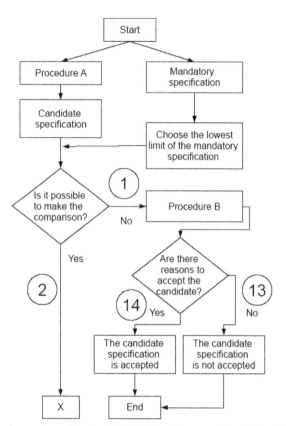

Fig. 1. Procedure for each analyte (part 1). Circles with a number inside identify the points of the algorithm.

The final point of each pathway and the analytes included are shown in **Table 2**. Only 10 analytes followed procedure A:

- For albumin (urine) and calcium (urine) our results were higher than the mandatory specifications, so they were accepted by the committee (pathway 2/5/7 in **Figs. 1** and **2**).
- For bilirubin, creatinine, fibrinogen, high-density lipoprotein cholesterol, lithium, and activated partial thromboplastin time (seconds), prior consensual specifications had been published (see **Table 1**, PS column) that were different from those obtained in this work (see **Table 1**, PA column). These specifications were higher than the mandatory specifications (in the United States and Germany, so they were selected by this committee (pathway 2/3/6/7 in **Figs. 1** and **2**).
- For phenytoin and prothrombin time, pathway 2/3/4 was applied, because our previously published specifications did not differ from those obtained by using procedure A.

Procedure B was applied in the other 72 analytes:

- For α-amylase (urine), functional antithrombin, chloride (urine), erythrocyte sedimentation rate, factor VIII, glycated hemoglobin (Hb), HbA2, fetal Hb, reticulocytes, and absolute reticulocytes, there were no mandatory specifications with

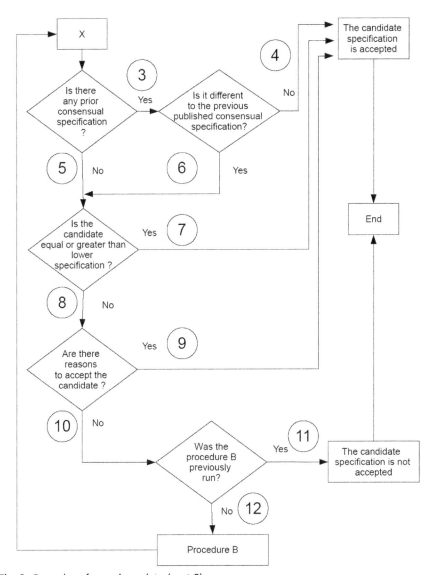

Fig. 2. Procedure for each analyte (part 2).

which to compare the result of the calculated specification. Procedure B was therefore directly applied and the results obtained were accepted by consensus (pathway 1/14 in **Fig. 1**).
- For creatinine (urine), glucose (urine), phosphate (urine), potassium (urine), sodium (urine), urate (urine), and urea (urine), specifications calculated by procedure A were lower than the mandatory specifications in the United States and Germany, so it was decided to apply procedure B (pathway 2/5/8/10/12/5/8/9 in **Figs. 1** and **2**).
- For alanine aminotransferase, alkaline phosphatase, α-amylase, aspartate aminotransferase, chloride, immunoglobulin A, immunoglobulin M, iron, lactate

Table 1
Analytes, comparison specifications, resulting specifications, flow way, chosen process and final specification

Order	Analyte	CLIA	RILI	HS	PA (%)	PB (%)	PS (%)	FW	CP	FS (%)
1	Activated partial thromboplastin time, ratio	—	—	—	15	15	20	2/3/6/8/10/ 12/3/6/8/9	B	15
2	Activated partial thromboplastin time, seconds	15	18	18	27	29	26	2/3/6/7	A	27
3	Alanine aminotransferase	20	21	21	18	23	20	2/3/6/8/10/ 12/3/6/7	B	23
4	Albumin	10	20	20	11	14	13	2/3/6/8/10/ 12/3/6/8/9	B	14
5	Albumin (urine)	—	26	26	38	72	—	2/5/7	A	38
6	Alkaline phosphatase	30	21	30	24	31	28	2/3/6/8/10/ 12/3/6/7	B	31
7	α-Amylase	30	—	30	26	35	33	2/3/6/8/10/ 12/3/6/7	B	35
8	α-Amylase (urine)	—	—	—	29	35	—	1/14	B	35
9	Alfa fetoprotein	—	24	24	17	20	22	2/3/6/8/10/ 12/3/6/8/9	B	20
10	Aspartate aminotransferase	20	21	21	18	21	—	2/3/6/8/10/ 12/3/6/7	B	21
11	Antithrombin functional	—	—	—	20	43	19	1/14	B	43
12	Bilirubin	20	22	22	24	32	23	2/3/6/7	A	24
13	Calcium	14	10	14	9	11	10	2/3/6/8/10/ 12/3/6/8/9	B	11
14	Calcium (urine)	—	17	17	30	28	—	2/5/7	A	30
15	Carcinoembryonic antigen	—	24	24	16	16	21	2/3/6/8/10/ 12/3/6/8/9	B	16
16	Chloride	5	8	8	7	9	8	2/3/6/8/10/ 12/3/6/7	B	9
17	Chloride (urine)	—	—	—	11	12	—	1/14	B	12
18	Cholesterol	10	13	13	9	11	10	2/3/6/8/10/ 12/3/6/8/9	B	11
19	Cortisol	25	30	30	23	28	25	2/3/6/8/10/ 12/3/6/8/9	B	28
20	Creatine kinase	30	20	30	19	24	20	2/3/6/8/10/ 12/3/6/8/9	B	24
21	Creatinine	15	20	20	20	25	28	2/3/6/7	A	20
22	Creatinine (urine)	—	21	21	12	15	—	2/5/8/10/12/ 5/8/9	B	15
23	Digoxin	—	30	30	21	20	20	2/3/6/8/10/ 12/3/6/8/9	B	20
24	Red blood cells	6	8	8	4	4	5	2/3/6/8/10/ 12/3/6/8/9	B	4

(continued on next page)

Table 1
(continued)

Order	Analyte	CLIA	RILI	HS	PA (%)	PB (%)	PS (%)	FW	CP	FS (%)
25	Erythrocyte sedimentation rate	—	—	—	43	54	—	1/14	B	54
26	Estradiol	—	35	35	22	26	25	2/3/6/8/10/ 12/3/6/8/9	B	26
27	Factor VIII	—	—	—	35	49	—	1/14	B	49
28	Ferritin	—	25	25	21	21	22	2/3/6/8/10/ 12/3/6/8/9	B	21
29	Fibrinogen	20	—	20	24	32	28	2/3/6/7	A	24
30	Follitropin	—	—	—	14	14	16	2/3/6/8/10/ 12/3/6/8/9	B	14
31	Free thyroxine	—	24	24	16	16	23	2/3/6/8/10/ 12/3/6/8/9	B	16
32	γ-Glutamyl transferase	—	21	21	17	22	22	2/3/6/8/10/ 12/3/4	B	22
33	Glucose	10	15	15	9	11	10	2/3/6/8/10/ 12/3/6/8/9	B	11
34	Glucose (urine)	—	22	22	10	12	—	2/5/8/10/ 12/5/8/9	B	12
35	HDL cholesterol	30	—	30	33	35	34	2/3/6/7	A	33
36	Hematocrit	6	9	9	6	8	7	2/3/6/8/10/ 12/3/6/8/9	B	8
37	Hb	7	6	7	4	5	5	2/3/6/8/10/ 12/3/4	B	5
38	Glycated Hb (HbA1c)	—	—	—	9	12	—	1/14	B	12
39	HbA2	—	—	—	27	37	—	1/14	B	37
40	Fetal Hb	—	—	—	27	39	—	1/14	B	39
41	Immunoglobulin A	—	20	20	14	21	24	2/3/6/8/10/ 12/3/6/7	B	21
42	Immunoglobulin G	25	18	25	13	16	20	2/3/6/8/10/ 12/3/6/8/9	B	16
43	Immunoglobulin M	—	26	26	17	28	33	2/3/6/8/10/ 12/3/6/7	B	28
44	International Normalized Ratio	—	—	—	21	24	28	2/3/6/8/10/ 12/3/6/8/9	B	24
45	Iron	20	—	20	19	24	22	2/3/6/8/10/ 12/3/6/7	B	24
46	Lactate dehydrogenase	20	18	20	17	26	25	2/3/6/8/10/ 12/3/6/7	B	26
47	Leukocytes	15	18	18	9	9	11	2/3/6/8/10/ 12/3/6/8/9	B	9
48	Lutropin	—	—	—	16	17	19	2/3/6/8/10/ 12/3/6/8/9	B	17
49	Lithium	—	12	12	18	23	19	2/3/6/7	A	18

(continued on next page)

Table 1
(continued)

Order	Analyte	CLIA	RILI	HS	PA (%)	PB (%)	PS (%)	FW	CP	FS (%)
50	Mean corpuscular Hb	—	—	—	4	5	6	2/3/6/8/10/12/3/6/8/9	B	5
51	Mean corpuscular Hb concentration	—	—	—	6	8	9	2/3/6/8/10/12/3/6/8/9	B	8
52	Mean corpuscular volume	—	—	—	5	7	7	2/3/6/8/10/12/3/4	B	7
53	Phenobarbital	—	20	20	14	15	18	2/3/6/8/10/12/3/6/8/9	B	15
54	Phenytoin	—	20	20	13	13	13	2/3/4	A	13
55	Phosphate	—	16	16	13	17	15	2/3/6/8/10/12/3/6/7	B	17
56	Phosphate (urine)	—	20	20	13	16	15	2/5/8/10/12/5/8/9	B	16
57	Platelet	25	18	25	14	16	16	2/3/6/8/10/12/3/4	B	16
58	Potassium	14	8	14	6	8	7	2/3/6/8/10/12/3/6/8/9	B	8
59	Potassium (urine)	—	15	15	10	12	—	2/5/8/10/12/5/8/9	B	12
60	Progesterone	—	35	35	25	26	29	2/3/6/8/10/12/3/6/8/9	B	26
61	Prolactin	—	—	—	19	22	28	2/3/6/8/10/12/3/6/8/9	B	22
62	Protein	10	10	10	9	12	10	2/3/6/8/10/12/3/6/7	B	12
63	Protein (urine)	—	24	24	19	34	—	2/8/10/12/5/7	B	34
64	Prothrombin time (%)	—	—	—	29	30	29	2/3/4	A	29
65	Prothrombin time ratio	—	23	23	16	17	25	2/3/6/8/10/12/3/6/8/9	B	17
66	Reticulocytes (%)	—	—	—	30	35	—	1/14	B	35
67	Reticulocytes, absolute ($\times 10^9$/L)	—	—	—	30	39	—	1/14	B	39
68	Sodium	3	5	5	4	5	5	2/3/6/8/10/12/3/4	B	5
69	Sodium (urine)	—	12	12	9	10	—	2/5/8/10/12/5/8/9	B	10
70	Testosterone	—	35	35	22	23	35	2/3/6/8/10/12/3/6/8/9	B	23
71	Theophylline	25	24	25	11	12	15	2/3/6/8/10/12/3/6/8/9	B	12
72	Triiodothyronine	—	24	24	20	24	24	2/3/6/8/10/12/3/4	B	24
73	Thyrotropin	—	24	24	14	15	17	2/3/6/8/10/12/3/6/8/9	B	15

(continued on next page)

Order	Analyte	CLIA	RILI	HS	PA (%)	PB (%)	PS (%)	FW	CP	FS (%)
	Table 1 *(continued)*									
74	Total prostate-specific antigen	—	25	25	16	17	17	2/3/6/8/10/12/3/4	B	17
75	Total thyroxine	—	24	24	18	24	20	2/3/6/8/10/12/3/6/7	B	24
76	Triglyceride	25	16	25	14	18	15	2/3/6/8/10/12/3/6/8/9	B	18
77	Urate	17	13	17	13	17	14	2/3/6/8/10/12/3/6/7	B	17
78	Urate (urine)	—	23	23	14	15	—	2/5/8/10/12/5/8/9	B	15
79	Urea	9	20	20	15	19	17	2/3/6/8/10/12/3/6/8/9	B	19
80	Urea (urine)	—	21	21	16	19	—	2/5/8/10/12/5/8/9	B	19
	Total acid phosphatase	—	—	—	57	78	—	2/3/6/8/10/12/3/6/8/10/11	—	—
	Antithrombin concentration	—	—	—	42	133	—	1/13	—	—

Abbreviations: CLIA, Clinical Laboratory Improvement Amendments (highest specification, if there is more than 1); CP, chosen procedure (A or B); FS, final specification; FW, flow way; Hb, hemoglobin; HDL, high-density lipoprotein; HS, highest specification considered as reference (the least strict specification of mandatory specifications); PA, resulting specification from procedure A application; PB, resulting specification from procedure B application; PS, previous specification; RILI, Richtlinie (Rilibak; highest specification, if there is more than 1).

dehydrogenase, phosphate, protein, total thyroxine, and urate, the calculated specifications (see **Table 1**, PB column) were higher than the previously released specifications (see **Table 1**, PS column) and lower than the mandatory specifications. Procedure B was therefore applied (see **Table 1**, FS column) (pathway 2/3/6/8/10/12/3/6/7 in **Figs. 1** and **2**).

- A similar pathway was followed for the following analytes: gamma-glutamyl transferase, hemoglobin, mean corpuscular volume, platelets, sodium, triiodothyronine, and total prostate-specific antigen. However, the results were similar to those previously published by our committee, so they were accepted (pathway 2/3/6/8/10/12/3/4 in **Figs. 1** and **2**).
- For protein (urine) the result obtained by procedure A was lower than the mandatory specifications, so it was decided to recalculate using procedure B (pathway 2/8/10/12/5/7 in **Figs. 1** and **2**).
- In addition, for all other analytes the 2/3/6/8/10/12/3/6/8/9 pathway was applied, because although the results obtained after applying procedure B were lower than the mandatory specifications, we found no reasons to reject them.

By implementing the algorithm (see **Figs. 1** and **2**), the Expert Committee had to manage the acceptance or rejection of the candidate specification for 72 analytes (the selection is based on points 1 or 8 from **Figs. 1** and **2**) of the 82 possible. The remainder (10 analytes) were automatically accepted. Only 2 cases (total acid phosphatase and antithrombin concentration) from the 72 analytes were not accepted.

Table 3 summarizes the comparison of our MQSs (procedures A and B) with those of CLIA and Richtlinie, expressed as number of analytes.

Table 2
Pathway final point, number of analytes resulted and analytes included in each pathway

Pathway	Analytes (N)	Analytes
4	9	Hemoglobin, mean corpuscular volume, phenytoin, platelet, prothrombin time, sodium, triiodothyronine, total prostate-specific antigen, γ-glutamyl transferase
7	22	Activated partial thromboplastin time, alanine aminotransferase, albumin urine, alkaline phosphatase, aspartate aminotransferase, bilirubin, calcium urine, chloride, creatinine, fibrinogen, HDL cholesterol, immunoglobulin A, immunoglobulin M, iron, lactate dehydrogenase, lithium, phosphate, protein, protein urine, total thyroxine, urate, α-amylase
9	39	Activated partial thromboplastin time ratio, albumin, calcium, carcinoembryonic antigen, cholesterol, cortisol, creatine kinase, creatinine urine, digoxin, estradiol, ferritin, follitropin, free thyroxine, glucose, glucose urine, hematocrit, immunoglobulin G, international normalized ratio, leukocytes, lutropin, mean corpuscular Hb concentration, mean corpuscular hemoglobin, phenobarbital, phosphate urine, potassium, potassium urine, progesterone, prolactin, prothrombin time ratio, red blood cells, sodium urine, testosterone, theophylline, thyrotropin, triglyceride, urate urine, urea, urea urine, alfa fetoprotein
11	1	Total acid phosphatase
13	1	Antithrombin concentration
14	10	α-Amylase urine, antithrombin functional, chloride urine, erythrocyte sedimentation rate, factor VIII, fetal Hb, glycated Hb, HbA2, reticulocytes (%), reticulocytes ($\times 10^9$/L)

DISCUSSION

The calculation model used in this work may be reproduced by other EQAP organizers, and may be expanded to all quantitative tests involved in EQAPs.

It uses an innovative concept that takes into account not only the individual results but also the whole results obtained by each laboratory during a cycle period.

Table 3
Comparison between minimum quality specification, Clinical Laboratory Improvement Amendments, and Richtlinie, expressed as number of analytes resulting in each group

Classification	cMQS vs CLIA		cMQS vs Richtlinie	
	Procedure A	Procedure B	Procedure A	Procedure B
Less restrictive	9	20	6	20
Same	1	1	2	5
More restrictive	21	10	49	32
No comparison[a]	51	51	25	25
Total	82	82	82	82

[a] No data in CLIA or in Richtlinie.

The high number of results considered gives the work a high statistical robustness. The results are based on an international consensus (Stockholm-Milan) that has been reinforced by the combination of 2 state-of-the-art calculations (procedures A and B). In addition, they are subjected to a review by the Expert Committee, and so 69 of them (that go through step 1 or step 8 on the flow chart) have been modified to adapt them to legislative criteria applied in other countries that have a prolonged experience with mandatory minimum quality requirements. Note that the acceptance or not of the candidate specification is based on the practicality of the criteria described by the algorithm, and not simply by the arbitrary judgment of the committee.

The practical uses of these MQSs are:

- They give a single numerical quality specification for each analyte studied in accordance with the total error concept
- They are easy to use by accreditation and certification bodies, and well accepted by laboratories, as has been shown in our country, where 55% of laboratories show awareness of the existence of these consensus MQSs and 49% agree that they should become mandatory)[14]
- They can be applied as the mandatory minimum level of quality, as is done in other countries
- They should not be used as goals, but as the minimum quality, and laboratories that cannot reach these goals are obliged to take action

As a positive experience, the authors would like to point in value the collaborative work performed with potential competitors, which enriches all of us and promotes harmonization of results within a country.

REFERENCES

1. Buño Soto A, Calafell Clar R, Morancho Zaragoza J, et al. Consensus on the minimum specifications of the analytical quality. Rev Lab Clin 2008;1(1):35–9.
2. Kenny D, Fraser CG, Hyltoft Petersen P, et al. Consensus agreement conference on strategies to set global quality specifications in laboratory medicine. Stockholm. Scand J Clin Lab Invest 1999;1999:585.
3. International Organization for Standardization. ISO/TR 15196: 2001. Identification and determination of analytical and clinical performance goals for laboratory methodologies. Geneva (Switzerland): ISO; 2001.
4. Sandberg S, Fraser CG, Horvath AR, et al. Defining analytical performance specifications: consensus statement from the 1st Strategic Conference of the European Federation of Clinical Chemistry and Laboratory Medicine. Consensus statement. Clin Chem Lab Med 2015;53:833–5.
5. Prada E, Blázquez R, Gutiérrez Bassine G, et al. Internal quality control vs external quality control. Rev Lab Clin 2016;9(2):54–9.
6. International Organization for Standardization. ISO/IEC 17043:2010 Conformity assessment - General requirements for proficiency testing. 1st edition. Geneva (Switzerland): ISO; 2010.
7. Guidelines for the requirements for the competence of EQAP organizers IFCC/EMD/C-AQ. Version 3. 2002.
8. International Organization for Standardization. ISO 9001:2008. Quality management systems. Requirements. Geneva (Switzerland): ISO; 2008.
9. Calafell Clar R, Gutiérrez Bassini G, Jou Turallas JS, et al. Consensus on the minimum analytical quality specifications for haematology and special biochemistry parameters. Rev Lab Clin 2010;3(2):87–93.

10. Ricós C, Ramón F, Salas A, et al. Minimum analytical quality specifications of in-terlaboratory comparisons: agreement among Spanish EQA organizers. Clin Chem Lab Med 2012;50(3):455–61.

11. Morancho J, Prada E, Gutiérrez-Bassini G, et al. Updates of analytical quality specifications 2014. Consensus of national scientific societies. Rev Lab Clin 2014;7(1):3–8.

12. Richtlinie der Bundesärztekammer zur Qualitätssicherung laboratoriumsmedizi-nischer Untersuchungen. Dtsch Ärztebl 2008;105:341–5.

13. Clinical Laboratory Improvement Amendments (CLIA). CLIA requirements for analytical quality. 2003. Available at: http://www.westgard.com/clia.htm. Ac-cessed May 1, 2016.

14. Morancho J, Prada E, Gutiérrez-Bassini G, et al. Level of implementation of analytical quality specifications in Spain. Rev Lab Clin 2015;8(1):19–28.

Six Sigma Quality Management System and Design of Risk-based Statistical Quality Control

CrossMark

James O. Westgard, PhD[a,b,*], Sten A. Westgard, MS[b]

KEYWORDS

- Six Sigma • Quality management system • Process capability • SQC
- Analytical run • Frequency of QC

KEY POINTS

- The traditional error model provides the basis for development of a scientific quality management system (QMS) that adheres to the Deming Plan-Do-Check-Act process for objective decision making based on data.

- Incorporation of Six Sigma concepts and metrics provides a QMS that supports analytical quality management with tools for specifying quality goals, judging the acceptability of performance of examination procedures, designing statistical quality control (SQC) procedures to detect medically important errors, and evaluating quality from external quality assessment and proficiency testing surveys.

- Design of risk-based SQC procedures is practical using the traditional criterion of achieving 90% detection of the critical medically important systematic errors, P_{edc} (probability of detection of medically important systematic errors), along with the documented relationship between P_{edc} and the Parvin measure of the maximum expected number of final unreliable test results, which can be understood as the maximum number of unreliable final test results that might be reported in an analytical run.

- The number of patient samples in an analytical run bracketed by quality control (QC) events, or frequency of QC, can be optimized from information on P_{edc} to minimize the risk of reporting erroneous test results.

- Practical tools for daily quality management are the strength of the error model and show why the uncertainty model has yet to be widely accepted in medical laboratories.

[a] Department of Pathology and Laboratory Medicine, School of Medicine and Public Health, University of Wisconsin, Madison, WI 53705, USA; [b] Westgard QC, Inc, Madison, WI 53717, USA
* Corresponding author. Department of Pathology and Laboratory Medicine, School of Medicine and Public Health, University of Wisconsin, Madison 53705, WI.
E-mail address: james@westgard.com

Clin Lab Med 37 (2017) 85–96
http://dx.doi.org/10.1016/j.cll.2016.09.008
0272-2712/17/© 2016 Elsevier Inc. All rights reserved.

INTRODUCTION

Metrology challenges some of the traditional concepts and practices that have been developed for quality management in medical laboratories, as discussed in some of the earlier articles in this issue (See Theodorsson's article, "Uncertainty in Measurement and Total Error – Tools for Coping with Diagnostic Uncertainty"; and James O. Westgard and Sten A. Westgard's article, "Measuring Analytical Quality: Total Analytical Error vs Measurement Uncertainty", in this issue) as well as other recent articles in the literature.[1–6] Nevertheless, medical laboratories now depend on practices that have evolved from the initial establishment of statistical quality control (SQC) and the evolution to Total Quality Management and Six Sigma quality management. The theoretic rigor of metrology and the practical needs in medical laboratories must be reconciled and will likely require that the uncertainty model of metrology and the error model, now considered traditional practice, coexist for the foreseeable future.

TRADITIONAL ERROR MODEL IS THE FOUNDATION FOR SIX SIGMA QUALITY MANAGEMENT SYSTEM

First and foremost, the concept of total analytical error (TAE) and the related quality goal in the form of allowable total error (ATE) seem to be contentious issues, even though they are well-established concepts with more than 40 years of widespread application in medical laboratories.[7,8] The practice of making a single measurement to report a test result is almost unique to medical laboratories, as opposed to metrology laboratories. That practice means that any test result may be in error because of both random error (imprecision, SD [standard deviation], or CV [coefficient of variation]) and systematic error (trueness, bias) and that a measure of accuracy, such as TAE, is necessary.[2] Likewise, quality goals in the form of ATE are needed for proficiency testing (PT) and external quality assessment (EQA) programs in which only a single measurement is generally performed on proficiency samples. Such ATE goals are also useful for validating method performance, selecting SQC procedures, prioritizing controls for risk-based quality control (QC) plans, and measuring and monitoring the quality achieved over time and distance.

Many tools and techniques are available to support the traditional quality management practices, as part of a Six Sigma quality management system (QMS),[9,10] whereas metrology tools and techniques are often more suitable for manufacturers of medical devices. Metrology emphasizes the use of reference methods and reference materials to provide a traceability chain that should provide comparability of test results (See Armbruster's article, "Metrological Traceability of Assays and Comparability of Patient Test Results", in this issue). The measure of quality of the traceability chain is the associated measurement uncertainty (MU), which is estimated from the components or sources of variation in the process. A bottom-up methodology is appropriate for use by manufacturers, but is too complicated for most applications in medical laboratories. A top-down methodology using intermediate-term precision data from routine SQC is recommended for medical laboratories by ISO (International Standards Organization) 15189.[11]

For quality management in medical laboratories, a Six Sigma QMS is recommended that follows the Deming Plan-Do-Check-Act cycle to implement a scientific management process, as shown in **Fig. 1** (plan, steps 1–2; do, steps 3–4; check, steps 5–9; act, steps 10–12):

- Plan: quality goals are the starting point in step 1 and ATE is the most common and useful format. The selection of an analytical examination procedure in step 2 should consider traceability and harmonization, along with the reference

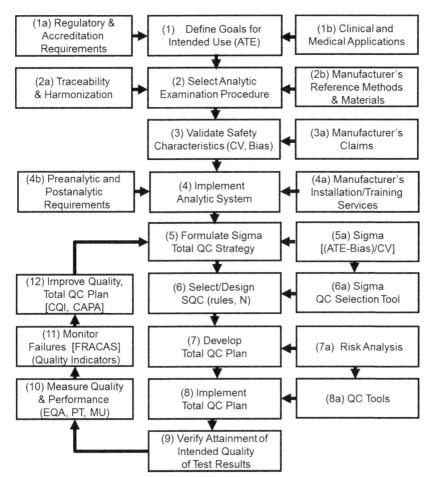

Fig. 1. Six Sigma QMS. CAPA, corrective and preventive action; CQI, continuous quality improvement; EQA, external quality assessment; FRACAS, failure reporting and corrective action system; MU, measurement uncertainty; PT, proficiency testing.

materials and methods available from the manufacturer. Metrology is important here, but the burden is on the manufacturer because the laboratory lacks the capability to implement reference methods and often cannot afford the expense of reference materials.

- Do: validation of safety characteristics for precision, trueness, and so forth, in step 3 is a critical function in the laboratory. Acceptable performance can be evaluated by determining quality on the sigma scale using a method decision chart prepared for the defined ATE and applied by plotting an operating point whose y coordinate represents the observed trueness (percentage bias) and x coordinate the observed imprecision (percentage CV). Ideally, sigma quality should be 5 or higher; 4 sigma is acceptable, but requires more QC; 3.5 sigma is the lowest quality that is practical for implementation; examination procedures less than 3.5 sigma quality should be rejected unless their performance can be improved. Implementation of an analytical system must consider the preanalytical and postanalytical requirements followed by thorough in-service training for analysts.

- Check: formulation of a total QC strategy based on the sigma quality provides general guidance for the QC plan that should be implemented to monitor the quality of routine production. The selection/design of a statistical QC procedure in step 6 should ensure detection of medically important errors. Practical tools include a sigma-metric SQC selection chart, the Chart of Operating Specifications, and the Westgard Sigma Rules graphic. Right-sizing the SQC procedure is the most important part of developing an effective total QC plan. To monitor the total testing process, preanalytical and postanalytical controls should be added to the right-size SQC procedure. Risk assessment may be useful to identify specific failure modes and specific controls to mitigate their risks. The total QC plan is then implemented in step 8 and applied routinely in step 9 to verify the attainment of the intended quality of test results.
- Act: quality and performance must be measured and monitored to ensure that the intended quality is being achieved. Important measures include results from PT/EQA surveys, which can also be used to determine sigma quality using a sigma quality assessment chart. MU is a requirement of ISO 15189 and may be determined from intermediate-term precision data as represented by routine QC results. Other quality indicators should be selected to monitor the critical failure modes. In addition, the laboratory must review these quality and performance metrics, compare with the goals for intended use, and make the necessary improvements in the QMS process and/or total QC plan.

SIGMA-METRIC IS A PROCESS CAPABILITY INDEX

A sigma-metric is calculated to compare the quality required for intended use to the performance observed for the examination procedure:

Sigma-metric $= (ATE - Bias_{obs})/SD_{obs}$

where *ATE* describes the tolerance limits and *Bias_{obs}* and *SD_{obs}* represent the observed trueness and imprecision of the examination procedure. Concentration units are preferred when a single reference material is analyzed following a protocol to estimate precision by the SD and bias by comparison of the observed mean with an assigned reference value. Alternatively, all terms may be in percentages:

Sigma-metric $= (\%ATE - \%Bias_{obs})/\%CV_{obs}$

Percentage figures are more reliable over a range of concentrations when the estimate of precision comes from a replication experiment or SQC data and the estimate of bias comes from a comparison of methods experiment or PT/EQA samples.

This sigma-metric is a process capability index whose use is well established for industrial process management.[12–14] For example, the industrial process capability index Cpk is related to the sigma-metric as follows:

Cpk $=$ (Tolerance specification − Off-centerness)/3 $\times$ Variation

If the tolerance specification is ATE, off-centerness is bias, and variation is SD, then:

Cpk $= (ATE - Bias)/3*SD$, and

Cpk*3 $= (ATE - Bias)/SD =$ Sigma-metric

For industrial production, the minimum Cpk that is acceptable is 1.0, which corresponds with 3 sigma. The ideal or desirable Cpk is 2.0, which corresponds with 6 sigma. Given that process capability indices have been used for many years in production operations (long before the introduction of Six Sigma concepts), the use of a sigma-metric as a process capability index provides an established approach for managing the production of laboratory testing processes. This metric corresponds with the long-term sigma in the Motorola Six Sigma methodology,[15] which was introduced in the 1990s, rather than the short-term sigma, which accommodates a systematic shift or bias equivalent to 1.5*SD. The long-term sigma accounts exactly for the bias observed for the process, thus is the preferred measure for an analytical examination process.

The origin of the sigma-metric as a process capability index shows that a quality requirement in the form of an ATE corresponds with the tolerance limits used in industrial production and that the off-centerness, or bias, of the production process is an important consideration for managing quality, along with the variation or precision of the process. Industrial tolerance limits apply to the individual products being produced, just like ATE applies to the individual test results being produced in a medical laboratory.

SIMPLE CALCULATION OF SIGMA-METRICS AT MEDICAL DECISION CONCENTRATIONS IS ADEQUATE

Given that the sigma-metric is such a critical measure of quality, there are some concerns about the best way to make the calculation. The established practice is to calculate sigma for each of the important medical decision concentrations; for example, 6.5% hemoglobin (Hb) for use of HbA1c for diagnosis, 7.0% Hb as the treatment goal, then select the most demanding sigma value or average the sigmas to guide the SQC design.

An alternative form of calculation has been proposed in the form of a patient-weighted sigma.[16] The argument here is that a patient-weighted sigma better represents the best single value for the observed patient population, rather than using sigma-metrics that are calculated for critical medical decision concentrations. The patient-weighted sigma is a much more complicated calculation and requires knowledge of the expected patient measurand distribution, the precision and bias profiles for the examination procedure, as well as the quality requirements throughout the observed patient range. The calculation is sufficiently complex and unique that it has been patented[17] and cannot be readily applied without proprietary software. The application of patient-weighted sigmas was shown in study of HbA1c methods to assess the risk and reliability of 6 different examination procedures commonly used in central laboratory testing.[18] Data for high and low controls (at 5% Hb and 10% Hb) were also provided, along with regression statistics for comparison with the NGSP (National Glycohemoglobin Standardization Program) reference method, thus permitting calculation of point estimates of sigma for HbA1c at the medical decision concentration of 6.5% Hb. Comparison of the point estimates and the patient-weighted sigmas shows small differences for 5 of the 6 methods studied (2.48 point estimate vs 2.29 patient-weighted sigma; 1.54 vs 1.43; 3.97 vs 3.90; 0.49 vs 0.36; 2.07 vs 2.36). For 1 method, the patient-weighted sigma was 1.57 versus the point estimate of 2.80; for this method, the bias for normal samples (low concentrations) was very high and likely reduced the patient-weighted sigma because of the preponderance of normal samples in a typical patient distribution. Thus, it is not clear that this more complicated patient-weighted sigma provides any practical improvement compared with the simple point estimates at medically important decision concentrations.

Recently, Coskun and colleagues[19] recommended the use of a z-transformation calculation to account for the exact tails when the distribution is shifted because of bias. When a shift occurs, 1 tail of the distribution may still be partially within the tolerance limits and represents some acceptable products or measurements. For 9 measurands studied by Coskun and colleagues,[19] the average difference between the sigma-metrics calculated by z-transformation minus the simple model was 0.16 sigma, with a maximum of 0.35 sigma, where the z-transformation calculations always provide higher values of sigma. Such small differences do not generally affect the decisions being made about the acceptability of performance and the selection of SQC procedures. Furthermore, the simple sigma-metric calculations provide conservative values, meaning that the decisions and judgments made are on the safe side, rather than misleading high values.

Another issue is whether or not to include bias in the calculation of sigma. Some analysts recommend that bias be assumed as zero because there is little that a laboratory can do to reduce or eliminate bias.[20] That assumption leads to higher sigmas and simpler SQC, which seems to be the objective:

The subtraction of bias may render sigmas so low that the chemist/technologist will attempt to use multiple control rules to manage assay quality, which will invariably increase the probability of false rejections. It is our belief that there is little that a laboratory system can do with bias once inter-instrument variation is minimized by using similar analytic systems and occasionally employ a conversion factor to make a test on one analyzer resemble the same test on a different analyzer...[20]

This practice assumes that reference ranges and critical decision levels have been developed internally and neglects the trend toward evidence-based medical treatment guidelines (eg, HbA1c) that are applied globally or nationally across laboratories and across examination procedures. Another serious problem is that the decision about the acceptability of an examination procedure must consider bias. When bias is large and sigma is low, the preferred decision should be to improve method performance or select another method, rather than to assume that those biases are not important as long as daily operation is stable.

SIGMA-METRIC IS A PREDICTOR OF RISK AND THE NEEDED STATISTICAL QUALITY CONTROL

The authors have long advocated the use of the sigma-metric as a predictor of risk. Sigma is inherently risk based and can readily be converted to the expected defect rates or expressed in terms of defects per million. It is therefore very useful for evaluating the performance of an examination procedure as well as for selecting/designing SQC procedures to detect medically important errors. To select appropriate SQC procedures, the rejection characteristics of different control rules and different numbers of control measurements can be described by power curves, or power function graphs.[21] Given a specification for ATE, the size of the medically important systematic error (ΔSE_{crit}) can be calculated as follows[22]:

$$\Delta SE_{crit} = [(ATE - Bias_{obs})/SD_{obs}] - 1.65$$

where 1.65 is the z-value for a 1-sided confidence limit, which allows a 5% risk of a medically important error.

To select SQC procedures, the calculated critical errors can be drawn over power curves.[23] With the introduction of Six Sigma concepts, the expression (ATE – Bias$_{obs}$)/SD$_{obs}$ can be replaced by the sigma-metric, thereby simplifying the calculation:

ΔSE_{crit} = Sigma-metric − 1.65

This relationship allows power function graphs to be rescaled in terms of the sigma-metric and makes it quicker and easier to select appropriate control rules and numbers of control measurements. An example is shown in **Fig. 2** for a 4-sigma testing process.

For goals in selecting an appropriate SQC procedure, the authors recommend achieving a probability of error detection (P_{ed}) of 0.90, or 90% chance, for the critical SE, while maintaining the probability for false rejection (P_{fr}) as low as possible. In the example in **Fig. 2**, that could be accomplished by selection of the $1_{3s}/2_{2s}/R_{4s}/4_{1s}$ multirule procedure with 4 control measurements per run. As shown in the key, P_{ed} is 0.91, which corresponds with the intersection of the vertical line and the top power curve. P_{fr} is 0.03, which corresponds with the y-intercept of that power curve.

STATISTICAL QUALITY CONTROL ANALYTICAL RUN, OR FREQUENCY OF QUALITY CONTROL, CAN BE RELATED TO ERROR DETECTION

A limitation of this design approach is the lack of a specification for the size of the analytical run or the frequency of QC. Parvin[24] developed a complimentary design approach based on the estimation of the number of unreliable, defective, or erroneous test results that might be accepted and reported in an analytical run with an undetected error condition. This parameter has been termed the maximum expected number of unreliable final test results [MaxE(N_{UF})[24]; pronounced max-enough]. The

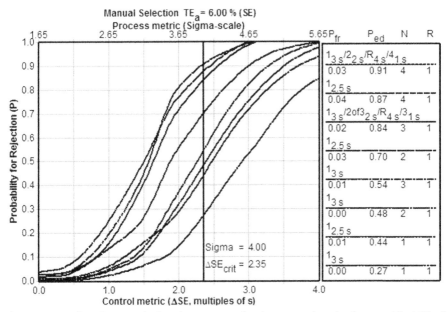

Fig. 2. Power function graph showing an examination procedure having a critical SE of 2.35*SD or a sigma-metric of 4.0. Probability of rejection is plotted on the y-axis versus the size of a ΔSE_{crit} on the lower x-axis and the sigma-metric on the upper x-axis. Power curves (top to bottom) correspond with the control rules and total number of control measurements (top to bottom) in the key at the right. Probability for false rejection (P_{fr}) in the key corresponds with the y-intercept of the power curve; probability of error detection (P_{ed}) corresponds with the intersection of the vertical line with the power curve.

approach was described in detail in a previous issue.[25] More recently, Yago and Alcover[26] showed how to integrate the classic Westgard approach with the Parvin approach to improve the SQC design process. They provide nomograms that show the relationship between sigma, various control rules, and the maximum expected number of erroneous results. They also show that the maximum expected number of erroneous results is related to the P_{ed} for the critical-sized systematic error (P_{edc}). **Fig. 3** shows this relationship and permits the estimation of the maximum number of unreliable or erroneous results from the probability of error detection, or vice versa:

> *The plot shows that the relationships between these performance measures are very similar for all rules considered, especially for rules with the same N value, so that 1 can estimate the value of 1 from the other with a relatively small margin of error, almost regardless of the QC procedure considered... To obtain an average of less than 1 unacceptable patient result as a consequence of an out-of-control condition, the plot shows that a QC procedure with a P_{edc} of about 0.8 is needed, assuming that 100 patient samples are analyzed between QC events...*[26]

This last statement suggests a goal of less than or equal to 1 erroneous result per run, which is also consistent with Parvin's[24] recommendation and examples. This goal can be used to assess run size in terms of the number of patient samples for

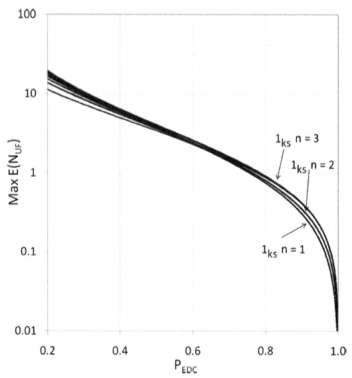

Fig. 3. Relationship between MaxE(N_{UF}) on the y-axis versus P_{edc} on the x-axis for families of SQC procedures with Ns from 1 to 3. (*From* Yago M, Alcover S. Selecting statistical procedures for quality control planning based on risk management. Clin Chem 2016;62:963. Published May 19, 2016. Reproduced with permission from the American Association for Clinical Chemistry.)

bracketed QC, in which a continuous production process is quality controlled period-ically and patient results released when both the initial and final QC events in a bracket are in control. If the goal of less than or equal to 1 erroneous result per run cannot be met with the current SQC procedure, changes in the control rules and number of con-trol measurements (N) may be able to increase P_{edc}, or the run size may be reduced and the frequency of QC increased.

As an example, Yago and Alcover[26] assess the length of the analytical run that would be appropriate for the classic design approach:

The selection of SQC procedures has been done classically with the objective of having 90% detection of the critical systematic errors, while maintaining false re-jections as low as possible. Fig. 3 shows that values for Max $E(N_{UF})$ in the range of 0.3 to 0.4 are obtained when simple QC procedures with P_{edc} = 0.90 are used to control an analytical process. This means that up to about 300 patient samples could be analyzed between QC events for reporting less than 1 erroneous result during an out-of-control condition, which represents a typical daily workload for many tests performed in a small or medium-sized laboratory. Therefore, use of P_{edc} = 0.90 as a general criterion appears to be quite reasonable for selecting QC procedures that reduce the probability of harming the patient to a level that could be considered acceptable for many tests conducted in a laboratory.

In this example, the size of the analytical run is calculated as $100/MaxE(N_{UF})$; for example, 100/0.3 would be 333 and 100/0.4 would be 250, which Yago and Alcover[26] summarize as "about 300 patient samples."

As another example, consider the 4-sigma process in which P_{edc} has been deter-mined in **Fig. 2**. Use of a $1_{3s}/2_{2s}/R_{4s}/4_{1s}$ multirule with N = 4 provides a P_{edc} of 0.91, which means that performance is equivalent to the example given earlier and the size of the analytical run could be 300 patient samples. Remember this means both the QC events at the beginning and end of the bracket require a multirule proced-ure with 4 control measurements. If the end-of-bracket QC event is out of control, then the quality of all 300 patient samples must be reassessed and the necessary patient samples repeated. In determining when a problem occurs during the run, it would be helpful to space the second set of 4 controls throughout the run, every 75 patient samples, rather than waiting until the end of the run. That would provide additional in-formation about when the problem began and the patient samples that need to be repeated, and might also provide earlier detection.

To see the effect of P_{edc} on the length of the analytical run for this 4-sigma testing process, consider the use of a $1_{3s}/2of3_{2s}/R_{4s}/3_{1s}$ multirule with N = 3, which provides a P_{edc} of 0.84. From **Fig. 3**, approximately 125 patient samples (100/0.80) would be appropriate to maintain a goal of less than or equal to 1 erroneous result being re-ported. If a 1_{3s} rule with N = 3 were used, P_{edc} would be 0.54, $MaxE(N_{UF})$ about 3.0, and the analytical run should be reduced to about 30 to 35 samples for a brack-eted continuous production operation. That would mean a total of 6 controls for 30 to 35 samples, which would be expensive but necessary to achieve the goal of less than or equal to 1 erroneous result per run.

Table 1 provides some estimates for the size of an analytical run as a function of P_{edc}, based on the estimation of $MaxE(N_{UF})$ from **Fig. 3**. The number of patient sam-ples is calculated as $100/MaxE(N_{UF})$ based on the goal of producing less than or equal to 1 erroneous result in a reported analytical run. These estimates are approximate because they depend on interpolation of the graphical results and assume that the general relationship between P_{edc} and $MaxE(N_{UF})$ also holds for multirule QC proced-ures and Ns as high as 4.

Table 1
Relationship between probability of error detection for critical sized systematic error, maximum expected number of final unreliable test results, and quality control frequency, expressed as the number of patient samples in an analytical run bracketed by control events. Values are interpolated from the relationship between ability of error detection for critical sized systematic error and maximum expected number of final unreliable test results, as documented by Yago and Alcover

P_{edc}	$MaxE(N_{UF})$	QC Frequency or Size of Run
1.00	0.01	10,000
0.99	0.02	5000
0.95	0.20	500
0.90	0.30	333
0.85	0.50	200
0.80	0.80	125
0.75	1.00	100
0.70	1.50	67
0.65	2.00	50
0.60	2.50	40
0.55	3.00	33
0.50	4.00	25
0.45	5.00	20
0.40	6.00	17
0.35	7.00	14
0.30	8.00	13
0.25	11.00	9
0.20	15.00	7

Data from Yago M, Alcover S. Selecting statistical procedures for quality control planning based on risk management. Clin Chem 2016;62:959–65.

SUMMARY

The design of risk-based SQC procedures shows the importance and practical value of the error model for quality management in medical laboratories. Metrology strangely ignores the uncertainty caused by the instability of an examination process as well as the uncertainty in the detection of medically important errors by SQC procedures. Selection of an adequate SQC procedure is an important task in developing QC plans that ensure the analytical quality of laboratory test results.

Our design approach, now considered traditional or classic, focuses on achieving 90% detection of a critical systematic error by selecting appropriate control rules and the number of control measurements, while also aiming for a low probability of false rejections. This design approach lacks a parameter for determining the frequency of QC or the size of an analytical run. Parvin[24] recommends the calculation of a parameter that represents the maximum expected number of unreliable final test results that may be reported in a run with an undetected error condition. This number of possible erroneous patient test results directly relates to the risk of patient harm, which makes this parameter particularly useful for risk-based SQC. This parameter is called $MaxE(N_{UF})$ and represents a concept that is difficult to understand and difficult to calculate. Its practical usefulness has also been limited by the need for specialized computer support for calculation.[27]

Yago and Alcover[26] simplified the Parvin approach by development of nomograms for the selection of control rules and Ns as a function of a method's sigma-metric and MaxE(N$_{UF}$). Both Parvin[24] and Yago and Alcover[26] suggested a design goal of less than or equal to 1 erroneous test result per run. The practical meaning is that there will be a maximum of 1 erroneous result reported in an analytical run, even when an error has occurred and gone undetected. This goal can be achieved by optimizing the SQC rules and number of control measurements or by changing the size of the analytical run or the frequency of QC.

Yago and Alcover[26] show that there is a close relationship between MaxE(N$_{UF}$) and P$_{edc}$, the probability of error detection for the critical sized systematic error that is medically important. The ready availability of power function graphs makes it easy to determine P$_{edc}$, which can then be used to look up MaxE(N$_{UF}$), which in turn can be used to determine the appropriate number of samples for the analytical run, which also defines the frequency of QC.

The overall design approach is to (1) define ATE, (2) measure the precision and bias of the examination procedure, (3) calculate a sigma-metric, (4) use a power function graph that has a sigma scale to assess P$_{edc}$ and identify the appropriate control rules and number of control measurements, (5) use the Yago-Alcover relationship to convert P$_{edc}$ to MaxE(N$_{UF}$), (6) determine the number of samples in the analytical run as 100/MaxE(N$_{UF}$) to achieve a goal of less than or equal to 1 erroneous test result per run.

There remain some practical issues with implementation of bracketed control of a continuous production process. The SQC design must be applied at the beginning and end of the bracket so it generally increases the cost of QC compared with current practices. The patient results must be held and not reported until the end of the bracket QC event is known to be in control, and if out of control there must be a corrective action strategy for repeating patient samples. Because it is helpful to identify when a problem occurs in an analytical run, it is generally useful to space out the controls for the second QC event throughout the run. If the hold time for results is too long, or the repeat costs are too great, the size of the run should be reduced and the frequency of control increased. Many factors may influence the practicality of the final SQC strategy and require careful assessment and judgment.

Tools for the design of risk-based SQC are but one example of the practical benefits of the error model versus the uncertainty model. It is possible that similar tools will become available in a metrology toolbox, but for now the practical tools are found only in the total-error toolbox. The continued development and improvement of these tools, as shown by the work of Parvin[24] and Yago and Alcover,[26] further show the priority of the error model for practical quality management in medical laboratories.

REFERENCES

1. Sandberg S, Fraser CG, Horvath AR, et al. Defining analytical performance specifications: consensus statement from the 1st strategic conference of the European Federation of Clinical Chemistry and Laboratory Medicine. Clin Chem Lab Med 2015;53(6):833–5.
2. Westgard JO. Useful measures and models for analytical quality management in medical laboratories. Clin Chem Lab Med 2016;54:223–33.
3. Panteghini M, Sandberg S. Total error vs. measurement uncertainty: the match continues. Clin Chem Lab Med 2016;54:195–6.
4. Oosterhuis WP, Theodorsson E. Total error vs. measurement uncertainty: revolution or evolution. Clin Chem Lab Med 2016;54:235–9.

5. Farrance I, Badrick T, Sikaris KA. Uncertainty in measurement and total error – are they so incompatible? Clin Chem Lab Med 2016;54:1309–11.
6. Kallner A. Is the combination of trueness and precision in one expression meaningful? On the use of total error and uncertainty in clinical chemistry. Clin Chem Lab Med 2016;54:1291–7.
7. Westgard JO, Carey RN, Wold S. Criteria for judging precision and accuracy in method development and evaluation. Clin Chem 1974;20:825–33.
8. Westgard JO, Westgard SA. Assessing quality on the sigma-scale from proficiency testing and external quality assessment surveys. Clin Chem Lab Med 2015;53:1531–5.
9. Westgard JO, Westgard SA. Quality control review: implementing a scientifically based quality control system. Ann Clin Biochem 2016;53:32–50.
10. Westgard JO, Westgard SA. Basic quality management systems. Madison (WI): Westgard QC; 2014.
11. ISO 15189. Medical laboratories – particular requirements for quality and competence. Geneva (Switzerland): ISO; 2012.
12. Westgard JO, Burnett RW. Precision requirements for cost-effective operation of analytical processes. Clin Chem 1990;36:1629–32.
13. Chesher D, Burnett L. Equivalence of critical error calculations and process capability index Cpk. Clin Chem 1997;43:1100–1.
14. Bais R. Use of capability index to improve laboratory analytical performance. Clin Biochem Rev 2008;29(Suppl 1):S27–31.
15. Harry M, Schroder R. Six sigma: the breakthrough management strategy revolutionizing the World's top corporations. New York: Currency; 2000.
16. Kuchipudi L, Yundt-Pacheco J, Parvin CA. Computing a patient-based sigma metric [Abstract]. Clin Chem 2010;56:A35.
17. Yundt-Pacheco J, Parvin CA. System and method to determine sigma of a clinical diagnostic process. US Patent 8,589,081 B2. 2013.
18. Woolworth A, Korpi-Steiner N, Miller JJ, et al. Utilization of assay performance characteristics to estimate hemoglobin A1c result reliability. Clin Chem 2014; 60:1073–9.
19. Coskun A, Serteser J, Kilercik M, et al. A new approach for calculating the sigma metric in clinical laboratories. Accred Qual Assur 2015;20:147–52.
20. Cembrowski GS, Cervinski MA. Demystifying reference sample quality control [Editorial]. Clin Chem 2016;62:907–9.
21. Westgard JO, Falk H, Groth T. Influence of a between-run component of variation, choice of control limits, and shape of error distribution on the performance characteristics of rules for internal quality control. Clin Chem 1979;25:394–400.
22. Westgard JO, Barry PL. Cost-effective quality control: managing the quality and productivity of analytical processes. Washington, DC: AACC Press; 1986.
23. Koch DD, Oryall JJ, Quam EF, et al. Selection of medically useful quality-control procedures for individual tests done in a multitest analytical system. Clin Chem 1990;36:230–3.
24. Parvin CA. Assessing the impact of the frequency of quality control testing on the quality of reported patient results. Clin Chem 2008;54:2049–54.
25. Yundt-Pacheco J, Parvin CA. Validating the performance of QC procedures. Clin Lab Med 2013;33:75–88.
26. Yago M, Alcover S. Selecting statistical procedures for quality control planning based on risk management. Clin Chem 2016;62:959–65.
27. Parvin CA, Yundt-Pacheco J. System and method for analyzing a QC strategy for releasing results. US Patent 8,938,409 B2. 2015.

Sigma Metrics Across the Total Testing Process

Navapun Charuruks, MD, FRCPath (Thailand)

KEYWORDS

- Statistical quality control (SQC) • Sigma verification program (SVP) • Sigma metrics
- Defect per million (DPM) • Individualized quality control plan (IQCP)
- Risk management • Laboratory processes

KEY POINTS

- The total testing process has traditionally been separated into 3 phases (preanalytical, analytical, and postanalytical), and in the last decade the prepreanalytical and postpostanalytical phases have been added to understand and manage the errors and risks that occur in the laboratory process.
- Laboratory quality control has been developed for several decades to ensure patient safety from a statistical quality control focus on analytical phase to risk management in order to cover the total laboratory processes, which include extra-analytical phases.
  - The number of errors that occur during laboratory processes are easily estimated by the method of estimating defects per million, whereas analytical performance can be calculated by the sigma metric equation.
  - Participation in a sigma verification program, which operates as an external independent third party to quantitate the sigma scale, is a convenient way to monitor analytical performance using continuous quality improvement and the sigma scale.
  - The sigma value not only shows the performance, it also provides the universal benchmark for continuous improvement of the laboratories. It is the objective quality datum for communication with physicians, patients, and customers, and useful feedback for manufacturers about their products' performance.
- The individualized quality control plan (IQCP), which mainly is involved with risk management of total laboratory processes, has recently been developed as an alternative or optional practice for laboratory quality control.
- The sigma concept can be applied to achieve high-quality requirements such as defining quality specifications to design IQCP, which is a difficult task for laboratories and an optional requirement in current quality standards.
- With the recent IQCP approach, new tools and techniques are required for integration. There has never been a single tool that is able to eliminate all errors or risks in laboratories. The appropriate combination of tools, such as failure modes and effect analysis, fishbone, and sigma metrics, has been introduced to meet this need.

Laboratory Department, Bumrungrad International Hospital, 33 Sukhumvit 3, Bangkok 10110, Thailand
E-mail address: navapun@bumrungraddoctor.com

Clin Lab Med 37 (2017) 97–117
http://dx.doi.org/10.1016/j.cll.2016.09.009   labmed.theclinics.com
0272-2712/17/© 2016 Elsevier Inc. All rights reserved.

INTRODUCTION

The total testing process has traditionally been separated into 3 phases (preanalytical, analytical, and postanalytical), and for several decades analytical quality has been the focus. In the 1930s, Shewhart[1] quality control (QC) was introduced, and around the 1950s the Levey and Jennings[2] chart or L-J Chart was developed. Since then the L-J Chart (first-generation QC) has been widely used. Quality has never been at a standstill, which is evident because QC was continuously developed to become statistical QC (SQC). To leverage SQC efficiency, Westgard[3–6] multirule (second-generation QC, in the 1980s) and sigma metrics (in the 1990s), which later developed to multistage QC (fifth-generation QC), are practiced worldwide. It is obvious that estimation of the sigma metric of a laboratory method is useful to understand the real quality that is being achieved by the analytical testing process.[7–9]

Several reviews show that the analytical phase has the best performing process compared with the 2 extra-analytical phases. It is often claimed that 62% of errors are preanalytical, 15% are analytical, and 23% are postanalytical. Regardless of the phase, errors have remained a challenge for laboratory performance improvement.[10,11] In preanalytical and postanalytical processes, errors are usually counted in numbers or percentages and are recorded for corrective and preventive actions. In analytical process, the examination procedure performances are typically evaluated in terms of precision and accuracy (bias).[12] For laboratories, information about these common laboratory practices consists of internal data for the laboratory's own improvements and are not generally understood by clinicians and patients. In several instances there are questions about laboratory performance and there are no clear scaling data to present.

Most clinicians and patients believe laboratory results have no errors; however, in real practice there are no processes with zero defects. For this reason, there are allowable total errors (TEa) for laboratories to manage.[13,14] Errors may occur at any time; it is the laboratorians' duty to do their best to control and monitor these errors, to follow quality standard regulations, and to keep TEa limited and in check for the patients' safety.

To provide a convenient way to assess and compare the quality that is required and intended for use with the precision and bias observed in a laboratory's[15] performance, the sigma scale is proposed. This scale measures the degree to which any process deviates from the target. The sigma value indicates how often defects are likely to occur; the higher the sigma value, the less likely the process will generate defects. Average services or products, regardless of their complexity, have a quality performance value of about 4-sigma. The best, or world-class, performance has a level of 6-sigma.[8]

The errors that occur during laboratory preanalytical, analytical and postanalytical processes are easily estimated by the method of defects per million (DPM)[16,17] and the analytical performances of tests can be calculated by equation: sigma metric = (TEa − bias)/precision (all values expressed as percentages). Sigma values can be widely explained to clinicians and patients so they can perceive the laboratories' performances.[7,18,19]

The challenges of laboratory quality improvement are never-ending. During the last decade the prepreanalytical and postpostanalytical phases were introduced to understand and manage the errors and risks that occur in the laboratory process. The idea is to identify activities associated with the initial selection of tests and, together with the interpretation by clinicians, to differentiate them from traditional general laboratory activities such as specimen collection, handling, and transportation (preanalytical phase), and result verification and reporting (postanalytical phase).[20] More recently, the risk management concept is being applied to improve laboratory quality. On

March 9, 2012, the Centers for Medicare and Medicaid Services (CMS) announced that the new laboratory quality policy of the Clinical Laboratory Improvement Amendments (CLIA), called the Individualized Quality Control Plan (IQCP),[21] which is mainly involved with risk management of total laboratory processes, will be an option for laboratory QC (alternative QC, sixth-generation QC).[22]

The laboratory quality concern is expanding beyond SQC and particularly emphasizes management's responsibilities and commitments to eliminate all errors in the total testing process. Risk management requires many tools and techniques that should be integrated with quality laboratory practice. The laboratories are expected to combine different types of controls to monitor different failure modes or different sources of errors to consistently achieve quality claims for their services from preanalytical, analytical, to postanalytical processes and eventually pushing them to design and define their IQCP.[21] This article shows that the implementation of the sigma concept not only benchmarks the laboratory performance and pushes for continuous quality improvement but also allows the integration of sigma metrics across the total testing process to be managed as a part of the IQCP of the individual laboratory.

Sigma Metrics in the Analytical Phase

The experts' opinion
The experts' opinion in several reviews mentioned that a better analytical quality should be achieved by setting and implementing evidence-based analytical quality specifications in everyday practice, thus requiring rules for internal QC (IQC) and external quality assessment procedures that are more appropriate.[8,23–25] There is a compelling need for standardized programs designed to improve metrological traceability and correcting biases and systematic errors. In addition, the experts suggest that more stringent metrics, such as 6-sigma, should be widely introduced in clinical laboratories to further improve analytical quality.[26]

Sigma verification program
In April 2014, a sigma verification program (SVP) for examination of procedures in medical laboratories was introduced.[27] It was designed to facilitate, support, and provide an evidence-based data-driven approach to quantify the quality being achieved by a laboratory method. Quantification of improvement in laboratory performance is essential for continuous quality improvement (CQI) programs, thus participation in an SVP to quantitate the sigma scale is a convenient way to implement analytical performance CQI.

From program to practice
At the beginning, data from 28 clinical chemistry assays (34 tests, including 6 urine assays) performed at the Laboratory Department, Bumrungrad International Hospital, Bangkok, Thailand, by the Laboratory Automation System, Abbott ACCELERATOR a3600 component, Abbott Laboratory Ltd, Thailand, during July to September (quarter 3 [Q3]), 2014, were collected and analyzed by WSVP (Westgard Sigma Verification Program) (**Fig. 1, Table 1**). The data were verified and certified by the SVP program on October 30, 2014. It was a continuous process and ran parallel with the proficiency testing (PT) program.

One difference from the SVP was that we used the TEa targets from the College of American Pathologists (CAP) instead of the SVP's recommended TEa values, most of them provided by CLIA. Our reasons were:

1. Our laboratory has participated in CAP PT
2. With CAP TEa, our laboratory could monitor and use CQI to improve our performance more consistently with our quality activities

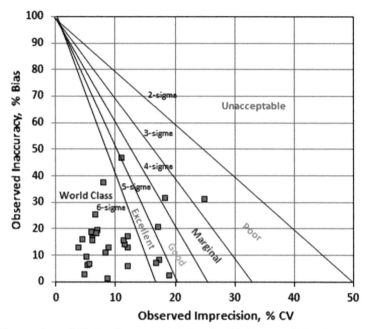

Fig. 1. Sigma values of 28 chemistry assays during the third quarter (Q3, July to September) of 2014 show there were 21 assays (75.0%) with performance equal to or better than 6-sigma level, 3 assays (10.7%) with 5-sigma to 6-sigma level, 2 assays (7.1%) had 4-sigma to 5-sigma level, 1 assay (3.6%) had 3-sigma to 4-sigma level, and 1 assay (3.6%) had lower than 3-sigma level. CV, coefficient of variation.

An SVP operates as an external independent third party requiring participating laboratories to submit annual or semiannual updates of sigma performance to maintain continuing certification. However, we initially decided to monitor the performance closely, then include the analysis of the results of Q4 (October to December 2014) to let our team get used to the SVP, do an early comparison (**Fig. 2**, **Table 2**), and proceed with the semiannual updates of sigma performance.[28,29]

From practice to continuous quality improvement process
In order to leverage the practice to implement CQI, the performances of each quarter were analyzed. Examples of the analysis are shown in **Table 3**. More than 70% of assays (20 of 28) maintained performance at or greater than 6-sigma and less than 5% of assays (1 of 28) had performance less than 3-sigma (see **Table 3**) during both Q3 and Q4 of the study. In Q3, it was observed that gamma-glutamyl transferase (GGT), glucose, and total protein assays had improved performance to more than 6-sigma. For GGT, the bias for CAP PT was unacceptable using the calibration factor set by the International Federation of Clinical Chemistry and Laboratory Medicine (IFCC) program, thus we opted to apply a non-IFCC calibration factor[30] that was recommended for laboratories that participate in the CAP PT program. The application of this factor significantly improved the GGT performance from 3.7-Sigma to greater than 6-sigma. The performance of blood urea nitrogen had not improved meaningfully (5.6-sigma to 5.8-sigma) because of little improvement of %CV (0.15–0.14). The small variation in sigma for chloride and sodium between Q3 and Q4 was noticed; personnel skills and performance were target concerns for improvement and consistency in performance for these assays.

Table 1
Sigma-metric worksheet during Q3, 2014, for core chemistry analytes running controls as recommended

Test	TEa Source	TEa	Group or Peer Mean (CAP PT)	BI Result (CAP PT)	Bias Units	Bias (%)	CV	Sigma	QC Rules Recommendation
				Instrument Information					
Albumin	10%	10.00	2.36	2.4	0.04	1.7	0.6	13.9	1:3s N = 2
Alkaline phosphatase	0.3	30.00	120.7	115.2	5.50	4.8	1.8	14.0	1:3s N = 2
ALT	0.2	20.00	104.4	110	5.60	5.1	1.3	11.5	1:3s N = 2
Amylase	30%	30.00	161.5	160	1.50	0.9	1.4	20.8	1:3s N = 2
AST	0.2	20.00	95.4	98	2.60	2.7	2.4	7.2	1:3s N = 2
Bilirubin, direct	0.4 mg/dL or 20%	44.44	0.75	0.9	0.15	16.7	3.5	7.9	1:3s N = 2
Bilirubin, total	0.4 mg/dL or 20%	20.00	4.13	4.2	0.07	1.7	3.5	5.3	1:3s/2:2s/R:4s N = 2
Calcium	1 mg/dL	8.08	12.354	12.37	0.02	0.1	0.7	11.4	1:3s N = 2
Chloride	0.05	5.00	101.3	101	0.30	0.3	0.6	7.8	1:3s N = 2
Cholesterol	10%	10.00	175.695	174	1.69	1.0	0.5	18.1	1:3s N = 2
CO_2	±3 SD	25.00	25.8	28	2.20	7.9	6.2	2.8	MAX QC: CONSIDER METHOD IMPROVEMENTS
CK	30%	30.00	245.1	255	9.90	3.9	1.1	23.7	1:3s N = 2
Creatinine	0.3 mg/dL or 15%	30.30	0.971	0.99	0.02	1.9	1.6	17.7	1:3s N = 2
GGT	±3 SD	22.00	102.2	95.5	6.70	7.0	4.0	3.7	1:3s/2:2s/R:4s/4:1s/8:x N = 4
Glucose	6 mg/dL or 10%	10.00	142.83	136.4	6.43	4.7	1.1	4.8	1:3s/2:2s/R:4s/4:1s N = 4
HDL	30%	30.00	60.007	57.2	2.81	4.9	1.3	19.3	1:3s N = 2

(continued on next page)

Table 1
(continued)

Test	TEa Source	TEa	Group or Peer Mean (CAP PT)	BI Result (CAP PT)	Bias Units	Bias (%)	CV	Sigma	QC Rules Recommendation
				Instrument Information					
Iron	20%	20.00	73.8	71	2.80	3.9	1.4	11.6	1:3s N = 2
LDL	0.3	30.00	90.632	85.8	4.83	5.6	2.0	12.2	1:3s N = 2
LDH	20%	20.00	195.3	201	5.70	2.8	2.3	7.5	1:3s N = 2
Lipase	30%	30.00	48.6	47	1.60	3.4	2.5	10.6	1:3s N = 2
Magnesium	25%	25.00	2.458	2.38	0.08	3.3	2.2	9.9	1:3s N = 2
Phosphorous	0.3 mg/dL or 10.7%	10.70	4.513	4.48	0.03	0.7	0.6	16.6	1:3s N = 2
Potassium	0.5 mmol/L	15.15	3.22	3.3	0.08	2.4	1.7	7.5	1:3s N = 2
Protein, total	10%	10.00	4.9	4.8	0.10	2.1	1.7	4.7	1:3s/2:2s/R:4s/4:1s N = 4
Sodium	4 mmol/L	3.17	126.1	126	0.10	0.1	0.6	5.2	1:3s/2:2s/R:4s N = 2
Triglycerides	25%	10.00	117.704	115.7	2.00	1.7	1.2	6.9	1:3s N = 2
Urea nitrogen	2.0 mg/dL or 9%	9.00	27.78	27.6	0.18	0.7	1.5	5.6	1:3s/2:2s/R:4s N = 2
Uric acid	0.17	17.00	2.58	2.5	0.08	3.2	1.0	13.8	1:3s N = 2

Sigmas at critical medical values are indicated by italic. Bias was calculated as the difference between an assayed/target mean and observed mean, or difference between PT/peer mean and observed mean.

Abbreviations: ALT, alanine transaminase; AST, aspartate transaminase; CK, creatinine kinase; GGT, gamma-glutamyl transferase; HDL, high-density lipoprotein; LDH, lactate dehydrogenase; LDL, low-density lipoprotein; PT, proficiency testing.

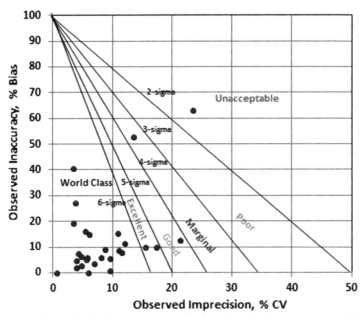

Fig. 2. Sigma values of 28 chemistry assays during the fourth quarter (Q4, October to December) of 2014 show there were 23 assays (82.1%) with performance equal or better than 6-sigma level, 2 assays (7.1%) had 5-sigma to 6-sigma level, 1 assay (3.6%) had 4-sigma to 5-sigma level, 1 assay (3.6%) had 3-sigma to 4-sigma level, and 1 assay (3.6%) had lower than 3-sigma level.

The apparent deterioration in performance for total bilirubin and CO_2 were also noticed. For bilirubin, analyte photosensitivity should be monitored by medical technologists. All staff members should also be trained to handle labile analytes appropriately. Other contributing factors included putative preanalytical issues such as delays in delivery of PT samples from the customs service, which is a complicated process. With stable analytes, there should be no effect; however, with labile analytes such as CO_2 and bilirubin, degradation could occur. Although our %CV for total bilirubin and CO_2 were improved in Q4, percentage bias was higher than in Q3 (see **Tables 1** and **2**). The stability of labile analytes such as bilirubin, electrolytes, and CO_2 could also be affected by transportation and environmental factors. Moreover, the labile analytes such as CO_2 highlighted operational practices for improvement, such as closing machine covers and acclimatizing new reagents to room temperature for 30 minutes before loading into instruments. After identifying the best practices to mitigate operational risks relating to CO_2, our laboratory CAP performance in January 2015 showed that our percentage bias was 0 at the medical decision level (25 mmol/L, see **Table 3**) and sigma was 4.2.

In addition, the instrument's ion-selective electrode module is designed for an operational life of 20,000 tests or 3 months usage. End-of-life performance deterioration may thus have an impact on the QC data used for SVP certification, so we have implemented replacement of this module every 3 months.

Lesson learn from sigma verification program
Our laboratory found participation in the SVP aided the laboratory in understanding its specific analytical quality performance. It allowed us to target weaker assays and

Table 2
Sigma-metric worksheet during Q4, 2014 for core chemistry analytes running controls as recommended

Test	TEa Source	TEa	Group or Peer Mean (CAP PT)	BI Result (CAP PT)	Bias Units	% Bias	CV	Sigma	QC Rules Recommendation
Albumin	0.1	10.00	2.7	2.7	0.00	0.0	0.6	16.7	1:3s N = 2
Alkaline phosphatase	0.3	30.00	146.9	143	3.90	2.7	2.6	10.4	1:3s N = 2
ALT	0.2	20.00	88	87	1.00	1.1	1.6	11.6	1:3s N = 2
Amylase	30%	30.00	147.1	145	2.10	1.4	1.2	23.8	1:3s N = 2
AST	0.2	20.00	64.3	70	5.70	8.1	0.7	16.9	1:3s N = 2
Bilirubin, direct	0.4 mg/dL or 20%	400.00	0.1	0.1	0.00	0.0	2.2	181.8	1:3s N = 2
Bilirubin, total	0.4 mg/dL or 20%	20.00	3.04	3.4	0.36	10.6	2.7	3.5	1:3s/2:2s/R:4s/4:1s/8:x N = 4
Calcium	1 mg/dL	12.64	7.859	7.91	0.05	0.6	0.7	16.9	1:3s N = 2
Chloride	0.05	5.00	102.5	103	0.50	0.5	0.9	5.2	1:3s/2:2s/R:4s N = 2
Cholesterol	0.1	10.00	162.302	159.9	2.40	1.5	0.6	13.9	1:3s N = 2
CO_2	±3 SD	25.00	22	19	3.00	15.8	5.9	1.6	MAX QC: CONSIDER METHOD CHANGE
CK	30%	30.00	218.2	220	1.80	0.8	1.4	20.7	1:3s N = 2
Creatinine	0.3 mg/dL or 15%	15.00	2.544	2.62	0.08	2.9	0.5	23.3	1:3s N = 2
GGT	±3 SD	22.00	84.8	80.0	4.80	6.0	0.8	19.5	1:3s N = 2
Glucose	6 mg/dL or 10%	10.00	116.79	118.6	1.81	1.5	1.1	7.8	1:3s N = 2

Analyte									Control Rules
HDL	0.3	30.00	60.414	59.1	1.31	2.2	1.3	*21.4*	1:3s N = 2
Iron	0.2	20.00	75.5	75	0.50	0.7	1.4	*13.9*	1:3s N = 2
LDL	30%	30.00	78.161	76.8	1.36	1.8	1.7	*16.4*	1:3s N = 2
LDH	0.2	20.00	194.6	198	3.40	1.7	2.2	*8.3*	1:3s N = 2
Lipase	30%	30.00	45.1	45	0.10	0.2	2.9	*10.4*	1:3s N = 2
Magnesium	25%	25.00	2.767	2.69	0.08	2.9	3.0	*7.3*	1:3s N = 2
Phosphorous	0.3 mg/dL or 10.7%	10.70	3.983	3.95	0.03	0.8	1.2	*8.0*	1:3s N = 2
Potassium	0.5 mmol/L	22.73	2.19	2.2	0.01	0.5	0.9	*25.0*	1:3s N = 2
Protein, total	10%	10.00	4.37	4.3	0.07	1.6	0.5	*15.5*	1:3s N = 2
Sodium	4 mmol/L	3.28	121.5	122	0.50	0.4	0.7	*4.1*	1:3s/2:2s/R:4s/4:1s N = 4
Triglycerides	25%	10.00	126.412	125.7	0.71	0.6	1.0	*9.9*	1:3s N = 2
Urea Nitrogen	2.0 mg/dL or 9%	9.00	40.76	40.4	0.36	0.9	1.4	*5.8*	1:3s/2:2s/R:4s N = 2
Uric Acid	17%	17.00	4.65	4.6	0.05	1.1	0.8	*19.4*	1:3s N = 2

Sigmas at critical medical values are indicated by italic. Bias was calculated as the difference between an assayed/target mean and observed mean, or difference between PT/peer mean and observed mean.

Table 3

Tests with recommended medical decision levels. CAP Tolerance limits are used to calculate Sigma and analytical performances are presented as quarter period: Q3 for July to September and Q4 for October to December 2014

Test	CAP Tolerance Limit TEa	Recommended Medical Decision Level	Sigma Values July-September (Q3), 2014	Sigma Values October-December (Q4), 2014	Difference Between Q3 and Q4, 2014	Remark
Albumin	10%	Near 2.5 g/dL	13.9	16.7	2.8	≥6-sigma
Alkaline phosphatase	30%	Near 150 U/L	14.0	10.4	−3.6	≥6-sigma
ALT	20%	Near 95 U/L	11.5	11.6	0.1	≥6-sigma
Amylase	30%	Near 145 U/L	20.8	23.8	3.0	≥6-sigma
AST	20%	Near 40 U/L	7.2	16.9	9.7	≥6-sigma
Bilirubin, direct	0.4 mg/dL or 20%	Near 0.3 mg/dL	7.9	181.8	173.9	≥6-sigma
Bilirubin, total	0.4 mg/dL or 20%	Near 3.0 mg/dL	5.3	3.5	−1.8	Investigation is needed
Calcium	1 mg/dL	Near 13.0 mg/dL	11.4	16.9	5.5	≥6-sigma
Chloride	5%	Near 100 mmol/L	7.8	5.2	−2.6	Investigation is needed
Cholesterol	10%	Near 180 mg/dL	18.1	13.9	−4.2	≥6-sigma
CO_2	±3 SD	Near 25 mmol/L	2.8	1.6	−1.2	Investigation is needed
CK	30%	Near 275 U/L	23.7	20.7	−3.0	≥6-sigma
Creatinine	0.3 mg/dL or 15%	Near 2.0 mg/dL	17.7	23.3	5.6	≥6-sigma
GGT	±3 SD	Near 85 U/L	3.7	19.5	15.8	World-class performance
Glucose	6 mg/dL or 10%	Near 120 mg/dL	4.8	7.8	3.0	World-class performance

HDL	30%	Near 50 mg/dL	19.3	21.4	2.1	≥6-sigma
Iron	20%	Near 75 mg/dL	11.6	13.9	2.3	≥6-sigma
LDL	30%	Near 100 mg/dL	12.2	16.4	4.2	≥6-sigma
LDH	20%	Near 170 U/L	7.5	8.3	0.8	≥6-sigma
Lipase	30%	Near 45 U/L	10.6	10.4	-0.2	≥6-sigma
Magnesium	25%	Near 2.5 mg/dL	9.9	7.3	-2.6	≥6-sigma
Phosphorus	0.3 mg/dL or 10.7%	Near 4.0 mg/dL	16.6	8.0	-8.6	≥6-sigma
Potassium	0.5 mmol/L	Near 2.5 mmol/L	7.5	25.0	17.5	≥6-sigma
Protein, total	10%	Near 5.7 g/dL	4.7	15.5	10.8	World-class performance
Sodium	4 mmol/L	Near 115 mmol/L	5.2	4.1	-1.1	Investigation is needed
Triglycerides	25%	Near 130 mg/dL	6.9	9.9	3.0	≥6-sigma
Urea nitrogen	2.0 mg/dL or 9%	Near 40 mg/dL	5.6	5.8	0.2	Excellent performance
Uric acid	17%	Near 3.3 mg/dL	13.8	19.4	5.6	≥6-sigma

develop a coherent plan for CQI. The sigma metrics provided a convenient way to compare the quality required for intended use with the precision and bias observed in the laboratory, and also provided guidance for selecting appropriate SQC (see **Tables 1** and **2**) to monitor performance. In addition, the selection of appropriate TEa limits had a significant impact on the comparison of performance between laboratories.[31] One important lesson learned from the SVP is that quality means not just performing and passing QC but providing the best quality performance for patients' safety.

The pros and cons of implementation of SVP were analyzed (**Table 4**). The biggest disadvantage of SVP is the additional resources required and the advantage is the amount of quality improvement. It is said that quality costs, but poor quality costs more, thus if the laboratory's main aim is patient safety, improvement of laboratory quality should be a priority. In the near future we plan to integrate sigma metrics across the total testing process as a part of our IQCP.

A further step beyond sigma verification program

For CQI, we took a step beyond SVP by expanding sigma metrics to include 43 clinical chemistry and 25 immunoassay tests.[32] Most of our assays, both chemistry and immunoassay, were between 3-sigma and 6-sigma. Approximately 87.0% of chemistry tests were greater than or equal to 4-sigma, whereas only about 48.0% of immunoassays were greater than or equal to 4-sigma (**Table 5**). About 74.5% of chemistry and 20.0% immunoassay tests were greater than or equal to 6-sigma. Fewer than 4.2% of chemistry and 20.0% of immunoassay tests were less than 3-sigma. The OPSpec (operating specification) charts showing the performance of 47 clinical chemistry and 25 immunoassay tests are presented in **Figs. 3** and **4**. No assays were less than 2-sigma or unacceptable. Although this is good, better performance is required. We compared some of our results with previous studies[7,9] and they were better than those reported in the literature, possibly because of the improvement of current technology and reagents. In addition, the tolerance limits of CAP are continuously adjusted to make them conform to the updated technology.

Sigma values of potassium, chloride, and sodium in urine were 39.6, 31.5, and 25.6 respectively, which were much better than in serum (9.6, 5.0, and 3.2, respectively). This finding could be explained by the differences in TEa for these tests: the urine assays have larger TEa values than the same tests in serum (TEa for potassium, chloride, and sodium in urine were ±29%, ±26%, and ±26%, respectively, whereas in serum they were ±0.5 mmol/L or 13.4%, ±5%, and ±4.0 mmol/L or 2.9%, respectively.) Other urine tests, such as albumin, creatinine, glucose, protein, and uric acid, have higher TEa targets than the same tests in serum; however, the sigma values of these tests are not significantly different (see **Fig. 3**).

Table 4	
Pros and cons WSVP	
Pros	**Cons**
Perceive laboratory analytical performance as presented in sigma scores	Add WSVP work into the daily services
Stimulate the CQI of quality performance in analytical process	Add WSVP cost into the laboratory budget
Gain improvement of personal competency and confidence	Need FTE (full-time equivalent) to perform WSVP

Table 5
The distribution of sigma metrics of performance of 43 clinical chemistry and 28 immunoassay tests are presented

Sigma Level	Chemistry		Immunology	
	Number	Percentage	Number	Percentage
≥6-sigma	35	74.5	5	20.0
≥5-sigma to ≤6-sigma	2	4.25	0	0.0
≥4-sigma to ≤5-sigma	4	8.5	7	28.0
≥3-sigma to ≤4-sigma	4	8.5	8	32.0
≥2-sigma to ≤3-sigma	2	4.25	5	20.0
Total tests	47	100.0	25	100.0

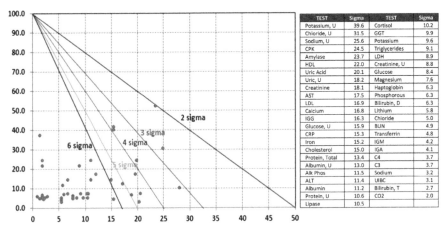

Fig. 3. The distribution of sigma metrics performance of 47 chemistry tests using normalized method decision chart. Approximately 87.0% of tests are at higher than 4-sigma. IGA, immunoglobulin A; IGM, immunoglobulin M.

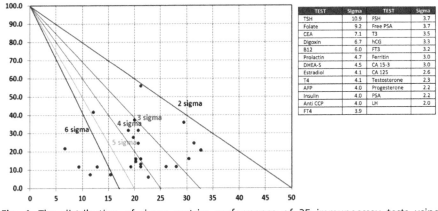

Fig. 4. The distribution of sigma metrics performance of 25 immunoassay tests using normalized OPSpec chart. Around 48.0% of tests are at higher than 4-sigma.

Sigma Metrics in the Extra-analytical Phases

The sigma values of processes such as errors in requests, errors in specimen collection, inappropriate specimens, and reporting error were estimated and normalized in terms of DPM. The calculated DPM values were converted to the sigma scale using the standard sigma table (**Table 6**).[17] In addition to these extra-analytical phases, process errors in the analytical phase, such as IQC out and unacceptable PT, were included. The 1.5 S shift is generally acceptable for the presence of short-term process variation. DPM with 1.5 S shift was chosen for this study.[33] The sigma values for preanalytical, analytical, and postanalytical processes are presented in **Table 7**. Laboratory processes (see **Table 7**) were more than 4-sigma. Only IQC failures for chemistry, immunoassay, and report delay were lower than 4-sigma, at 3.2-sigma, 3.3-sigma, and 3.1-sigma respectively.

A study on sigma assessment in clinical laboratories analyzed the performance of common laboratory processes and found that most laboratory processes were between 3-sigma and 6-sigma.[9] Most of our performances were between 3-sigma and 6-sigma as well. However, our performances were better; for example, the order or request errors of the previous study showed 3.6 sigma,[9] compared with our performance of 4.5-sigma (see **Table 7**). Our PT was also better at 4.3-sigma for chemistry tests and 4.0-sigma for immunoassays compared with 3.9-sigma (chemistry combined with immunology) of the previous study.[9] For reporting errors, our performance for report delay was 3.1-sigma, keying in wrong data was 6.3-sigma, and error from the LIS was 4.6-sigma compared with reporting errors of 4.8-sigma in the previous study.[9] More details of our process performances in DPM are shown in **Table 7**.

From another study,[34] we found that the sigma values were similar: error in test request was 3.4-sigma compared with our performance of 4.5-sigma (see **Table 7**), error in sample volume was 4.4-sigma to 5.0-sigma compared with our 4.2-sigma, clotted sample was 4.3-sigma to 5.0-sigma compared with 4.7-sigma, hemolysis sample was 4.1-sigma compared with 4.4-sigma, error in handling was 5.0-sigma compared with 6.1-sigma, unacceptable PT was 3.4-sigma compared with 4.0-sigma to 4.3-sigma, and delay in result report was 2.8-sigma to 4.1-sigma compared with 3.1-sigma.

These results not only inform us of the quality of our services but also provide data for improvement priority. The sigma metrics reported here also reflect assay

| Table 6 | | |
| Standard sigma table used for converting defects per million to sigma value | | |
Sigma Metric	DPM Without Shift	DPM with 1.5 S Shift
1.0	317,311	697,672
1.5	133,614	501,350
2.0	45,500	308,770
2.5	12,419	158,687
3.0	2700	66,811
3.5	465	22,750
4.0	63.3	6210
4.5	6.8	1350
5.0	0.57	233
5.5	0.038	32
6.0	0.002	3.4

Table 7
Preanalytical, analytical, and postanalytical errors

Items	% Error	DPM	Sigma Level	σ Nevalainen et al,[8] 2000	σ Llopis et al,[34] 2011
I. Preanalytical process	0.13	7662	4.5	—	—
1. Request errors	0.17	1700	4.5	3.6	3.4
2. Sample: collection errors	0.00	2	6.1	—	—
3. Sample: inappropriate volume	0.37	3676	4.2	—	4.4–5.0
4. Sample: clotted	0.06	634	4.7	—	4.3–5.0
5. Sample: hemolysis, turbid, icteric	0.16	1648	4.4	—	4.1
6. Handling errors	0.00	2	6.1	—	5.0
II. Analytical process	2.12	21,260	3.5	—	—
1. IQC out: chemistry	4.05	40,470	3.2	—	—
2. IQC out: immunology	3.43	34,297	3.3	—	—
3. PT unacceptable: chemistry	0.29	2934	4.3	3.9	3.4
4. PT unacceptable: immunology	0.73	7337	4.0		
III. Postanalytical process	1.78	17,775	3.6	—	—
1. Report: delay	5.21	52,125	3.1	4.8	2.8–4.1
2. Report: errors from key in results	0.00	1	6.3	—	
3. Report: LIS problem	0.12	1200	4.6		—
Average of total laboratory process	1.12	11,233	3.8	—	—

Abbreviation: LIS, Laboratory Information System.
Data from Nevalainen D, Berte L, Kraft C, et al. Evaluating laboratory performance on quality indicators with six sigma scale. Arch Pathol Lab Med 2000;124:516–9; and Llopis MA, Trujillo G, Llovet MI, et al. Quality indicators and specifications for key analytical-extranalytical processes in the clinical laboratory. Five years' experience using the Six Sigma concept. Clin Chem Lab Med 2011;49(3):463–70.

performance at the time the data were collected and thus represent a moment or snapshot in time. Performance, in general, can change over time for a variety of reasons (eg, reagent lot-to-lot variation, equipment condition, new personal). Periodic calculation of sigma metrics is appropriate to determine whether assay quality has been maintained, has decreased, or has improved. The sigma metrics thus represent another quality assurance tool that should be monitored periodically to assess changes in assay quality.

Sigma Services Across the Entire Laboratory Process

Sigma concept

Attainment of 6-sigma is envisaged as the gold standard for world-class quality. Although sigma metrics allow comparison of different processes with each other, across different institutions and with different industries, in health care the sigma performance of common processes is less well known. The 6-sigma concept concentrates on regulating a process to 6 standard deviations (SD), which represents 3.4 DPM opportunities (see **Table 6**).[35] World-class quality is generally recognized as a

6-sigma process. Average services or products, regardless of their complexity, have a quality performance value of about 4-sigma. The minimum performance needed for a process to be considered for routine operation is usually set at 3-sigma.[8,17] A higher sigma metric means fewer analytical errors and fewer questionable test results are accepted and reported, and fewer acceptable test results are falsely rejected and not reported. In addition, all assays with performance greater than 6-sigma can implement a similar QC procedure (typically wider control limits, fewer rules, and fewer control materials are needed).

With this concept, the area under the 6-sigma line in a method decision chart or 6-sigma region is considered world class; excellent, good, marginal poor, and unacceptable are applied for 5-sigma, 4-sigma, 3-sigma, and 2-sigma regions (**Table 8**), respectively.[17,19] The 6-sigma idea asserts an association between the numbers of product defects, wasted operating costs, and levels of customer satisfaction. It can be inferred that, as sigma increases, the consistency and steadiness of the test improves, thereby reducing the operating costs.[26] The goal of 6-sigma, in its simplest distillation, is to eliminate or reduce all variation in a process. Variation in a process leads to wasted effort and resources; for example, on retesting and workarounds. Reducing defects reduces costs, and improves performance and profitability. A process that achieves the goal of 6-sigma delivers both quality and efficiency. Those services that achieved less than 6-sigma still have room for improvement.

Sigma metrics in all laboratory phases
The errors occurred in the preanalytical, analytical, and postanalytical phases are 62%, 15%, and 23% respectively. However, our study showed that most activities in the extra-analytical phase are greater than 4-sigma, and only result report delay in the postanalytical phase was less than 4-sigma. Errors of IQC out failures and unacceptable PT in the analytical phase are around 3-sigma to 4-sigma, with IQC failures at less than 4-sigma. The information showed that the error in the analytical phase is still a challenge for laboratory quality. The errors in the analytical phase may be higher than we have perceived. More studies and investigations in total laboratory process are required. In addition, good information collection system support by information technology is necessary for convenience and complete data collection for analysis. Software for quality work in the laboratory is necessary to address these increasing demands.

There are several activities in the laboratory that involve different phases, personnel, types of errors, and so forth, and high-quality performance in every activity is necessary. A QC program that is only good enough to be compliant is not sufficient for CQI. Risk

Table 8 Description of criteria for each sigma level	
Sigma Level	**Criteria of Performances**
<2-sigma	Unacceptable, not valid as routine measuring procedure
≥2-sigma to <3-sigma	Poor, a quality improvement scheme must be applied
≥3-sigma to <4-sigma	Moderate, it needs a QC procedure with more than 1 analytical run (R), and multiple measurements per run (N)
≥4-sigma to <5-sigma	Good, the clinical utility of results is ensured by multiple rules
≥5-sigma to <6-sigma	Very good or excellent, the clinical utility of the results is ensured by single rule
≥6-sigma	World class

management and error reduction close to zero defects for patients' safety are the goals of current health care services. It is obvious that the integration of sigma metrics into laboratory work provides information and direction for laboratories performing CQI.

Sigma Metrics in Clinical Laboratory at Glance

Sigma and continuous quality improvement

These findings provide important information about performance and can be used for CQI. The appropriate rules can also be planned and selected to control and monitor analytical tests in a more cost-effective fashion. Because our laboratory participates in the CAP PT program, the TEa values used in our study were obtained from CAP. Our results are consistent because of different sources of TEa. In addition, though bias is usually difficult to estimate realistically, our approach is to estimate our performance biases as the difference between our PT results and mean values from peer groups of CAP PT participants. Therefore, the observed bias is only relative instead of absolute. Our precisions are based on a typical 20-day performance of IQC. For further management, we considered an even more robust precision estimate to be made from long-term QC data; for example, over a 6-month or 1-year period. Although it is expected that a long-term data estimate would result in a larger %CV, which can provide greater variability over a longer time period, %CV is more typical of long-term analytical performance variation. Using precision calculated over a shorter period of time could result in a more optimistic estimate and in a higher sigma metric.

Sigma metrics between chemistry and immunology

From the data, these analytical sigma metric findings suggested that chemistry methods are more robust than immunoassays. In addition, although it seemed that immunoassay performance is just a little lower than that of chemistry (see **Table 5**), the TEa provided for immunoassays are much wider than the TEa provided for chemistry. Thus these sigma metrics may give unwarranted assurance for immunoassay performance. There is still ample room for improvement for immunoassays.

One important thing that all laboratorians should keep in mind is the importance of TEa.[12] The TEa is intended to be an estimate of the quality of a measurement procedure; its practical value depends on a comparison with the quality required for the intended use of a test result. The definition refers to the amount of error that is allowable without invalidating the interpretation of a test result. Most laboratories are comfortable applying TEa from their PT providers or even CLIA. The best TEa to meet patients' need is a TEa calculated from clinical decision making.[36] However, TEa calculated from clinical decision making is still too subjective, does not comply with current laboratory practice, and is hard to achieve effectively with the current technology. One example of a TEa that meets the requirement is the TEa for hemoglobin A1c (Hb A1c). The TEa of 6% for Hb A1c does not come from the peer group or technology performance, but it from standardization and a target from a limit of 6% error accepted by clinicians.[37]

Sigma metrics between laboratory and manufacturer

Those tests or methods less than 3-sigma are analyzed for internal processes improvement as well as becoming issues for discussion with manufacturers as having room for improvement, such as bilirubin and bicarbonate for chemistry and cancer antigen 125, testosterone, progesterone, prostate-specific antigen, and luteinizing hormone for immunology.

Laboratory service is now essential for patients' care and safety; thus the best performance service is necessary. Laboratories should be responsible for driving the improvements in QC and voicing the need for better quality technology as one of their requirements from manufacturers and suppliers. Performance limitation from production can be identified for the manufacturers so they can improve their products. In addition, laboratories frequently assume that simply following the manufacturer's directions is enough to ensure the quality of the tests, but this is not true because there is always room for manufacturers to improve.

Sigma Metrics and Individualized Quality Control Plan

From January 1, 2016, all laboratories in the United States performing nonwaived testing are required to (1) follow the default QC as required by the CLIAs of 1988, using 2 levels of external QC each day of testing or other specified frequency; or (2) implement an IQCP in order to monitor the accuracy and precision of the complete testing process.

IQCP is the new concept of doing QC by offering laboratory flexibility to meet QC requirements appropriate for a unique testing environment and patients. IQCP is voluntary and can be applied to all nonwaived testing, including existing and new test systems. All CLIA specialties and subspecialties except pathology are eligible for IQCP. IQCP considers the entire testing process: preanalytical, analytical, and postanalytical; thus, a laboratory needs to consider the corresponding risks in each of these phases and applicable regulatory requirements. An IQCP has 3 requirements: (1) a risk assessment (RA) evaluation to identify errors or problems in the test process. The results of RA are used to create (2) a customized QC plan and establish (3) a quality assessment program to monitor whether the QC plan ensures accurate test results.

Compared with the current laboratory QC performed worldwide, the scope of an IQCP has a more conclusive approach to ensuring the quality of the entire testing process of preanalytical, analytical, and postanalytical phases. IQCP provides a framework for customizing a QC program for individual test systems and an individual laboratory's unique environment. Thus it is necessary to keep up to date and be familiar with IQCP, because it seems that individualized or personalized medicine will be the trend in all medical fields.

IQCP is an acceptable QC option that provides laboratories with the framework for its implementation, when appropriate, and offers flexibility to design a QC plan that meets the needs of the laboratory. There are no specific forms required when creating an IQCP. A laboratory may develop its own model and form or may adapt models and forms from available resources. Our laboratory plans to integrate the sigma metrics concept to IQCP and starts with IQCP qualified tests. At least 5 areas mentioned by CLIA (specimen, test system, reagent, environment, and personnel)[38] will be risk assessed to create IQCP, then quality assessment will be done to perform CQI for IQCP. Risk analysis can be conducted by failure modes and effect analysis (FMEA).[39] Meanwhile, the sigma concept approach can provide a quantitative estimate of risk as well as performance, which can be easily benchmarked, as already mentioned.[40]

With the use of a type of FMEA called 2-factor models of risk acceptable matrix (ISO [International Standards Organization] 14971), which ranks for severity and probability of occurrence of harm, at least 2 dimensions of harm can be assessed at the same time,[41] whereas the use of sigma metrics can provide information about risk. Thus, combination of sigma metrics with FMEA should provide useful information to the laboratory for quality improvement.

DISCUSSION

The authors found that participation in an SVP helps laboratorians understand the performance of each assay as well as plan for CQI. However, comparing between laboratories, TEa use in the sigma metrics calculation has a major impact on sigma values. In the future, we plan to implement multi-stage SQC designs to ensure quality throughout the analytical run. In addition, although the quantitative measurement of laboratory processes using the sigma scale may be challenging, the authors found that application of sigma concepts to determining DPM is a powerful method to identify targets for improvement in laboratory operational performance. The baseline sigma measurement of laboratory performance represents the basis for our laboratory's drive to achieve higher quality goals for CQI.

In conclusion, it is possible to estimate and evaluate laboratory performance using DPM and the sigma metric calculation. Although determination and comparison of the quality requirement of a laboratory test is not simple, these quality requirements can be measured as DPM and by the sigma concept to express laboratory performance. Knowledge of the laboratory performance position can be used as a baseline for laboratory improvement. Furthermore, the sigma scale can be applied as a universal benchmark for the comparative evaluation of performance between tests, methods, equipment, and laboratories. In addition, the sigma concept can be applied to achieve high quality, such as when defining quality specifications to design IQCP, which is a difficult task for laboratories and a requirement in current quality standards.

SUMMARY

Quality management in preanalytical, analytical, and postanalytical processes in laboratory services are still the great challenge for laboratory quality management. Expectations of current QC should not only be about analytical methods or process but should extend to cover all laboratory processes. The number of errors that occur during laboratory processes are easily estimated by the method of estimating defects per million and analytical performance can be calculated by the sigma metric equation.

The sigma value not only shows the performance of an individual activity; it also provides the universal benchmark for continuous improvement of laboratories. It represents understandable quality data for communication with physicians, patients, and customers, and useful feedback information to manufacturers about their products' performance. Risk management is increasing in health care and requires new tools and techniques for integration, but there has never been a single tool that is able to eliminate all errors or risks in laboratories, thus an appropriate combination of tools, such as FMEA, fishbone, sigma metrics, is required.

ACKNOWLEDGMENTS

I would like to express my deepest appreciation to the Medical Director/CEO, Num Tanthuwanit, MD, and the executive administrative team for their support with all necessary resources to complete these activities.

Other acknowledgments include my deep gratitude to all the laboratory staff members for their excellent work. My sincere thanks to Cherrie Yee Sithichaisawad, MD, for assisting with the English. My special thanks to Abbott Laboratories Limited, Thailand, for all the kind cooperation and support provided.

REFERENCES

1. Shewhart WA. Economic control of quality of manufactured product. New York: D Van Nostrand Company; 1931.

2. Levey S, Jennings ER. The use of control charts in the clinical laboratory. J Clin Pathol 1950;20:1059–66.
3. Westgard JO. QC past, present and future. Available at: https://www.westgard.com/history-and-future-of-qc.htm, Accessed April 15, 2016.
4. Westgard JO, Groth T, Aronsson T, et al. Performance characteristics of rules for internal quality control: probabilities for false rejection and error detection. Clin Chem 1977;23:1857–67.
5. Westgard JO, Barry PL, Hunt MR, et al. A multi-rule Shewhart chart for quality control in clinical chemistry. Clin Chem 1981;27:493–501.
6. Westgard JO. Six sigma quality design & control: desirable precision and requisite QC for laboratory measurement processes. Madison (WI): Westgard QC; 2001.
7. Westgard JO, Westgard S. The quality of laboratory testing today: an assessment of σ metrics for analytic quality using performance data from proficiency testing surveys and the CLIA criteria for acceptable performance. Am J Clin Pathol 2006; 125:343–54.
8. Nevalainen D, Berte L, Kraft C, et al. Evaluating laboratory performance on quality indicators with six sigma scale. Arch Pathol Lab Med 2000;124:516–9.
9. Singh B, Goswami B, Gupta VK, et al. Application of sigma metrics for the assessment of quality assurance in clinical biochemistry laboratory in India: a pilot study. Indian J Clin Biochem 2011;26(2):131–5.
10. Bonini P, Plebani M, Ceriotti F, et al. Errors in laboratory medicine. Clin Chem 2002;48:691–8.
11. Carraro P, Plebani M. Errors in a stat laboratory: types and frequencies 10 years later. Clin Chem 2007;53:1338–42.
12. Westgard JO, Carey RN, Wold S. Criteria for judging precision and accuracy in method development and evaluation. Clin Chem 1974;20:825–33.
13. Westgard JO, Seehafer JJ, Barry PL. Allowable imprecision for laboratory tests based on clinical and analytical test outcome criteria. Clin Chem 1994;40:1909–14.
14. Chinchilli VM, Miller WG. Evaluating test methods by estimating total error. Clin Chem 1994;40:464–71.
15. Westgard JO. Charts of operational process specifications ("OPSpecs charts") for assessing the precision, accuracy, and quality control needed to satisfy proficiency testing performance criteria. Clin Chem 1992;38:1226–33.
16. Lasky FD, Boser RB. Designing in quality through design control: a manufacturer's perspective. Clin Chem 1997;43:866–72.
17. Westgard JO. Six sigma quality design and control. 2nd edition. Madison (WI): Westgard QC; 2006.
18. Westgard JO. Six sigma risk analysis; designing analytical QC plans for medical laboratory. Madison (WI): Westgard QC; 2011.
19. Westgard JO, Westgard SA. Basic quality management systems: essentials for quality management in the medical laboratory. Madison (WI): Westgard QC; 2014.
20. Laposata M, Dighe A. "Pre-pre" and "post-post" analytical error: high-incidence patient safety hazards involving the clinical laboratory. Clin Chem Lab Med 2007;45:712–9.
21. CLSI. Laboratory quality control based on risk management; approved guideline. CLSI document EP23-A™. Wayne (PA): Clinical and Laboratory Standards Institute; 2011.
22. CMS memorandum: implementing the individualized quality control plan (IQCP) for Clinical Laboratory Improvement Amendments (CLIA); 2012. Available at: https://www.cms.gov/Medicare/Provider-Enrollment-and-Certification/SurveyCertification GenInfo/Downloads/SCLetter12_20-.pdf. Accessed November 11, 2016.

23. Plebani M. The CCLM contribution to improvements in quality and patient safety. Clin Chem Lab Med 2013;51:39–46.
24. Coskun A. Six sigma and calculated laboratory tests. Clin Chem 2006;52:770–1.
25. Tetrault G. Evaluating laboratory performance with the six sigma scale. Arch Pathol Lab Med 2000;124(12):1748–9.
26. Westgard JO. Quality control. How labs can apply six sigma principles to quality control planning. Clin Lab News 2006;32:10–2.
27. Sigma verification for examination procedures in medical laboratories. Madison (WI): Westgard QC; 2014.
28. Charuruks N, Thanudpasa S, Kedsomboon P, et al. Westgard Sigma Verification Program, as a tool to improve laboratory performance. Poster Number B-169, Poster presentation at the 2015 AACC Annual Meeting. Atlanta, GA, July 26–30, 2015.
29. Charuruks N. Implementation of Westgard Sigma Verification Program. Oral Presentation, the 8th Annual Asia Pacific & Japan Scientific Symposium: turning science into caring. Bali, Indonesia, December 1–3, 2015.
30. Clinical Chemistry ARCHITECT GAMMA GULTAMYL TRANSFERASE Ref 7D65, 304645/R02, reagent package insert for ARTHITECT c systems. Abbott Park (IL): Abbott Laboratories; 2012.
31. Hens K, Berth M, Armbruster D, et al. Sigma metrics used to assess analytical quality of clinical chemistry assays: importance of the allowable total error (TEa) target. Clin Chem Lab Med 2014;52(7):973–80.
32. Charuruks N, Thanudpasa S, Kedsomboon P, et al. Six sigma clinical laboratory services at Bumrungrad International Hospital, Thailand. Poster Code W109, Poster presentation at the IFCC-EFLM Euro Med Lab Paris 2015 Congress. Paris, June 21–25, 2015.
33. Kubiak TM. Perusing process performance metrics selecting the right measures for managing processes. Available at: http://asq.org/quality-progress/2009/08/34-per-million/perusing-process-performance-metrics.html. Accessed December 24, 2014.
34. Llopis MA, Trujillo G, Llovet MI, et al. Quality indicators and specifications for key analytical-extranalytical processes in the clinical laboratory. Five years' experience using the Six Sigma concept. Clin Chem Lab Med 2011;49(3):463–70.
35. Revere L, Black K. Integrating Six Sigma with total quality management; a case example for measuring medication errors. J Healthc Manag 2003;48:377–91.
36. Fraser CG. General strategies to set quality specifications for reliability performance characteristics. Scand J Clin Lab Invest 1999;59:487–90.
37. Woodworth A, Korpi-Steiner N, Miller JJ, et al. Utilization of assay performance characteristics to estimate hemoglobin A1c result reliability. Clin Chem 2014;60(8):1073–9.
38. CLIA Brochure #13 CLIA Individualized Quality Control Plan. What is an IQCP? November 2014. Available at: https://www.cms.gov/Regulations-and-Guidance/Legislation/CLIA/Downloads/CLIAbrochure13.pdf. Accessed November 11, 2016.
39. McDermott RE, Mikulak RJ, Beauregard MR. The basics of FMEA. 2nd edition. New York: CRC Press; 2009.
40. Westgard S. Prioritizing risk analysis quality control plans based on sigma metrics [In: Westgard JO, Westgard S. Ed., Clinics in laboratory medicine: quality control in the age of risk management]. Clin Lab Med 2013;33(1):41–53.
41. Westgard JO. Perspectives on quality control, risk management, and analytical quality management. Clin Lab Med 2013;33(1):1–14.

Metrological Traceability of Assays and Comparability of Patient Test Results

David Armbruster, PhD, DABCC

KEYWORDS

- Metrology • Traceability • Standardization • Harmonization • Comparability

KEY POINTS

- As of 2003, metrological traceability of assay calibrators has been a regulatory requirement and necessary to ensure accuracy and comparability of patient test results.
- Calibrator traceability and comparability of test results from different assays are necessary for the use of electronic health records and optimal patient care.
- Calibrator traceability is one significant aspect of the standardization of clinical laboratory practice, which includes standardization of other facets, including reporting units, test nomenclature, and evidence-based laboratory medicine guidelines.

INTRODUCTION

The clinical laboratory field is experiencing globalization. Laboratory practice is moving toward harmonization and the ability to produce comparable patient test results. Greenberg observed, "An increasingly important objective in laboratory medicine is ensuring the equivalency of test results among different measurement procedures, different laboratories and health care systems, over time."[1,2] Metrological traceability is required to provide equivalence of results from diverse analytical systems.[3] Laboratories no longer work in isolation, and harmonization of laboratory testing is far-reaching, including all aspects of the total testing process (TTP).[4] The goal is "Right result, Right patient, Right time, Right form, Right test choice, Right interpretation, and Right advice." Test results must be equivalent to use universal clinical guidelines for disease diagnosis and patient management. Impediments to harmonization include inadequate measurand (analyte) definition, lack of analytical specificity, non-commutability of reference materials, lot-to-lot variability of reference materials and

Conflict of Interest: D. Armbruster is an employee of Abbott Diagnostics.
Clinical Chemistry, Abbott Diagnostics, Department 09AC, Building CP1-5, 100 Abbott Park Road, Abbott Park, IL 60064, USA
E-mail address: david.armbruster@abbott.com

Clin Lab Med 37 (2017) 119–135
http://dx.doi.org/10.1016/j.cll.2016.09.010
0272-2712/17/© 2016 Elsevier Inc. All rights reserved.

labmed.theclinics.com

assay reagents, and a lack of systematic approaches to standardization. These issues affect patient care because physicians fail to understand the limitations of laboratory measurements, including the lack of interchangeability of results from different analytical methods.[5]

Generating comparable results remains a holy grail due to use of multiple assays for the same analyte, potentially causing different clinical interpretations.[5,6] Clinical decision values (cutpoints) are decided by international expert groups without consideration of analytical disparity. Even advances in technology are not always an improvement. As noted by White, "frustration at the lack of significant progress…was captured in the title 'Accuracy in Clinical Chemistry — Does anybody care?', in which Tietz identified that the accuracy of many routine laboratory methods had declined as use of faster, automated methods and instrumentation increased. Since Tietz's *cri de coeur*, there has been significant progress with both the theory and the practice of implementing a coherent reference system for measurements in clinical laboratories."[6] Harmonization was not possible historically due to a lack of established reference materials and methods. Miller and Myers[7] noted, "True and precise routine measurements of quantities of clinical interest are essential if results are to be optimally interpreted for patient care. Additionally, results produced by different measurement procedures for the same measureand must be comparable if common diagnostic decision values and clinical research values are to be broadly applied."

A patient's test history would be consistent if only one laboratory performed all testing (same methodology, analyzer, and so forth), so a significant change in concentration would signal a meaningful clinical change. But patients are increasingly mobile and multiple laboratories may test their samples so results may not be consistently interpreted.[8] Harmonization can produce essentially equivalent results (not quantitatively equal but clinically equivalent) and changes in concentration can be correctly interpreted.[9] Harmonization needs to include nomenclature, units of measurement, and other factors for use of evidence-based clinical practice guidelines.[8,10] Physicians expect results to be interchangeable even though analytes can be measured by multiple methods. Many clinicians do not realize tests performed by one method cannot be reliably compared with those from another method. This lack of comparability creates barriers to sharing laboratory results across health care systems and can have adverse patient consequences.[11] For some analytes, reference materials do not exist or there is a limited supply, and new lots may not be identical to the original material.[10] It is even difficult to know which molecule is actually being measured given structural variability, for example, the various forms of human chorionic gonadotropin (HCG).

Lack of harmonization has real adverse clinical consequences, and prostate-specific antigen (PSA) is a prime example.[6,12–14] An early PSA assay (Hybritech, San Diego, CA) used the manufacturer's calibrator, and the standard 4.0 mg/L PSA cutoff for prostate cancer was established. Other assays use calibrators traceable to World Health Organization (WHO) international reference material (WHO 96/670 and 96/668). A 2004 study of 2304 patients compared PSA results from assays using the Hybritech or the WHO calibrator. Of 288 patients, 55 (19%) exceeded the PSA 4.0-mg/L cutoff based on the Hybritech calibrator result but were not candidates for prostate biopsy by the WHO-calibrated results. In another PSA study, 106 men were tested using both the Hybritech and WHO traceable calibrators and WHO calibrator results were 20% lower. Depending on the assay, some men are candidates for prostate biopsy (a definitely invasive procedure) and others are not. Many clinicians are unaware, however, that different PSA results are produced for the same patient sample if tested by assays using different calibrators, resulting in different clinical interpretation and adverse patient consequences. Lack of comparability is a concern for immunoassays, such as thyroid and fertility hormones and cancer markers. Traceability/standardization of immunoassays is a special problem because internationally accepted clinical protocols and common reference intervals (RIs) depend on it, and "free" hormones and heterogeneous polypeptide hormones are difficult.[15]

Cholesterol is a prime example of successful harmonization. A cholesterol reference measurement system (RMS) was created over approximately 30 years (1970–2000) and produced a major reduction in mortality rates for coronary heart disease in the United States, achieving a huge savings in health care dollars.[1] Consequences of the lack of harmonization were detailed in a National Institute of Standards and Technology (NIST) report on calcium (Ca) that estimated the cost of a 0.1-mg/dL Ca bias can mean an additional $8 to $31 cost for unnecessary patient follow-up testing.[16] A Ca bias of 0.5 mg/dL could result in an additional $34/patient to $89/patient, and on an annual basis, a 0.1-mg/dL bias could translate into $75 million/y to $250 million/y (adjusted for 2016 dollars) for approximately 3.55 million patients screened for Ca.

EHRs contain a wealth of laboratory data on patients but the benefit is negated if the values for the same analyte are not comparable. It has been suggested that laboratory data account for approximately 70% of clinical decisions. Hallworth[17] has challenged that blanket statement but allows, "The value of laboratory medicine in patient care is unquestioned. That value is greatly diminished without comparability of test results."

HARMONIZATION AND STANDARDIZATION

Assay harmonization is a high priority but so is harmonization of terminology, reporting units, and even the pre-preanalytical and the post-postanalytical phase.[1] Clinicians expect to receive the "right test at the right time for the right patient" and also assume the "same results and interpretation for a sample irrespective of the laboratory that produced the result."[18]

In this discussion, *harmonization* is used interchangeably with *standardization*, although there is a distinction between the two.[9] Standardization means results are traceable to higher metrological order reference materials and/or methods and ideally can be reported in International System of Units (SI units). Harmonization means results are traceable to some declared reference but higher-order reference materials and/or methods are not available and SI units are not applicable. Harmonization ensures comparability of results, enables application of clinical best practice guidelines and RIs, increases patient safety, and decreases medical care costs. To achieve it requires the cooperation of laboratories, academia, professional societies, metrological institutes, government agencies, external quality assessment/proficiency testing (EQA/PT) providers, and industry.

Two standardization success stories are creatinine and glycated hemoglobin (hemoglobin A_{1c} [HbA_{1c}]).[3] Field assays for both analytes have complete traceability chains, firmly anchored by RMSs. In one HbA_{1c} study, reference samples with target values assigned by the International Federation of Clinical Chemistry and Laboratory Medicine (IFCC) reference method (European Reference Laboratory for Glycohemoglobin) were tested using an enzymatic method field assay.[19] The maximum systematic bias for the commercial assay was only 1.9%, and the mean bias ranged from −1.1 to 1.0 mmol/mol. Ironically, results for creatinine and HbA_{1c} assays are still reported in different units, creatinine in mg/dL (conventional units) and µmol/L (SI units), and HbA_{1c} in %HbA_{1c} (NGSP units) and mmol/mol (SI units). Beyond analytical traceability is the challenge of harmonization of the TTP, including use of identical reporting units. Ideally, a certification process for in vitro diagnostics (IVD) manufacturers could document and ensure harmonization.[3] It would likely be organized by national or international bodies, and stakeholders would include clinical and laboratory organizations, IVD manufacturers, government and regulatory agencies, journal editors, research organizations, metrology institutes, and standard setting organizations.

METROLOGICAL TRACEABILITY

As White[6] explains, "Metrology, the science of measurement, provides laboratory medicine with a structured approach to the development and terminology of reference measurement systems which, when implemented, improve the accuracy and comparability of patients' results." Metrological principles are relatively new in the clinical laboratory. The third edition of the *Tietz Textbook of Clinical Chemistry* made no mention of the metrology terms, *uncertainty* and *commutability*.[20] The fourth edition mentioned *uncertainty* and gave a definition of *commutability*.[21] The fifth edition includes a discussion of *uncertainty* along with *commutability*.[22] But as noted by De Bievre,[23] "Discussions with analytical chemists have revealed that basic concepts in metrology, including 'traceability' are generally not an integral part of university or college curricula and are not treated in most textbooks of analytical chemistry."

Full implementation of the IVD Directive (IVDD) (December, 2003) under European law requires calibration of quantitative IVD assays be traceable to available higher-order reference methods or materials.[24] The IVDD applies to Europe for the purposes of the Conformité Européenne [European Conformity] (CE) mark but has global implications. Manufacturers must establish metrological traceability for calibrators and controls and the uncertainty of kit calibrators. Assays have always been anchored by some kind of standards, but strict metrological traceability was not always in place or even necessarily appreciated. Powers[25] attributes the IVDD in part to European laboratory professionals striving for result accuracy and patient test result transferability, pointing to International Organization for Standardization (ISO) 17511 in which is found this statement: "It is essential that results reported to physicians and patients are adequately accurate (true and precise) to allow correct medical interpretation and comparability over time and space."[25] Metrological traceability satisfies basic clinical needs and improves patient care but the details for implementation of the process continue to be a challenge.[26]

The IVD field routinely performs measurements on an estimated 400, 600, or even 1000 different analytes, but full calibration systems with acceptable traceability currently exist for perhaps only 30 to 100 analytes.[24,25] Benefits for industry from traceability include interchangeability of data between products, competitiveness (levels the playing field), defined quality goals, lower long-term costs, clearer pathway to market access, transferable technology, and independent tools to ensure long-term performance stability. Trade-offs include diverting qualified people to participate in standards work versus other programs, risk of investing in standards not acceptable to all stakeholders, lengthy cycle time to achieve deliverables, costs of transition to new standards, less variety and fewer alternatives for customers, and barriers to innovation and market entry.[24]

Traceability originated in the metrological community and was first defined in 1993 in the International Vocabulary of Metrology — Basic and General Concepts and Associated Terms (VIM).[26] The VIM definition is the "property of a measurement result whereby the result can be related to a stated reference through a documented unbroken chain of calibrations, each contributing to the measurement uncertainty."[1,26] **Fig. 1** illustrates the hierarchical order of materials and measurement procedures for an unbroken traceability chain. It follows an alternating process of assigning target values to materials

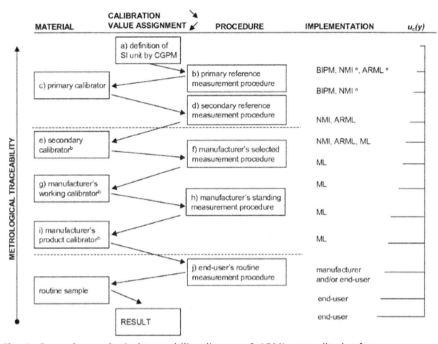

Fig. 1. General metrological traceability diagram. [a] ARML, accredited reference measurement laboratory (such a laboratory may be an independent or a manufacturer's laboratory); [b] SI unit of measurement; CGPM, General Conference on Weights and Measures; ML, manufacturer's laboratory; $u_c(y)$, combined standard uncertainty of measurement. (*From* ISO 17511. In vitro diagnostic medical devices—Measurement of quantities in biological samples—Metrological traceability of samples assigned to calibrators and control materials. International Organization for Standardization; 2003; with permission.)

used to calibrate the next lower-order measurement procedure.[26] Traceability is established using the ISO standards 17511, 15193, 15194, and 15195.[13,16,27]

The traceability to internationally recognized and accepted reference materials and measurements is the key element assuring accuracy and comparability of results.[28]

Diagnostic manufacturers must ensure analytical systems are traceable to certified reference materials and measurement procedures and that calibrator uncertainty is documented.[13] Analytes are either type A (well-defined chemical entities, traceable to SI units) or type B (heterogenous analytes in human samples and that are not directly traceable to SI units). Type A analytes represent a small number of well-defined compounds (approximately 65) belonging to classical clinical chemistry, for example, electrolytes, minerals, cholesterol, creatinine, steroid hormones, and vitamins. Type B analytes are all the rest, including most of the proteins (usually measured immunochemical methods) and more esoteric compounds whose results are expressed in terms of arbitrary units, for example, WHO international units or mass units.[13] The esoteric type B analytes measured by immunoassays are more challenging to standardize due to use of different calibrators by manufacturers because of internationally recognized reference material/measurement procedures not available, comparison of assays to different predicate devices, use of antibodies recognizing different antigens/epitopes on the same analyte, and use of different capture/detection antibodies in 2-step immunoassays for the same analyte.[14]

The IVDD requirements are incorporated in ISO 15189 (medical laboratories—particular requirements for quality and competence), the basis for many laboratory accreditation programs.[28] Metrologists are principally interested in accurate measurements and when ISO standards were drafted, committee debates about metrological principles and terminology, interesting on a philosophical level, often overshadowed concerns for the intended clinical use of assays, explaining the academic tone of the standards.[28] The standards meant a major shift for manufacturers away from using in-house materials and methods to the use of reference materials and methods vetted by metrology. Ideally, SI reporting units are used.[6] Broad implementation of SI units has facilitated scientific exchange and the Bureau international des poids et mesures [BIPM] provides a coherent system of measurements traceable to the SI, ensuring equivalence of measurements, including those used in laboratory medicine.[6]

Metrology theory introduces complications because a measurement result is an estimate of the true value of the measurand and, because the true value cannot be exactly known, the concept of measurement uncertainty (MU) was developed.[5,6] MU assumes significant bias in the reference material is eliminated and calculates an interval of values for the measurand (analyte) within which the true value lies with a stated level of confidence. Metrology defines MU as a non-negative parameter characterizing the dispersion of the quantity values being attributed to a measurand, based on the information used.[6] Clinical and Laboratory Standards Institute (CLSI) EP29 (expression of MU in laboratory medicine) is a recent guideline for estimating uncertainty.[29] "The GUM [Guide to the Expression of Uncertainty in Measurement] approach to uncertainty is rapidly gaining acceptance in metrological institutes and industry, and must be applied in ISO (International Organization for Standardization) and CEN (European Committee for Standardization) standards. It should be used in accredited laboratory work but chemists often find the implementation difficult and therefore hesitate. Additionally, sometimes, there is a fear that honest GUM uncertainty intervals, which may be wider than classical precision intervals, are bad for business."[30]

Metrology must be adapted to clinical laboratory science for harmonization but in a practical manner due to the differences between the disciplines. Metrology is a pure science in contrast to the mixed science of clinical chemistry that combines diverse disciplines and technologies. National metrology institutes (NMIs) are ivory towers in comparison to clinical laboratories, which are more like the trenches. Metrologists test pure, well-defined analytes in simple matrices whereas clinical laboratorians test complex, ill-defined analytes in challenging matrices (serum, plasma, urine, and so forth). Metrology uses expanded uncertainty (with bias eliminated) to set accuracy goals whereas clinical laboratories tend to use a total error allowable (TEa) methodology (TEa = bias + imprecision). Metrology seeks "absolute scientific truth" by reference method analysis but clinical laboratories must deal with relative truth by field method analysis. Good metrology does not necessarily equal good clinical laboratory science, but clinical laboratories need to adapt metrological concepts and adapt them for practical application.

THE PILLARS OF HARMONIZATION

The Treaty of the Meter (1875) enabled comparability of measurements, and metrology is the science of measurement.[1] Metrology is a separate science in its own right but its concepts are relevant to many other disciplines, including clinical laboratory science.[31] The IVDD calls for traceability of calibrators to higher-order reference materials and/or reference methods. But *higher-order* was not defined by the legislation beyond assigning responsibility for traceability to national notified bodies. The premise is manufacturers will be responsible for traceability, but manufacturers need to know which reference materials and methods can anchor assays.[14] The IVDD made it necessary to identify a final arbiter of traceability. Stenman noted that many organizations deal with standardization but it is not clear who is responsible for what and it is desirable that one international organization manage standardization.[14]

In anticipation of the IVDD, the Joint Committee for Traceability in Laboratory Medicine (JCTLM) was formed in 2002 (http://www.bipm.org/en/committees/jc/jctlm).[1,2,13] The JCTLM is an international consortium (government, clinical laboratory profession, and industry), sponsored by the BIPM, the IFCC, and the International Laboratory Accreditation Cooperation. Its mission is to support worldwide comparability, reliability, and equivalence of measurement results to improve health care.[32,33] The JCTLM established 3 pillars of traceability: (1) reference measurement procedures (RMPs), (2) reference materials, and (3) a network of reference measurement laboratories. The JCTLM maintains a searchable database for all 3 pillars on the BIPM Web site.[13,14,34] JCTLM Working Group 1 (reference materials and reference methods), and JCTLM Working Group 2 (reference measurement services) and their review teams judge database submissions for blood cell counting, coagulation factors, drugs, metabolites and substrates, microbial serology, nonelectrolye metals, nonpeptide hormones, nucleic acids, proteins, vitamins and micronutrients, electrolyte and blood gases, and enzymes.[1] The components of an RMS are definition of the analyte, RMPs that specifically measure the analyte, primary and secondary reference materials, and reference measurement laboratories. Analytes fall into 2 categories: type A (well defined, concentration in SI units, results not method dependent, and full traceability chain) and type B (not well defined, heterogeneous, present in both bound and free state, not traceable to SI, and rigorous traceability chain not available).

Primary and matrix-based secondary references are both needed.[35] Secondary reference materials (pooled human serum, plasma, and urine) are critical for IVD manufacturers to anchor calibrators. RMPs, such as isotope dilution mass spectrometry, are developed by metrology institutes but for analytes, such as enzymes, standardization is only possible by method-specific protocols. Metrology institutes do not have sufficient medical/clinical expertise to set ideal specifications for secondary reference materials and must develop them in close collaboration with laboratory experts (eg, American Association for Clinical Chemistry [AACC] and IFCC). Even then, success is not guaranteed. Studies performed using human pooled serum spiked with NIST SRM (Standard Reference Material) 2921 (human cardiac troponin complex) demonstrated this material does not behave like individual patient samples with elevated troponin I, probably due to lack of commutability.[35]

Even defining a measurand (analyte) is difficult.[6] Not all are well characterized with a known molecular structure and weight (eg, glucose or sodium). Complex molecules, such as proteins, may be structurally heterogeneous due to post-translational modification, glycosylation, complex formation, and so forth. A prime example is HCG with 7 significant isoforms. Relative concentrations of these isoforms can differ markedly depending on the clinical condition.

A special requirement for harmonization is commutability. Rej and colleagues[36] introduced the term in 1973 to designate the property that calibrators and controls should exhibit (ie, analytical response indistinguishable from that of authentic patient samples). Noncommutability was particularly noticeable for enzymes because of sample differences, for example, nonhuman animal sources, isoenzymes, stability, matrix differences, and effects of sample preparation procedures (eg, lyophilization and preservatives).[37] Other variables are differences in substrates, cofactors, pH, and reaction temperatures used by assays.

Commutability is equivalence of the mathematical relationships between the results of different measurement procedures for a reference material and for representative samples from healthy and diseased individuals.[9,38,39] Without commutability, results from routine methods cannot legitimately be compared to identify a calibration bias, and the reference material cannot be used as a calibrator without commutability, so traceability to the reference system is invalid. Fresh patient samples and calibrators need to provide an identical analytical response (**Fig. 2**). Many secondary reference materials are not commutable and have failed to achieve harmonized results. Non-commutable EQA/PT samples require peer group grading because they are not amenable to accuracy-based grading, that is, comparison of results reported by laboratories to a target value determined by reference method analysis. Commutability is not a universal property of reference materials and must be proved with every field method. Well recognized by metrology, commutability was not widely appreciated by clinical laboratories and commutability of calibrators was not routinely established. Noncommutability results in biases with field assays due to matrix effects, use of nonhuman forms of analyte, lack of antibody specificity, or other causes. Producing sufficiently large pools of commutable material for EQA/PT samples is a practical difficulty because of the large volume required.[38] JCTLM now requires a commutability assessment before listing a reference material in its database. CLSI EP30 (characterization and qualification of commutable reference materials for laboratory medicine) is a recent guideline providing commutability guidance.[40] Commutability of each calibrator in a calibration hierarchy is essential for traceability.[6] Noncommutability breaks traceability. During manufacture, secondary calibrators may suffer matrix modifications due to lyophilization, freeze-thawing, filtration, and so forth, and commutability may be lost.[6]

The JCTLM faces several challenges. Like many similar professional organizations, it depends on volunteers and their expertise. Many laboratory professionals and organizations (metrology institutes, governmental regulatory agencies, manufacturers, and so forth) are actively engaged in JCTLM activities and support involvement. But JCTLM participation is an "extracurricular activity" for the volunteers and not part of the day job or a top priority for employers. It is difficult for stakeholders to allocate human and other

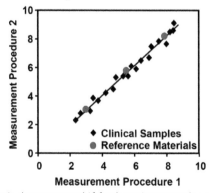

Commutable: same relationship for clinical samples and reference materials

Fig. 2. Commutability is demonstrated if fresh patient samples and reference materials, for example, calibrators, demonstrate an equivalent analytical response when tested by 2 methods.

resources to support the JCTLM.[14] NMIs providing reference materials and methods may have limited resources to maintain the necessary metrological infrastructure. The JCTLM operates by consensus and obtaining consensus among the members may require considerable discussion. After all, if agreement on internationally accepted reference materials and methods were simple, there would have been no need to form the JCTLM in the first place. There is not a fixed JCTLM budget and the participating organizations are expected to fund activities on a pay-as-you-go basis."[14]

In addition to the 3 pillars defined by the JCTLM, the laboratory community has identified 3 more: universal RIs and medical decision levels, EQA/PT programs to ensure traceability of field assays is maintained (eg, accuracy-based grading programs, such as the College of American Pathologists [CAP] requirement of ± 6% of the target value for HbA_{1c}), and harmonization of clinical laboratory practice and the TTP, for example, standardized nomenclature/terminology, reporting units, and evidence-based laboratory medicine.

The fourth pillar—universal RIs—cannot be erected without the adoption of RMSs and assay harmonization. RIs for some analytes are affected by various partitioning factors, for example, age, gender, ethnicity, and body mass index; thus, universal ranges may not be feasible. But such decisions cannot be made until harmonization has been achieved and study results are comparable.

The requirement for result trueness and comparability requires a fifth pillar: validation of manufacturers' traceability by EQA/PT. EQA/PT surveys were originally educational exercises to compare laboratories to their peers. Although still useful for this purpose, PT surveys now also serve a regulatory purpose.[38] Target values for PT samples should be determined using reference methods and materials because peer group comparison leaves open the question of the absolute accuracy because there can be multiple true values, each peer group mean value representing a relative true value. Comparison to the true value as determined by an RMP allows both an absolute and relative performance yardstick.[14]

Regulatory programs may have wider acceptance limits because it is undesirable for too many participant laboratories to fail challenges. Passing EQA/PT surveys means a laboratory meets some minimum regulatory requirement but does not guarantee clinically acceptable and desired performance. EQA/PT is a one–time point assessment subject to random error, and performance can vary from one survey cycle to another. EQA/PT programs using commutable samples with reference method target values allow accuracy-based grading.[41] Ideally, PT/EQA surveys should be sent to laboratories as blind samples indistinguishable from actual patient samples so they are handled as patient specimens, for example, survey samples should be analyzed only once.[38] Blind testing is a challenge. Horowitz[41] notes, "Far too many laboratories consider proficiency testing just a necessary evil, little more than periodic pass–fail exercises we perform solely to meet regulatory requirements" and "Even for central-laboratory techniques, traditional PT suffers from 'matrix effects,' in that samples used for testing often react differently from native patient samples. Therefore, comparisons must be made only to peer groups, rather than to the 'true value.' What if the peer group as a whole is wrong?"[41] EQA/PT has typically been used to measure proficiency at performing a test and not the trueness of the test method or its performance relative to other methods.[10] Miller and colleagues[42] conclude, "Traditional PT materials are not suitable for field-based postmarketing assessments of a method's trueness."

Collection and pooling of unaltered samples to prepare EQA/PT aliquots, stored frozen (≤70), is considered the best method for preparing commutable samples.[38] Target values should be assigned using reference methods. In the absence of an

RMS, all-participant means or median values may be used as the target value. Because EQA/PT can be driven by either regulatory, clinical decision considerations or by biological variability goals, passing EQA/PT challenges may indicate a laboratory meets minimum standards but it does not necessarily guarantee clinically acceptable performance. In a well-designed study using commutable samples with reference method target values for 10 analytes, glucose, iron, potassium, and uric acid methods exhibited the best performance, with all peer groups meeting the minimum and more than 87.5% of peer groups meeting the desirable, biological variability bias goals.[42] But the other 6 analytes did not meet bias goals. Accuracy-based EQA/PT is ideal but more demanding than peer group grading. EQA/PT results reflect laboratory performance at a given point in time and continuous participation in EQA/PT is necessary to ensure continual acceptable performance.

Interlaboratory comparability of EQA/PT results allows evaluation of calibration traceability.[43] In one study, commutable serum-based material assigned target values by reference methods for 6 enzymes (alanine aminotransferase [ALT], aspartate aminotransferase [AST], creatine kinase [CK], γ-glutamyltransferase [GGT], lactate dehydrogenase [LD], and amylase) was tested by 70 laboratories using 6 field methods.[44] Results were graded on accuracy using biological variability targets. For ALT, results were deemed acceptable for greater than 94% of 6 commercial assays. Performance for the other 5 enzymes was variable and all methods demonstrated significant bias for CK. It was concluded method bias should be reduced by improved traceability to internationally accepted reference systems. Tacrolimus is measured by liquid chromatography–mass spectrometry (LC-MS) and immunoassays and all methods are calibrated without traceability to a recognized reference method or material.[45] Tacrolimus results thus may not be comparable between methods, with potential risks to cancer patients monitored by therapeutic drug monitoring. A global comparability study conducted to assess analytical variability found an immunoassay (ARCHITECT, Abbott, Chicago, IL, USA) demonstrated the best precision (coefficients of variation [CVs] of 3.9%–9.5%) whereas CVs for another immunoassay (Dade Dimension, Dade, Glasgow, DE, USA) and LC-MS methods ranged from 5% to 48.1% and 11.4% to 18.7%, respectively. Higher LC-MS imprecision was primarily due to between-laboratory variability. An advantage of the commercial immunoassays is they use the same extraction procedure, instrumentation, detection systems, and calibration, whereas the LC-MS method parameters varied. Even the use of a common calibrator did not harmonize the LC-MS results. No LC-MS tacrolimus method has yet been listed in the JCTLM database, and thus none is recognized as defining analytical truth for the analyte.

The sixth harmonization pillar is the TTP. Plebani[46] observed, "Although the focus is mainly on the standardization of measurement procedures, the scope of harmonization goes beyond method and analytical results: it includes all other aspects of laboratory testing, including terminology and units, report formats, reference intervals and decision limits, as well as test profiles and criteria for the interpretation of results." Harmonization of reporting units seems easy, but is it not. A UK survey revealed 80% of laboratories reported hemoglobin using grams per deciliter although grams per liter is the recommended unit.[46] Harmonization of basic terminology and units is necessary but the international laboratory community has yet to reach agreement. See **Table 1** for examples of disharmony.

CHALLENGES TO HARMONIZATION

Thienpont[47] has lamented that major IVD manufacturers have not agreed to a new measurement paradigm in clinical chemistry and moved to accuracy-based assays,

Table 1 Examples of disharmony		
Analyte	Conventional Units	SI Units
ALT	U/L	mkat/L
Bilirubin	mg/dL	mmol/L
Cl	mEq/L	mmol/L
Glucose	mg/dL	mmol/L
Creatinine	mg/dL	mmol/L
HbA$_{1c}$	% Hb A$_{1c}$	mmol/mol

demonstrating transparency by comparing assays with accepted RMPs. Embracing metrological harmonization is a paradigm shift for the IVD industry. Manufacturers traditionally sought to differentiate themselves from competitors (eg, claiming a greater dynamic range, lower limit of detection, better precision, smaller sample size, and so forth) and producing comparable patient results was not a priority. Lack of harmonization among field assays is evident from EQA/PT data, often requiring peer group reporting. Manufacturers are responding to the need for comparability by providing calibrator traceability/uncertainty information, restandardizing assays, establishing commutability, and so forth. Manufacturers play an integral role in educating laboratories about assay harmonization and modern clinical laboratory practice in general. But the old question remains, "Where do manufacturers' obligations end and the obligations of laboratory directors begin?" Manufacturers must provide fit-for-purpose tests, but laboratories must use the assays properly and effectively. When an assay failure occurs (and failure can apply to myriad issues and causes), does the fault lie with the manufacturer or with the laboratory and its use of the test?

A major manufacturer challenge is to choose a TEa goal from many available options: US-specific CLIA requirements, CAP, Royal College of Pathologists of Australasia, Guidelines of the Germany Federal Medical Society (RiliBÄK [Richtlinien der Bundesarztekammer]), or other EQA/PT provider specifications. Another popular source of TEa goals is biological variability, but there are 3 targets from which to choose:

$$\text{Minimum TEa} < 1.65 \, (0.75 \, CV_i) + 0.375 \, (CV_i^2 + CV_g^2)^{1/2}$$

$$\text{Desirable TEa} < 1.65 \, (0.5 \, CV_i) + 0.25 \, (CV_i^2 + CV_g^2)^{1/2}$$

$$\text{Optimum TEa} < 1.65 \, (0.25 \, CV_i) + 0.125 \, (CV_i^2 + CV_g^2)^{1/2},$$

where CV_i is individual biological variability and CV_g is group biological variability.

The IFCC Working Group on Allowable Error for Traceable Results (WG-AETR) was formed to define clinically acceptable limits for harmonization and better clinical application and to cooperate with manufacturers, regulatory bodies, and end-users.[48] WG-AETR concluded, "Although manufacturers are compelled by the European IVDD, 98/79/EC, to have traceability of the values assigned to their calibrators if suitable higher order reference materials and/or procedures are available, there is still no equivalence of results for many measurands determined in clinical laboratories." For some common analytes, such as sodium, current assays are too imprecise to meet TEa targets based on biological variation. Due to cost and limited resources, IVD manufacturers

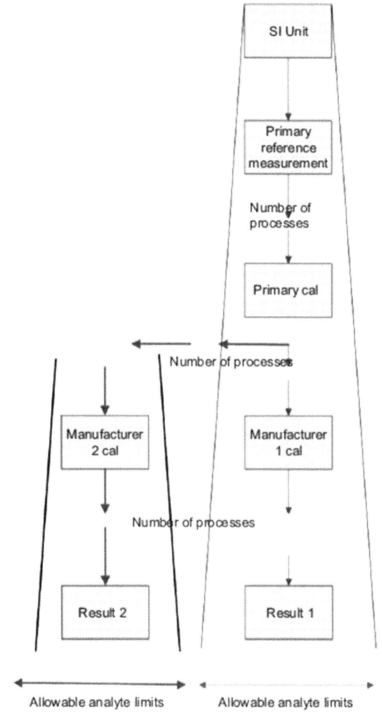

Fig. 3. Manufacturers may prepare calibrators (cal) starting with traceability to the same reference material and/or reference method but the calibrator manufacturing process

do not always follow the full traceability chain steps to value assign every new calibrator lot but rely on value transfer from an internally stored master calibrator material. In most cases, this procedure is probably valid, but a common complaint is calibrator lot-to-lot variability. WG-AETR noted when there are 2 traceability paths for a measurand, calibrators from different manufacturers may both be derived from valid traceability chains but produce nonequivalent results, as illustrated by **Fig. 3**. Equivalent results from 2 systems may only be possible by using a correction factor determined by a correlation study.

The international clinical laboratory community has embraced harmonization. A good example is the AACC International Consortium for Harmonization of Clinical Laboratory Results (ICHCLR).[3] The ICHCLR prioritizes analytes globally for harmonization and development of reference materials and RMPs. ICHCLR stakeholders include clinical laboratory and medical professional societies, IVD manufacturers, metrology institutes, public health organizations, regulatory agencies, and standard-setting organizations. A similar initiative is Pathology Harmony in the United Kingdom.[49] Pathology Harmony states, "As we the move towards full electronic reporting of pathology results, we appreciate more fully that variations in things such as test names, reference intervals and units of measurement associated with our results is something that hinders progress." In Australia, the Pathology Information, Terminology and Units Standardisation Project is dedicated to harmonization, in particular focusing on the interoperability of pathology test requesting and reporting.[50] Harmonization of report formats, RIs, and decision limits and best practice evidence for test requesting are also concerns.[51] Staff requesting and receiving test results and information system developers may be unaware of reporting differences, and clinicians often assume results from different methods are comparable and there is no risk of misinterpretation or adverse patient outcomes.

IN VITRO DIAGNOSTICS MANUFACTURERS AND HARMONIZATION

Clinical laboratories assume manufacturers have implemented calibrator metrological traceability and uncertainty. But full traceability may not be available or may lack sufficient detail, and calibrator uncertainty may be lacking or not be reasonable due to the variety of methods for calculating it.[33] IVD manufacturers have set aside traditional commercial competition for the goal of assay comparability and equivalent patient results. Even with rigorous calibrator traceability, manufacturers may be reluctant to provide full information for fear of disclosing proprietary data or opening themselves to technical criticism. Full disclosure of this information remains a challenge for Industry.[33]

Manufacturers all have substantial product development priority lists and requirements for which personnel and financial resources are committed over long-term periods. Reprioritization is possible and welcomed by industry to benefit clinicians, patients and health care systems, but global harmonization creates competing priorities for companies. As manufacturers support harmonization, timelines reflecting development cycles (years) require companies to simultaneously reprioritize

---

may diverge at some point, resulting in significantly different results for the same measurand in the same patient sample if tested by the 2 field methods, despite metrologically acceptable traceability for each assay's calibrators (cal). (*From* Bais R, Armbruster D, Jansen RT, et al. Defining acceptable limits for the metrological traceability of specific measurands. Clin Chem Lab Med 2013;51(5):975; with permission.)

resources while maintaining projects driving innovation and product portfolio development.

The IVD industry has readily accepted and supported the JCTLM.[13] Benefits from the JCTLM include realistic timelines to restandardize assays using traceability chains, an efficient source of traceability information (ie, the JCTLM database), and an effective communication forum on traceability and standardization. Manufacturers still face traceability challenges, including difficulty identifying reference materials and methods even with the JCTLM database, unavailability of some reference materials (eg, enzyme standards), lack of secondary reference materials for some measurands (eg, analytes in matrices, such as whole blood, serum, plasma, and urine), reference materials not expressed in SI units, noncommutable reference materials, reference methods not easily transferable or available (eg, definitive methods, such as isotope dilution–gas chromatography/mass spectrometry), time required to restandardize (often optimistically estimated at 18–24 months due to manufacturing process changes, labeling changes, inventory obsolescence, communications to customers/PT providers/regulatory agencies, changes in RIs, and so forth), producing assays compatible with evidence-based laboratory medicine, and laboratory medicine practice guidelines. Another consideration is whether harmonization always provides a benefit. Accuracy is important but there are situations in which existing assays may be relatively harmonized yet the reference method is very different from commercialized assays. The cost of harmonization, which includes physician education, patient safety, and investment in product redevelopment, should be weighed to prove the benefit of harmonization.

Health care consumers (physicians and patients) expect (take for granted) laboratory test that results are of high quality and suitable for diagnosis and management and that accurate results are produced by all laboratories at all times. But it is a daunting task for different laboratories to analyze the same patient specimens and generate equivalent results, within acceptable analytical tolerance limits, regardless of the measurement system used.[31]

Uncertainty is routine in metrology but a new concept in the clinical laboratory. Estimating uncertainty is valuable for manufacturers, allowing them to identify and minimize variability of calibrators. It remains unclear to what extent uncertainty is useful for clinical purposes and whether it should be reported with test results. For example, clinicians could be confused if ALT enzyme results are expressed in SI units with uncertainty as serum ALT; catalytic concentration = (1.15 ± 0.23 ukatal [kat]/L).[17]

SUMMARY

There is no doubt global harmonization of the clinical laboratory field is the next frontier and efforts to achieve this goal will continue in the twenty-first century. Success depends on creativity, such as creating the JCTLM as a new international organization devoted to assay traceability and bringing together a wide variety of stakeholders in this effort.[52] Analytical standardization to allow assays to produce clinically equivalent test results is only one facet of this movement. Success will be defined by harmonization of the TTP encompassing the preanalytical, analytical, and postanalytical phases.[53]

REFERENCES

1. Greenberg N. Update on current concepts and meanings in laboratory medicine: standardization, traceability and harmonization. Clin Chim Acta 2014;432:49–54.
2. Armbruster D, Donnelly J. Harmonization of clinical laboratory test results: the role of the IVD industry. EJIFCC 2016;27:37–47.

3. Miller WG, Myers GL, Gantzer ML, et al. Roadmap for harmonization of clinical laboratory measurements procedures. Clin Chem 2011;57:1108–17.
4. Tate JR, Johnson R, Barth J, et al. Harmonization of laboratory testing- current achievements and future strategies. Clin Chim Acta 2014;432:4–7.
5. McLawhon RW. Patient safety and clinical effectiveness as imperatives for achieving harmonization inside and outside the clinical laboratory. Clin Chem 2011;57:936–8.
6. White GH. Metrological traceability in clinical biochemistry. Ann Clin Biochem 2011;48:393–409.
7. Miller WG, Myers GL. Commutability still matters. Clin Chem 2013;59:1291–3.
8. Beastall GH. Adding value to laboratory medicine: a professional responsibility. Clin Chem Lab Med 2013;51:221–7.
9. Gantzer ML, Miller WG. Harmonisation of measurement procedures: how do we get it done? Clin Biochem Rev 2012;33:95–100.
10. Malone B. A jumpstart on harmonization. Clinical Laboratory News 2010;36:12.
11. Hernandez JS, Dale JC, Bennet K, et al. Challenges and opportunities for medical directors in pathology and laboratory medicine. Am J Clin Pathol 2010;133:8–13.
12. Stephan C, Siemben K, Camman H, et al. Between-method differences in prostate-specific antigen assays affect prostate cancer risk prediction by nomograms. Clin Chem 2011;57:995–1004.
13. Panteghini M. Traceability as a unique tool to improve standardization in laboratory medicine. Clin Biochem 2009;42:236–40.
14. Armbruster D, Miller RR. The Joint Committee on Traceability in Laboratory Medicine (JCTLM): a global approach to promote the standardization of clinical laboratory results. Clin Biochem 2007;28:105–13.
15. Morris HA. Traceability and standardization of immunoassays: a major challenge. Clin Biochem 2009;42:241–5.
16. NIST. Planning report 04-1, the impact of calibration error in medical decision making. Gaithersburg (MD): National Institute for Standards and Technology; 2004.
17. Hallworth MJ. The '70% claim': what is the evidence base? Ann Clin Biochem 2011;48:487–8.
18. Tate JR, Johnson R, Barth JH. Harmonization of laboratory testing- a global activity [Editorial]. Clin Chim Acta 2014;432:1–3.
19. Teodoro-Morrison T, Janssen MJW, Mols J, et al. Evaluation of a next generation direct whole blood enzymatic assay for hemoglobin A1c on the ARCHITECT c8000 chemistry system. Clin Chem Lab Med 2015;53:125–32.
20. Burtis CA, Ashwood ER, editors. Tietz textbook of clinical chemistry. 3rd edition. Philadelphia: W.B. Saunders Co; 1999.
21. Burtis CA, Ashwood ER, Bruns DE, editors. Tietz textbook of clinical chemistry and molecular diagnostics. 4th edition. Philadelphia: W.B. Saunders Co; 2006.
22. Burtis CA, Ashwood ER, Bruns DE, editors. Tietz textbook of clinical chemistry and molecular diagnostics. 5th edition. Philadelphia: W.B. Saunders Co; 2011.
23. De Bievre P. Metrological traceability of measurement results in chemistry: concepts and implementation. IUPAC Technical Report. Pure Appl Chem 2011;83:1873–935.
24. Greenberg N. The IVD directive and availability of reference systems for IVD medical devices: a view from Industry. IVD Technology 2001;7:18–27.
25. Powers DM. Traceability of assay calibrators: the EU's IVD Directive raises the bar. IVD Technology 2000; July – August.
26. Vesper HW, Thienpont LM. Traceability in laboratory medicine. Clin Chem 2009;55:1067–75.

27. ISO 17511. In vitro diagnostic medical devices - measurement of quantities in biological samples - metrological traceability of values assigned to calibrators and control materials. Geneva, Switzerland: International Organization for Standardization; 2003.
28. ISO 15189. Medical laboratories — requirements for quality and competence. International Organization for Standardization; 2012.
29. CLSI EP21. Expression of measurement uncertainty in laboratory medicine. Wayne (PA): Clinical Laboratory Standards Institute; 2012.
30. Dybkaer R. From total allowable error via metrological traceability to uncertainty of measurement of the unbiased result. Accred Qual Assur 1999;4:401–5.
31. Armbruster D. Measurement traceability and US IVD manufacturers: the impact of metrology. Accred Qual Assur 2009;14:393–8.
32. Panteghini M. Traceability, reference systems and result comparability. Clin Biochem Rev 2007;28:97–104.
33. Braga F, Panteghini M. Verification of in vitro medical diagnostics (IVD) metrological traceability: responsibilities and strategies. Clin Chim Acta 2014;432:55–61.
34. Available at: www.bipm.org/jctlm. Accessed March 19, 2016.
35. Bunk DM. Reference materials and reference measurement procedures: an overview from a national metrology institute. Clin Biochem Rev 2007;28:131–7.
36. Fasce CF, Rej R, Copeland WH, et al. A discussion of enzyme reference materials: applications and specifications. Clin Chem 1973;19:5–9.
37. Rej R. Accurate enzyme activity measurements. Arch Pathol Lab Med 1993;117:352–64.
38. Miller WG, Jones GRD, Horowitz GL, et al. Proficiency testing external quality assessment: current challenges and future directions. Clin Chem 2011;57:1670–80.
39. Miller WG, Myers GL, Rej R. Why commutability matters. Clin Chem 2006;52:553–4.
40. CLSI EP30. Characterization and qualification of commutable reference materials for laboratory medicine. Wayne (PA): Clinical Laboratory Standards Institute; 2010.
41. Horowitz GL. Proficiency testing matters. Clin Chem 2013;59:335–7.
42. Miller WG, Myers GL, Ashwood ER, et al. State of the art in trueness and interlaboratory harmonization for 10 analytes in general clinical chemistry. Arch Pathol Lab Med 2008;132:838–46.
43. Miller WG. The role of proficiency testing in achieving standardization and harmonization between laboratories. Clin Biochem 2009;42:232–5.
44. Jansen R, Schumann G, Baadenhuijsen H, et al. Trueness verification and traceability assessment of results from commercial systems for measurement of six enzyme activities in serum: an international study in the EC4 framework of the Calibration 2000 project. Clin Chim Acta 2006;368:160–7.
45. Levine DM, Maine GT, Armbruster DA, et al. The need for standardization of tacrolimus assays. Clin Chem 2011;57:1739–47.
46. Plebani M. Harmonization in laboratory medicine: the complete picture. Clin Chem Lab Med 2013;51:741–51.
47. Thienpont LM. Accuracy in clinical chemistry- Who will kiss Sleeping Beauty awake? Clin Chem 2008;46:1220–2.
48. Bais R, Armbruster D, Jansen RTP, et al. Defining acceptable limits for the metrological traceability of specific measurands. Clin Chem Lab Med 2013;51:973–6.
49. Berg J, Lane V. Pathology Harmony; a pragmatic and scientific approach to unfounded variation in the clinical laboratory. Ann Clin Biochem 2011;48:195–7.

50. Legg M. Standardisation of test requesting and reporting for the electronic health record. Clin Chim Acta 2014;432:148–56.
51. Tate JR, Johnson R, Legg M. Haromonisation of laboratory testing. Clin Biochem Rev 2012;33:81–4.
52. Jones GRD, Jackson C. The Joint Committee for Traceability in Laboratory Medicine (JCTLM)- Its history and operation. Clin Chim Acta 2016;453:86–94.
53. Aarsand AK, Sandberg S. How to achieve harmonization of laboratory testing-the complete picture. Clin Chim Acta 2014;432:8–14.

A Total Quality-Control Plan with Right-Sized Statistical Quality-Control

James O. Westgard, PhD[a,b,]*

KEYWORDS

- Risk-based QC • Individualized QC plan • Total QC plan • Hazard identification
- Risk assessment • Westgard Sigma Rules

KEY POINTS

- US CLIA regulations allow use of risk-based QC plans (called individualized quality control plans [IQCP]) as an option for compliance beginning January 1, 2016.
- An IQCP requires performance of a risk assessment, development of a QC plan, and implementation of a quality assessment program to monitor ongoing performance.
- Laboratories may instead develop a total QC plan that implements a "right-sized" SQC procedure to detect medically important errors and complies with the CLIA requirement of analyzing a minimum two levels of controls per day. This total QC plan should include preanalytic and postanalytic controls to monitor the total testing process.
- Determination of a Sigma-metric provides a good index of the risk of a laboratory testing process and guidance for selecting the right-sized SQC.
- Westgard Sigma Rules provides a new and simpler tool for selecting the right control rules and the right number of control measurements to detect medically important errors.

INTRODUCTION

Risk-based thinking has been a recent trend in International Organization for Standardization (ISO) standards and has also been adopted by Centers for Medicare and Medicaid Services (CMS) in the new Clinical Laboratory Improvement Amendments (CLIA) guidance for risk-based quality control (QC) (called individualized QC plan [IQCP]). The background for this development and approach were discussed previously in detail,[1] including an overview of the principles and approach for risk-based QCPs,[2] a review of the Clinical and Laboratory Standards Institute (CLSI) EP23-A

[a] Department of Pathology and Laboratory Medicine, School of Medicine and Public Health, University of Wisconsin, Madison, WI 53705, USA; [b] Westgard QC, Inc, Madison, WI 53717, USA
* Department of Pathology and Laboratory Medicine, School of Medicine and Public Health, University of Wisconsin, Madison, WI.
E-mail address: james@westgard.com

Clin Lab Med 37 (2017) 137–150
http://dx.doi.org/10.1016/j.cll.2016.09.011
0272-2712/17/© 2016 Elsevier Inc. All rights reserved.

proposal for developing risk-based QCPs,[3] and a discussion of the US CLIA regulations and options for QC compliance.[4]

Before January 1, 2014, the CLIA regulations provided three options for QC compliance: (1) default QC, (2) right statistical QC (SQC), and (3) equivalent QC (EQC)[5]:

- Default QC: Analyze a minimum testing of two levels of controls each day of patient testing, as specified in §493.1256(d) (3i).
- Right SQC: Establish QC procedures to monitor the accuracy and precision of the complete analytical process; establish the number, type, and frequency of testing control materials based on the performance (precision, bias) verified by the laboratory; detect immediate errors that occur because of test system failure, adverse environmental conditions, and operator performance; and monitor over time the accuracy and precision of test performance that may be influenced by changes in test system performance and environmental conditions, and variance in operator performance, as described in §493.1256(a-c).
- EQC: Implement a procedure for equivalent quality testing as stated in §493.1256(d), in accordance with the CMS requirements for EQC found in Appendix C of the State Operations Manual.[6]

As of January 1, 2016, the option for EQC was eliminated and replaced by a new option called IQCP.[7]

- IQCP: Implement IQCPs based on risk assessment, which CMS describes in the State Operations Manual.[6]

The simplest way to comply with CLIA is to analyze a minimum of two levels of controls each day (CLIA default QC). If the laboratory wishes to satisfy the ISO 15189 requirement for QC,[8] that is, design internal QC procedures that verify the attainment of the intended quality of test results, then the laboratory should optimize the detection of medically important errors by using available SQC planning/design tools. This also satisfies CLIA right SQC option and should be the preferred approach for implementing the QC necessary to guarantee the quality required for patient care, which is the intended use of test results produced by a medical laboratory. If a laboratory's interest is to reduce the frequency of SQC, then the laboratory may consider implementing IQCP.

UNDERSTANDING INDIVIDUALIZED QUALITY CONTROL PLAN

CMS describes an IQCP as follows[6,7]:

An IQCP is comprised of three parts, a risk assessment (RA), a Quality Control Plan (QCP), and a Quality Assessment (QA) plan. The RA is the identification and evaluation of potential failures and errors in a testing process. A QCP is a laboratory's standard operating procedure that describes the practices, resources, and procedures to control the quality of a particular test process. The QA is the laboratory's policy for ongoing monitoring of the effectiveness of their IQCP.

Risk Assessment

Risk assessment is the starting point. Possible sources or errors, or failure modes, should be identified for the particular measurement procedure and the operating conditions in the laboratory. The risk posed by each error source is then assessed based on how likely it is that the error will happen (occurrence), the chance that the error can be identified (detectability), and the potential impact of the error on the patient (severity). Occurrence, detection, and severity determine risk. High-risk failure modes need to be "mitigated" by preventive actions, by detection by control mechanisms followed by corrective actions, and finally by provision of information for patient safety to physicians and caregivers.

A Quality Control Plan

A QCP is a document that describes the practices, resources, and procedures to control the quality of a particular test process. The QCP must ensure the accuracy and reliability of test results and that test result quality is appropriate for patient care.[6,7] It should summarize the laboratory's activities for preventing errors from occurring, detecting errors if they occur, and taking corrective actions when necessary. The QCP should cover the total testing process and consider preanalytic, analytical, and postanalytic sources of errors, particularly those related to specimens, environment, reagents, test systems, and testing personnel. To detect errors, the laboratory must implement control mechanisms that are appropriate for the error conditions of interest. In principle, that allows the laboratory to specify different controls for different error conditions, which provides flexibility in the control mechanisms that can be used by the laboratory. Whereas traditional QC practices have depended heavily on SQC to monitor many possible error sources, the QC plan allows the laboratory to identify different control mechanisms that are useful for specific failure modes, then assemble those controls as a QCP.

A Quality Assessment Policy or Program

A quality assessment policy or program is needed to monitor the ongoing quality of the testing process and identify problems, initiate additional preventive actions, and prioritize improvements that are needed to ensure the quality meets the needs for patient care. Typically this involves performing root cause analysis when problems are observed, participating in proficiency testing, assessing operator competency, and monitoring quality indicators, such as specimen rejection rates and corrective actions, stable performance from QC data, unstable performance caused by analytical run rejections, including corrective actions and causes of failures, patient error reports, turnaround time distributions, and customer complaints.

GUIDANCE FOR DEVELOPING A QUALITY CONTROL PLAN

Although use of risk management is widespread in the diagnostic industry, there have been few formal, quantitative applications in medical laboratories. That means experience is lacking and there is a wide divergence of opinions and recommendations on how to perform a risk assessment for an IQCP. CMS requires no formal methodology, nor use of any of the common tools, such as failure mode effects analysis, which is a standard tool in industrial applications.

Clinical and Laboratory Standards Institute Guidance

With the sponsorship of CMS, CLSI developed the EP23-A consensus guideline for use of risk management in laboratory QC, which was published in 2011.[9] To understand the approach, definitions of some of the important terms are as follows:

- Risk: combination of the probability of occurrence of harm and the severity of that harm.
- Risk assessment: overall process comprising a risk analysis and a risk evaluation.

- Risk analysis: systematic use of available information to identify hazards and to estimate the risk.
- Risk estimation: process used to assign values to the probability of occurrence of harm and the severity of that harm.
- Risk evaluation: process of comparing the estimated risk against given risk criteria to determine the acceptability of risks.

The CLSI risk assessment methodology includes the following steps:

- Collect information about the test and test system, which involves the medical requirements for the test, knowledge of regulatory and accreditation requirements, and a thorough review of all the manufacturer's labeling and instructions for use.
- Identify potential hazards, also called failure modes, or more commonly, sources of error. Flow-charting the testing process is often helpful and other tools, such as a fishbone diagram, can be used to graphically summarize sources of errors.
- Estimate risk by assigning weights or values to the risk factors for each potential failure mode. CLSI identifies a two-factor risk model that involves the probability of occurrence of harm and the severity of harm, even though three-factor models that add detectability are more common in most industries. The guidance recommends use of a scale from 1 to 5 to assign weights to the risk factors.
- Evaluate risk to determine whether each failure mode is adequately controlled or needs an additional control mechanism to reduce risk.

The remaining steps focus on risk control, or risk mitigation, whereby control mechanisms are selected from the laboratory QC tool box to reduce risk of failures. Those controls are assembled in a QC plan, the residual risks evaluated, and the resulting plan implemented and monitored over time to ensure the quality and safe use of test results.

Centers for Medicare and Medicaid Services/Centers for Disease Control and Prevention Guidance

It was expected that the CLSI guidance would be adopted by CMS because an early CMS memo referenced the CLSI EP23-A document.[7] However, later guidance largely ignores the EP23-A methodology in favor of a much simpler approach, which is described in the workbook on "Developing an IQCP: A step-by-step Guide," available free for download from the Centers for Disease Control and Prevention (CDC) Web site.[10] The document is 62 pages long, describes an example application, and includes worksheets that can be used by the laboratory to create the three components required for an IQCP: (1) Risk Assessment Worksheet, (2) Quality Control Plan Worksheet, and (3) Quality Assessment Worksheet. **Tables 1–3** provide a description and contents of these worksheets.

The approach is even more qualitative and subjective than that recommended by CLSI. The risk assessment worksheet involves addressing three questions: (1) what are our possible sources of error, (2) can our identified sources of error be reduced, and (3) how can we reduce the identified sources of errors. These questions must be considered for the total testing process (preanalytic, analytic, and postanalytic phases) and specifically for possible sources of errors from the specimen, test system, reagent, environment, and testing personnel.

There is a clear focus on identification of possible sources of errors, which is the starting point for risk assessment, but what follows is simply a question of whether one can do anything to reduce those errors, and if yes, what can actually be done.

Table 1
CMS/CDC risk assessment worksheet

Risk Assessment Component	What Are Our Possible Sources of Errors?	Can Our Identified Sources of Errors Be Reduced?	How Can We Reduce Identified Sources of Error?
Specimen			
Test system			
Reagent			
Environment			
Testing personnel			

From CDC, CMS, US Department of Health and Human Services. Developing an IQCP: a step-by-step guide. Available at: wwwn.cdc.gov/CLIA/Resources/IQCP/.

Table 2
CMS/CDC quality control plan worksheet

Type of Quality Control	Frequency	Criteria for Acceptability

From CDC, CMS, US Department of Health and Human Services. Developing an IQCP: a step-by-step guide. Available at: wwwn.cdc.gov/CLIA/Resources/IQCP/.

Table 3
CMS/CDC quality assessment worksheet

QA Activity to Monitor	Frequency	Assessment of QA Activity (Variation from Policy?)	Corrective Action (When Indicated)

Abbreviation: QA, quality assessment.
From CDC, CMS, US Department of Health and Human Services. Developing an IQCP: a step-by-step guide. Available at: wwwn.cdc.gov/CLIA/Resources/IQCP/.

That is fine and good, but that is not risk assessment. This is simply hazard identification followed by a decision whether or not to do something about the hazards, regardless of their potential impact on the patient.

Risk, by definition, relates to the probability or frequency of failures that cause harm, and the severity of that harm. Failures occur because of hazards or failure modes that are present in the testing process. Identification of hazards is the first step of risk analysis. Estimation of risk should then follow, which means assigning values to the probability of occurrence of harm and the severity of harm. Once those values have been assigned, risk can be evaluated by comparison of the estimated risk with criteria for acceptable risk. Unacceptable risks should then be mitigated by prevention (to reduce occurrence), detection (by implementing controls), and providing physicians with information for safe use (to reduce severity).

In the CMS/CDC guide for developing an IQCP, there is no assessment of probability of occurrence or severity of harm, there is no assignment of values for risk factors, no evaluation of the expected risk, and no comparison with criteria for acceptable risk. There is actually no assessment of risk. This is CMS's practical solution to the difficulties of risk assessment.

DEVELOPING A TOTAL QUALITY CONTROL PLAN

The concept of a QCP is good, but it is difficult to perform a proper risk assessment to implement a risk-based IQCP. There is an alternative approach in the form of a total QCP that is more widely applicable, particularly for applications other than point-of-care testing. We recommend the general application of total QCPs whenever SQC procedures can be implemented for daily control.

We use the term "total QCP" for our approach to identifying and assembling control mechanisms to monitor the total testing process, which includes preanalytic, analytical, and postanalytic phases of the process. Critical to this approach is optimizing or "right-sizing" the SQC procedure to ensure detection of medically important errors, which can be accomplished with the application of available SQC planning/design tools. Compliance with the CLIA QC requirements is achieved by analysis of control materials and does not depend on formal risk assessment. Nonetheless, a total QCP can provide an effective approach for controlling the total testing process by adding preanalytic and postanalytic controls to the right-sized SQC procedure.

The decision to develop a total QCP or IQCP should be made based on review of current QC practices and their compliance with the CLIA QC options, review of the manufacturer's QC instructions and performance claims, and determination of the Sigma quality of the test and test system. The laboratory director must be involved in this decision because CMS specifically assigns the responsibility to the director[6,7]:

Per the existing CLIA regulations, the laboratory director is responsible for deciding whether the laboratory will utilize IQCP for some or all of its tests and for ensuring that the QCP he/she develops effectively meets the IQCP requirements. It is also incumbent upon the laboratory director to consider the laboratory's clinical and legal responsibilities for providing accurate and reliable testing when approving and signing off on the QCP. Lastly, the laboratory director may assign, in writing, specific duties for the IQCP to qualified individuals in the laboratory but is still responsible overall for the entire testing process.

We recommend developing a total QCP whenever it is possible to analyze at least two levels of controls per day. The laboratory will then comply with the CLIA default option and can focus its attention on optimizing the SQC procedure to detect medically important errors. Preanalytic and postanalytic controls can be added to cover the total testing process, but a detailed risk assessment is not required, thus simplifying the development process.

GENERAL APPROACH

Fig. 1 describes a general approach for developing QCPs. The laboratory should begin by auditing current QC practices for compliance with the CLIA QC options. For those applications where a QCP is to be developed, it is important to identify potential hazards by reviewing the manufacturer's directions for use and QC instructions. Next, the laboratory should determine quality on the Sigma-scale from the manufacturer's performance claims, from performance validation studies in the laboratory (or

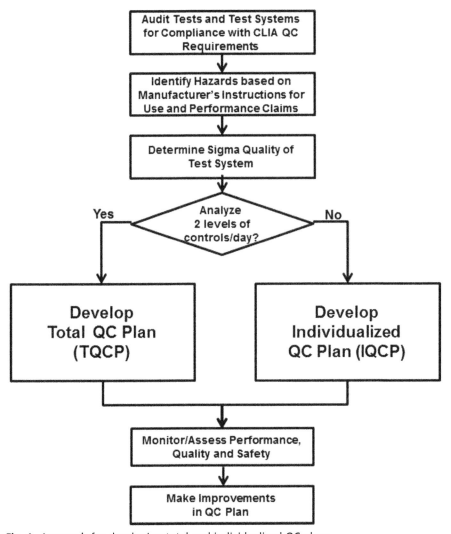

Fig. 1. Approach for developing total and individualized QC plans.

documented in the literature), or from ongoing performance from QC materials and proficiency testing surveys.

A Sigma-metric can be calculated from the quality requirement for the test expressed as an allowable total error (TEa or ATE) and the precision (SD [standard deviation], %CV [coefficient of variation]) and accuracy (bias) observed for the measurement procedure, as follows:

$$Sigma = (TEa - |Bias|)/SD$$

where all terms are expressed in concentration units. Percentage units may also be used, in which case the equation is typically written as follows:

$$Sigma = (\%TEa - |\%Bias|)/\%CV$$

Quality on the Sigma-scale is described as "world class" when Sigma is six or higher and "not fit for production" when Sigma is less than or equal to three. For SQC, methods with high Sigma quality are controlled with simpler rules and fewer control measurements. Methods with low Sigma quality require more control rules and more control measurements and ultimately may not be controllable by affordable SQC.

Based on this information, the laboratory should decide whether or not it can comply with the CLIA default option of analyzing a minimum of two levels of controls per day. If the answer is yes, then the laboratory should maintain the practice of using traditional control materials and adopt the strategy for developing a total QCP, as indicated on the left side of **Fig. 1**. If the answer is no, then the laboratory should develop an IQCP, as indicated by the right side of the figure.

STEP-BY-STEP PROCEDURE

As shown in **Fig. 2**, the approach typically involves a small project team (step 1) whose members have expertise about the preanalytic, analytical, and postanalytic phases or subprocesses. Hazard identification begins with review of manufacturer's instructions for use, QC instructions, claims for performance, and disclosures of limitations (step 2). This second step is consistent with the CMS/CDC guidance to identify hazards, therefore it is useful when developing either a total QCP or an IQCP.

In a total QCP, the emphasis is to optimize SQC and then prioritize other analytical controls on the basis of the Sigma quality determined for the method (step 3). The Sigma-metric is inherently risk-based because it predicts the number of defects produced by the testing process. With knowledge of Sigma, SQC procedures can be right-sized using planning tools, such as Westgard Sigma Rules (step 4). Other analytical controls can be prioritized based on the observed Sigma quality (step 5), followed by addition of preanalytic and postanalytic controls to monitor the total testing process (step 6).

The various controls that have been identified are then assembled into a total QCP, which should specify the frequency of applying the different controls, criteria for acceptance, and guidance on what to do if a control is not acceptable (step 7). A quality assurance program should also be prepared to monitor the actual performance achieved under routine operation (step 8). Finally, the QCP must be documented, including the development process and the data used (step 9).

RIGHT-SIZING STATISTICAL QUALITY CONTROL

Available SQC planning tools include the Sigma-metric SQC selection tool,[11] charts of operating specifications (OPSpecs Charts),[12] a computer program that prepares

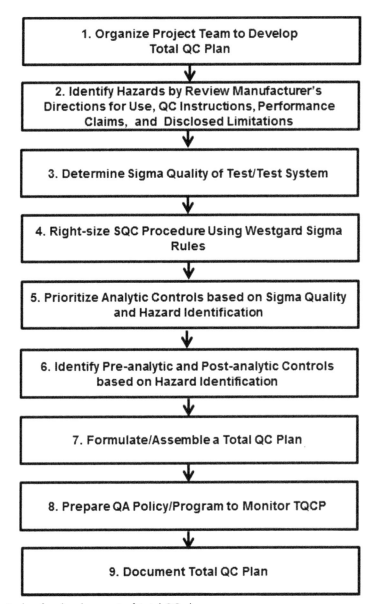

Fig. 2. A plan for development of total QC plans.

these graphs and charts and automatically selects appropriate control rules and the total number of control measurements (N),[13] and a new simple graphic tool called Westgard Sigma Rules.[14]

Westgard Sigma Rules are rules of thumb that identify the appropriate control rules and Ns as a function of the Sigma-metric determined for a test. See **Fig. 3** for the Westgard Sigma Rules for two levels of control materials. At first glance, this figure looks just like the traditional Westgard Rules diagram except there is no 2 SD warning rule. That is an important distinction, but the most important change is at the bottom of

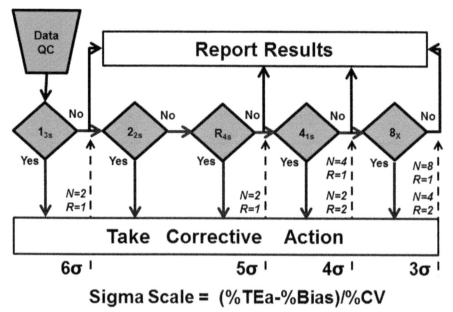

Fig. 3. Westgard Sigma Rules for two levels of controls. Note Sigma-scale at the bottom of the diagram. To apply, determine sigma-metric, locate on the Sigma-scale, identify rules *above* and to the *left*, find N and R *above* the sigma value.

the diagram where there is a Sigma-scale. That scale provides guidance for the rules that should be applied based on the Sigma quality of each assay determined in the laboratory.

The dashed vertical lines that originate at the Sigma-scale show the extent of the rules that should be applied based on the Sigma quality determined in the laboratory. For example:

- 6-Sigma quality requires only the 1_{3s} control rule. The notation N = 2 R = 1 (alongside the dashed arrow) indicates that a total of two control measurements (N = 2) are needed in a single run (R = 1).
- 5-Sigma quality requires three rules, $1_{3s}/2_{2s}/R_{4s}$, with two control measurements in each run (N = 2, R = 1). See **Fig. 4** for illustration of this application.
- 4-Sigma quality requires addition of a fourth rule and implementation of a $1_{3s}/2_{2s}/R_{4s}/4_{1s}$ multirule, preferably with four control measurements in each run (N = 4, R = 1), or alternatively, two control measurements in each of two runs (N = 2, R = 2), using the 4_{1s} rule to inspect the control rules across both runs. This second option suggests dividing a day's work into two runs and monitoring each with two controls.
- <4-Sigma quality requires a multirule procedure that includes the 8x rule, which can be implemented with four control measurements in each of two runs (N = 4, R = 2) or alternatively with two control measurements in each of four runs (N = 2, N = 4). The first option suggests dividing a days' work into two runs with four control measurements per run, whereas the second option suggests dividing a day's work into four runs and monitoring each with two controls.

A similar diagram in **Fig. 5** describes Westgard Sigma Rules for three levels of controls.

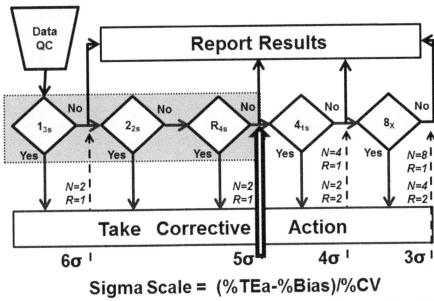

Fig. 4. Example of Cholesterol 5.0 sigma method, where TEa is 10%, bias is 0.0%, and CV (coefficient of variation) is 2.0%. Appropriate SQC procedure is $1_{3s}/2_{2s}/R_{4s}$ multirule procedure having a total of two control measurements per run (N = 2, R = 1).

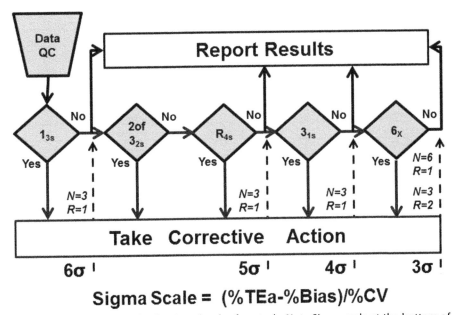

Fig. 5. Westgard Sigma Rules for three levels of controls. Note Sigma-scale at the bottom of the diagram. To apply, determine sigma-metric, locate on the Sigma-scale, identify rules *above* and to the *left*, find N and R *above* the sigma value.

- 6-Sigma quality requires only a 1_{3s} rule and one measurement on each of three levels of controls in a single run.
- 5-Sigma quality requires adding the $2of3_{2s}$ and R_{4s} rules for use with one measurement on each of three levels of controls in a single run.
- 4-Sigma quality requires adding a 3_{1s} rule for use with one measurement on each of three controls in a single run.
- <4-Sigma quality requires a multirule procedure that includes the 6x rule and a doubling of control measurements to a total of six, which suggests that the three levels of controls be analyzed in duplicate in one run (N = 6, R = 1) or the day's work divided into two runs with three control measurements per run (N = 3, R = 2). If a 9x rule were substituted for the 6x rule, then a day's work could be divided into three runs with three controls per run (N = 3, R = 3).

ASSEMBLING A TOTAL QUALITY CONTROL PLAN

After right-sizing the SQC procedure, one is in compliance with the CLIA requirements to analyze a minimum of two levels of controls and also the ISO 15189 requirement to verify attainment of the intended quality by detecting medically important errors. One should then add relevant preanalytic and postanalytic controls without the need for a formal risk assessment. The strategy is to satisfy the CLIA QC requirement without performing a risk assessment, but to still ensure quality testing by inclusion of the

Table 4
Example of a total QC plan that identifies control mechanisms, frequency of use, and acceptability criteria

Control Mechanism	Frequency	Criteria for Acceptance
Preanalytic controls		
Patient identification	Every patient	Correct ID
Specimen labeling	Every specimen	Correct name on label
Sample inspection	Every sample	No visible hemolysis or lipemia
Analytical operator controls		
Standard operating procedure	Yearly SOP review	Signed by technical supervisor
Operator training	Every operator	Proficiency by supervisor
Operator checklists	Daily	Supervisor review
System maintenance	Manuf. schedule	Supervisor review
Operator competency	Yearly	Proficiency assessment
Analytical test system controls		
Sample acceptability	Every sample	Instrument indices and volume limits
Calibration checks	Manuf./Reg.	Controls within limits
Statistical QC	Startup + monitor	Controls within limits
Proficiency testing	3 times per year	Acceptable scores
Analytical test review controls		
Limit checks	Every sample	Instrument working range check
Implausible values	Every sample	Critical limits
Postanalytic controls		
Confirm/call critical values	Each test result	Critical limits
Turnaround time	Each sample	60 min for Stats, 3 h other
Customer feedback	Each complaint	Supervisor review

most critical preanalytic, analytical, and postanalytic controls. One should identify those controls on the basis of experience, with help from others involved in the total testing process, guidance based on the Sigma quality of the test system, and guidance from the manufacturer's instructions for use.

An example total QCP is shown in **Table 4**. The minimum preanalytic control is to examine samples for acceptability for analysis (sample type, volume, potential interferences). Operator controls are essential, such as proper training and adherence to standard operating procedures (SOPs), checklists, and maintenance schedules. SQC is the essential analytical control and may be supplemented by other analytical controls, such as limit and implausible values checks. Proficiency testing or external quality assessment is important for long-term monitoring of the analytical quality of the testing process. Postanalytic controls should include the identification of critical values for immediate reporting and the monitoring of turnaround time.

SUMMARY

Medical laboratories can adopt the concept of a total QCP without the need to perform a formal risk assessment, adding preanalytic and postanalytic controls to right-sized SQC procedures to monitor the total testing process. Right-sized SQC is the key building block in a total QCP and can be relied on to detect many of the possible failure modes in the analytical process. Other controls can be added based on knowledge and experience, but there is no requirement to perform a formal risk assessment. Instead, the determination of Sigma quality provides a general assessment of risk that guides the selection of SQC procedures and the addition of other controls. A total QCP provides a good starting point for improving laboratory QC and a logical building block for developing IQCPs. Further details on the application of risk management principles for IQCPs is found in *Basic QC Practices*,[15] which describes a simplified risk assessment model that should be useful in medical laboratories and recommends the use of "patient test repeats" as controls in point-of-care settings. Risk-based thinking is good in principle, but requires considerable study and experience to develop quantitative QC applications in a medical laboratory.

REFERENCES

1. Westgard JO, Westgard SA. Quality control in the age of risk management. Clin Lab Med 2013;33(1):1–194.

2. Westgard JO. Perspectives on quality control, risk management, and analytical quality management. Clin Lab Med 2013;33:1–14.

3. Person NB. Developing risk-based quality control plans: an overview of CLSI EP23A. Clin Lab Med 2013;33:15–26.

4. Ehrmeyer SS. Satisfying regulatory and accreditation requirements for quality control. Clin Lab Med 2013;33:27–40.

5. US Centers for Medicare & Medicaid Services (CMS). Medicare, Medicaid, and CLIA programs: laboratory requirements relating to quality systems and certain personnel qualifications. Final rule. Fed Regist 2003;68(16):3640–714.

6. Appendix C of State Operations Manual, Regulations and Interpretive Guidelines for Laboratories and Laboratory Services. Available at: www.cms.gov/clia/appendc.asp. Accessed June 9, 2016.

7. CMS Memo of August 16, 2013: Individualized quality control plan (IQCP): a new quality control (QC) option. Available at: www.cms.gov/Regulations-and-Guidance/Legislation/CLIA/Downloads/IQCPbenefits.pdf.

8. ISO 15189. Medical laboratories – requirements for quality and competence. Geneva (Switzerland): International Organization for Standards; 2012.
9. CLSI EP23A. Laboratory quality control based on risk management. Wayne (PA): Clinical and Laboratory Standards Institute; 2011.
10. CDC, CMS, US Department of Health and Human Services. Developing an IQCP: a step-by-step guide. Available at: wwwn.cdc.gov/CLIA/Resources/IQCP/.
11. CLSI C24A3. Statistical quality control for quantitative measurement procedures: principles and definitions. Wayne (PA): Clinical and Laboratory Standards Institute; 2005.
12. Westgard JO. Charts of operational process specifications (OPSpecs Charts) for assessing the precision, accuracy, and quality control needed to satisfy proficiency testing criteria. Clin Chem 1992;38:1226–33.
13. Westgard JO. Assuring the right quality right. Chapter 11. How to use the EZ-Rules 3 computer program. Madison (WI): Westgard QC, Inc; 2007.
14. Westgard JO, Westgard SA. Basic quality management systems. Chapter 12. Designing SQC procedures. Madison (WI): Westgard QC, Inc; 2014.
15. Westgard JO, Westgard SA. Basic QC practices. 4th edition. Madison (WI): Westgard QC, Inc; 2016.

Accreditation of Individualized Quality Control Plans by the College of American Pathologists

CrossMark

Gerald A. Hoeltge, MD

KEYWORDS

- Laboratory accreditation • Laboratory inspection • Quality control
- Risk management • Clinical laboratory • Medical laboratory

KEY POINTS

- Accreditation of a laboratory that has implemented an individualized quality control plan (IQCP) is grounded in principles of risk management.
- Inspection of an IQCP activity evaluates process rather than outcome.
- All 3 elements of an IQCP must be documented: risk assessment, the laboratory's quality plan, and follow-up assessment.
- New accreditation requirements had to be written and old requirements related to equivalent quality control rewritten.
- Robust support systems, particularly training and communication, are essential to the success of the IQCP accreditation process.

When the Centers for Medicare and Medicaid Services (CMS) announced their plan to allow each laboratory to devise its own approach to analytical quality control (QC),[1] the Laboratory Accreditation Program (LAP) of the College of American Pathologists (CAP) was faced with a decision. Should the LAP follow suit and allow its participants to develop individual schemes for QC? QC is central to the reliability of laboratory testing. Structured requirements for inspecting QC, initiated 50 years earlier, had dismissed the notion of QC strategies that varied from laboratory to laboratory. A control system based on individualized risks, with the determination of those risks to be performed by the laboratory itself, seemed impossible to inspect.

At the same time, administrators of the program realized that at least some of its subscribers would seek to develop an individualized QC plan (IQCP) for 1 or more

---

Disclosure: The author has nothing to disclose.
College of American Pathologists, 325 Waukegan Road, Northfield, IL 60093-2750, USA
E-mail address: gahfcap@gmail.com

Clin Lab Med 37 (2017) 151–162
http://dx.doi.org/10.1016/j.cll.2016.09.012   labmed.theclinics.com
0272-2712/17/© 2016 Elsevier Inc. All rights reserved.

of its tests. To refuse to inspect a laboratory's IQCP implementation was in the best interest of neither the laboratory nor the program. A fundamental change in how the LAP would regard quality management was inevitable.

This article discusses that dilemma, how it was solved, and the inspection tools developed by the college for accreditation of a laboratory that chooses to follow its unique QC plan. It addresses the options imagined by the LAP and the resources amassed to sort through those options. Both the requirements for accreditation regarding IQCPs and the support systems available to participating laboratories are described.

BACKGROUND

The CAP accredits nearly 8000 laboratories in 50 countries. The CAP is deemed by the CMS as an accreditation organization (AO) under Clinical Laboratory Improvement Amendments (CLIA).[2] Most certified laboratories offering a range of specialty tests choose the CAP as their AO. CMS requires each AO to inspect for compliance with the CLIA regulations. An AO is allowed to impose additional requirements, but, at a minimum, on-site inspectors must compare the laboratory's performance with the CLIA regulations.

CAP accredits a wide variety of clinical laboratories. Some have thousands of employees, and others are small. Hospital laboratories integral to a health care delivery system are accredited, as are independent laboratories. The CAP's accreditation program spans all of the clinical laboratory specialties. The complete set of LAP checklist requirements in the 2015 edition totals 2890, although only those requirements defined by the laboratory's scope of activity are printed on its checklist, which is tailored to its on-site inspection. CAP inspectors are practicing laboratory professionals who volunteer their time and expertise in the spirit of peer review. It is critical that checklist requirements be written in precise language to avoid differences in interpretation but be sufficiently succinct to be managed within the time allotted. That CAP inspectors evaluate those requirements in a uniform manner is a tenet of the program. To introduce a requirement intended to be evaluated differently from site to site was unfamiliar territory.

The consensus process of the Clinical and Laboratory Standards Institute (CLSI) preceded the regulated IQCP option. CAP, a founding member of CLSI, participated in the development of those consensus documents. CLSI had developed EP18-A, *Quality Management for Unit-Use Testing*, in 2002.[3] EP18-A described how a manufacturer of an in vitro testing device and its users, particularly those self-contained devices that use cartridges used only once, identifies and controls the modes of failure specific to the use of that device. The subsequent version, EP18-A2, published as *Risk Management Techniques to Identify and Control Laboratory Error Sources*,[4] focused on the process of risk assessment.

EP18-A2 became the theoretic construct behind CLSI's EP23-A, *Laboratory Quality Control Based on Risk Management*.[5] EP23-A is a consensus guideline, not an evaluation protocol. It was developed by individuals broadly representative of the laboratory community: regulatory authorities, manufacturers of in vitro devices, and clinical laboratory professionals. Unlike traditional QC (most often described as 2 levels of external controls per test per day), the IQCP option expects the laboratory to identify and then control failure modes along the entire path of workflow (ie, from preanalysis, the assay itself, to postanalysis). Failure-mode analysis directs the user to consider personnel training, environmental conditions, patient populations, and logistical support systems as well as the analytical process.

The LAP recognized the challenges for inspection of an IQCP. How would the adequacy of a risk assessment be determined? Would manufacturers of in vitro diagnostics provide users with sufficient technical data to identify analytical failure modes? The EP18-A2 protocol lists 124 potential sources of failure in its appendix; would all of these potential source of failure need to be considered? These and other questions had to be answered rapidly. The LAP checklists are published in a new edition each year, and the IQCP regulatory option would take effect in 2016. The IQCP option had to be defined and announced early in 2015 to allow participants time to develop any plans for implementation.

THE VALIDATION CONUNDRUM

An inspection strategy defined by fixed standards, no matter how arbitrary, may be the basis for interlaboratory comparison. Traditional QC measures quality by periodic analysis of samples with measurands that have expected values. Measurements that differ from those expected values are labeled QC failures. The rate and size of such differences from what is expected permits comparison over time and between laboratories. A new method may be declared better than an old method if the results better approximate the expected results; that is, when there are fewer QC failures.

Individualized laboratory QC is not based on external standards. Moreover, an IQCP is impossible to validate. Each user's approach to systematic identification and mitigation of potential causes of failure is unique. The frequency with which the user chooses to test control samples is driven by the identified points of failure and an assessment of their risks. An IQCP's QC strategy goes beyond the number, type, and frequency of analytical control samples. Its criteria for acceptable performance are unique to that environmental setting. It includes the monitoring of the reagents and testing environment, specimen quality, instrument calibration and function, and the performance of the testing personnel. Traditional QC is not the benchmark. The familiar rules for interlaboratory comparison are not possible because of the lack of an external standard to define acceptable performance. A laboratory chooses the IQCP option on the reasonable but unproven assumption that quality improves when failure modes are controlled.

The assumption that a well-done risk assessment, a QC plan based on that assessment, and periodic metrics that gauge the test system along the entire path of work flow will be superior to one that measures analytical quality according to fixed or external standards may be unvalidated, but traditional QC as defined by regulatory and accrediting authorities is equally unvalidated. Traditional QC may miss out-of-control conditions because the intermittent periodicity of control samples exposes the testing process to out-of-control results between QC events.

External assessment by any regulatory body or an accrediting organization is grounded in measurable standards of performance. To inspect a laboratory's IQCP, or any other activity in the laboratory, requires objective criteria expressed in clear language, especially for an AO that has thousands of inspectors. If the CAP were to incorporate the CMS's IQCP option into its accreditation program, how would it determine the acceptability of a laboratory's individual and unique strategy? Would it require the laboratory to show that its IQCP was as good as or better than the standard approach to QC? Would it develop device-specific rules to hold all users of that particular device to the same accreditation criteria? Or would it accept the premise that a risk-based strategy built on a consensus model is an appropriate alternative to traditional QC?

The college chose to pursue the last of these alternatives, deferring to each laboratory director's judgment as to whether the data generated during the risk assessment justified the alternative strategy. The LAP's requirements for IQCP therefore target the process, not the decision. How the laboratory performs its assessment, what it includes, and who approves of the process became central elements of the inspection.

THE INDIVIDUALIZED QUALITY CONTROL PLAN DEVELOPMENT GROUP

The college convened a working group to develop an IQCP inspection strategy. Key members of the CAP's Point-of-Care Testing Committee and the LAP Checklists Committee met to create a workable proposal on an expedited schedule. It was understood that the working group's proposal would be vetted by the committees responsible for training of inspectors and by the college's specialists in communication.

The working group divided its project into 3 tasks:

1. Write the requirements inspectors are to use when evaluating a scheme for quality management as developed by the laboratory. The brochures on IQCP published by CMS were the group's basic resource,[6] because any IQCP option offered by an AO to its participants would require approval from CMS. CMS had directed its own inspectors to focus on laboratory process for mitigating risk rather than on the laboratory director's medical decision making. CAP's *Standards for Laboratory Accreditation*[7] vest ultimate responsibility for compliance with the laboratory director, which includes QC. Within the context of IQCP, requirements were written to document the director's review of the thoroughness of the risk assessment, the director's determination that the QC plan sufficiently mitigates the risks before implementation, and how the plan will be managed going forward.

   The working group decided to focus the requirements on point-of-care testing; specifically, those test systems that featured a manufacturer-supplied internal control (built-in, electronic, or procedural). Although a risk-management strategy could define an individualized approach to quality for any testing platform, it was predicted that most early adopters would choose it in settings with multiple, identical devices. The group further decided to limit those requirements to non-waived testing (ie, those classified by CMS as moderate or high complexity). In situ hybridization test systems were initially included as well in the initial strategy because most use procedural, internal controls. Generic requirements were to be written for the inspection of the laboratory's risk assessment, for its QC plan, and how it would assess the quality of the test system after implementation.

2. Part of the CMS's announcement allowing IQCPs was a critical corollary: its equivalent QC (EQC) regulation[8] would sunset at the end of 2015. The EQC alternative, which had been available since 2003, was written primarily for office laboratories operating single-use devices. EQC had allowed laboratories to reduce the frequency of external QC under specified conditions. The LAP had offered a modified version of the EQC option to its participants when a test system with adequate internal controls had been validated by the laboratory. Twenty-five checklist requirements detailed the EQC option. An additional 22 requirements supported the EQC option in related ways, such as quality management, corrective action, and instrument function checks. Each of these had to be deleted or altered for the 2015 edition.

3. In October 2014, CMS added new requirements for microbiology to its IQCP regulation.[9] This unexpected addition surprised the microbiology community. For many years, measurements of the quality of media, the use of microbial identification systems, and the practice of antimicrobial susceptibility testing (AST) had followed the

consensus standards of CLSI.[10-15] The data behind those standards were very extensive and had taken years to compile. It would be impossible for any laboratory to reproduce such resources. CMS's addition to the end of EQC prohibited AOs from incorporating CLSI publications as normative standards into their requirements for accreditation. CAP, CLSI, and the American Society for Microbiology (ASM) immediately began developing guidelines for those microbiologic laboratories that use commercially prepared media, use microbial identification systems, and perform AST. The LAP began to work with its Microbiology Resource Committee to convert those guidelines into checklist language.

All 3 writing tasks had to be completed by the summer of 2014 to allow time for stakeholders to review and revise any drafted requirements. The CMS required AOs to show that its requirements were at least as stringent as CMS's own inspection guidelines.[16] The CAP submitted its drafted checklist requirements on IQCP to the CMS in November 2014.

CHECKLIST LANGUAGE

The CAP working group developed 5 general requirements for a laboratory's IQCP to complete the first task and placed them within the All Common Checklist (COM). COM applies to every area of the laboratory. (A note excluded anatomic pathology and cytopathology to match the CMS guideline.) Only those IQCPs (1) that addressed non-waived testing, (2) that reduced external control analysis to a frequency less than the limits defined for standard QC (equivalent to those specified in the CLIA regulations) but not less than those indicated in the manufacturer's instructions, and (3) that targeted test platforms with an internal control system would be eligible for IQCP inspection. For convenience, a listing of all of the CLIA regulations related to QC was included.

Like all checklist items, each of the 5 new requirements featured a requirement number, a title, a declarative statement to summarize the requirement, explanatory notes, and literature references. The first 4 requirements cover risk assessment, the elements of the QC plan, how quality will be assessed following implementation, and plan approval. The fifth defines how the laboratory is to describe each of the IQCPs at the time of application. The entry, which follows a defined format, provides the assigned inspector with the specifications for the requirement. **Box 1** and **Fig. 1**, from the 2015 edition, provide examples. The complete set of IQCP requirements is available on the CAP Web site.[17]

The specialty checklists cross-reference the 5 general requirements in the COM checklist with a reminder that reads, "If an internal quality control process (eg, electronic/procedural/built-in) is used instead of an external control material to meet daily quality control requirements, the laboratory must have an individualized quality control plan."

Once an IQCP has been implemented, inspectors are instructed to determine whether the laboratory is monitoring appropriate metrics. For example, records of repeated QC failures may signal the need to revise the laboratory's risk mitigation practices. Each laboratory must monitor quality indicators that are specific for each of its IQCPs. The requirements for record keeping are specified. In addition, each IQCP must be assessed annually and be reapproved by the laboratory director or designee.

The editorial task in microbiology was greatly facilitated by guidance documents prepared by the ASM, the CLSI, and the CAP. Published on the ASM Web site, microbiology laboratories now had good examples of IQCPs for media control, organism identification, and AST.[18] The examples showed how the practice guidelines of the

---

Box 1
Example of a checklist requirement (2015 edition) for College of American Pathologists accreditation of a laboratory that has implemented an individualized quality control plan

Risk assessment

The IQCP for a test/device/instrument includes a risk assessment to evaluate potential sources of error to include all of the following:

- Preanalytical, analytical, and postanalytical phases of the testing process
- Intended medical uses of the test and impact if inaccurate results are reported (clinical risk)
- Components of the tests, including reagents, environment, specimen, testing personnel, and test system
- Variations in the components based on use of the tests (eg, use in different environments, by different personnel, or multiple identical devices)
- Data from the laboratory's own environment, instrument/equipment performance, and testing personnel
- Manufacturer's instructions and recommendations

Note: the risk assessment must include a process to identify the sources of potential failures and errors for a testing process, and evaluate frequency and impact of those failures and sources of error.

The laboratory director must consider the laboratory's clinical and legal responsibilities for providing accurate and reliable patient test results. Published data and information may be used to supplement the risk assessment, but is not a substitute for the laboratory's own studies and evaluation. The laboratory must involve a representative sample of testing personnel in the process of conducting the risk assessment. It is not necessary for all personnel to be involved.

The risk assessment for laboratories with multiple identical devices must show that an evaluation was performed if there are differences in testing personnel or environments in which testing is performed, with customization of the QC plan as needed.

The QC study performed to assess the performance and stability of the tests must support the QC frequency and elements defined in the laboratory's QC plan. The study must include data representing, at a minimum the maximum interval between runs of external QC. The laboratory may use historical data during the risk assessment for tests already in place.

For affiliated laboratories (eg, systems) with integrated procedures, each accredited laboratory must have its own IQCP approved by the laboratory director. There must be records showing that risks specific to the site were evaluated involving a representative sample of local testing personnel to conduct the risk assessment and that laboratory-specific QC data were used in the study to support the defined frequency of QC. Laboratories may use data from other sites to supplement risk assessments and to support their findings.

Requirement references.[5,23–26] *Courtesy of* College of American Pathologists, Washington, DC; with permission.

CLSI, which had been used by laboratories for many years, could be incorporated into a laboratory-developed QC plan. Doing so would allow current practice to continue, and formulating an IQCP added the benefit of individualized risk management.

PEER REVIEW OF THE CHECKLISTS' REQUIREMENTS

The CMS approved the IQCP updates to the CAP's checklists in March 2015. Between March and July, the entire 2015 checklist edition was vetted by peer reviewers. Thirty-one scientific resource committees reviewed the language of the final draft.

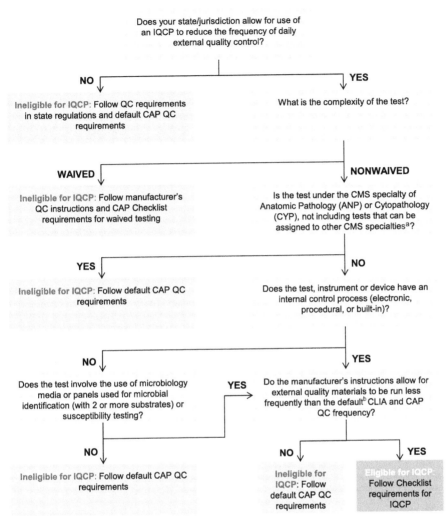

Fig. 1. Algorithm used by CAP inspectors to determine a test's eligibility for IQCP inspection. [a] ANP or CYP tests are ineligible for IQCP unless the testing can be billed under another CMS specialty. [b] The default CAP QC frequency for external QC materials is as follows. (1) Quantitative tests: 2 controls at different concentrations each day of patient testing, except for coagulation tests (2 levels every 8 hours) and blood gas testing (1 level every 8 hours). (2) Qualitative tests: positive and negative controls each day of patient testing. (*Courtesy of College of American Pathologists, Washington, DC; with permission.*)

Simultaneously, the final draft was sent to a panel of 89 participants in the LAP for their feedback. Every comment made by a reviewer was considered before the edition was published on July 28, 2015.

INTERIM CHANGES

To introduce an interim change to a published edition of the checklists is rare. Any change first must be approved by CMS. Because the working version of any participant's set of checklists is printed on demand, the most recent version is used for the on-site inspection.

The college did need to make an interim change to its IQCP requirements late in 2015. The CMS withdrew permission to construct an IQCP for certain molecular-based tests, including fluorescent in situ hybridization, microarrays, and next-generation sequencing. The phrase "internal control," although commonly used to refer to expected, microscopic signals from normal elements of the genome, is a different type of control than was intended when the EQC requirements were rewritten. Molecular-based assays that use a single-use cartridge continue to be eligible for the IQCP option. A CAP e-Alert (a bulletin to laboratories transmitted by e-mail) describing the interim change was sent to all accredited laboratories on December 23, 2015.

SUPPORT SYSTEMS

To supplement the checklist requirements on IQCP, a set of companion forms was constructed. On the first, the applicant laboratory lists all implemented IQCPs to help CAP inspectors manage their inspection activity. Each entry shows the title of the IQCP, its location in the laboratory, and the tests involved.

The second form is used to describe each IQCP in more detail. Although each laboratory is free to use the model of its choosing to construct its plan, inspectors need to see its key points in a structured summary for their audit to be efficient. The participant identifies the instrument or device, all tests covered by that plan, the number of identical devices in operation, each testing site where the plan has been implemented, and a brief statement about the control process used to monitor risk. Covering the categories of reagents, environment, specimen, test system, and testing personnel, the summary helps orient the inspector to the IQCP documents that are written in the laboratory's own style.

Table 1 lists the resources that the CAP provides to laboratories on its Web site to help subscribers understand the IQCP requirements.

Table 1 Individualized quality control plan resources provided to laboratories on the College of American Pathologists Web site	
Resource	**Comment**
Algorithm to determine IQCP eligibility	Graphical tool to aid in determining whether a test system is eligible for CAP accreditation
Changes to the microbiology requirements	Tabular display of changes to the MIC Checklist in the 2015 edition
Frequently Asked Questions Web page	Lists common questions and their answers regarding IQCP
IQCP in Microbiology Q & A	List of common questions specific to microbiology and developed by ASM, CLSI, and the CAP
Template for use with commercial AST systems and examples	Tool developed by ASM, CLSI, and the CAP
Link to online resources provided by CMS	Link to the CMS Web site
Link to online resources provided by ASM, CLSI, and CAP	Links to the CAP Web site
Recorded webinar	Webcast in August 2015 and available for replay on demand at the CAP Web site

TRAINING

Volunteer inspectors must be trained to apply the checklist requirements in a fair and objective manner. For a subject like IQCP, which alters basic processes in an inspection, special training is needed. Training programs are provided to inspectors by the CAP on its Web site. Completion of the introductory courses for team leaders and team members is awarded with 4 credit hours of Continuing Education or Continuing Medical Education credit. Follow-up programs are available for those who want detailed instruction in IQCP inspections, competency assessment, documentation, or detection of systemic deficiencies. **Table 2** lists the training resources provided to CAP inspectors.

CAP's technical staff were trained to manage the new IQCP requirements. Thirty-four technical specialists and staff inspectors field calls and messages regarding the LAP. Whether from laboratories preparing for inspection or from inspectors during an inspection activity, answers to subscribers' questions have to be authoritative and uniform. Subject matter for staff training accrues as participants ask questions. Information on the types of telephone calls and e-mails received is captured in a database. Novel questions and their optimal answers are shared during staff training sessions.

Key issues regarding IQCP extracted from that database have been framed as frequently asked questions (FAQ) and published on the CAP Web site. At the time of this writing, there are 59 questions and answers on that Web page but the number is growing. The FAQ page answers participants' questions about how the checklist describes IQCP inspections. The database of calls is reviewed as each edition of the checklists is prepared. The core requirements for accreditation are written by content experts; explanatory language is revised according to customer feedback.

INTERNATIONAL LABORATORIES

The college accredits 40 laboratories outside the United States and Canada, and 65 others are in the process of accreditation. Most are not CLIA certified. The CAP offers the IQCP option to all of its accredited laboratories regardless of location or CLIA certification. Non-CLIA laboratories were allowed an extra 6 months to prepare and implement their IQCPs.

Table 2
Web site resources for individualized quality control plan inspectors

Resource	Comment
Instructions to inspector	Detailed instructions for an IQCP inspection to supplement those printed in the checklists
IQCP requirements	Includes the 5 COM requirements and a listing of all discipline-specific checklist changes
Algorithm to determine IQCP eligibility	Identical to that provided to laboratories on the CAP Web site
Tip sheet	Identifies the key documents to review and what to look for on each
Online inspector training	Training modules for team leaders and team members on the CAP Web site
Inspection "Do's and Don'ts"	Addresses decisions often faced by inspectors during an on-site inspection
Fast Focus on Compliance: IQCP: "What it Means for an Inspector"	A training video specific to IQCP available on the CAP Web site

Table 3 Communication strategies	
Strategy	**Comment**
CAP TODAY	Monthly magazine with 48,000 subscribers
Webinar	Webcast in August 2015 and available for replay on demand at cap.org
National meetings	Seminars at conventions of the CAP and the CLMA
CAPcast	Streaming audio file on CAP's social network
FAQ sheet	Webpage available at cap.org for download on demand
e-Alert	Emailed notification of interim changes to checklist requirements
Hotline	Toll-free telephone consultations with a technical specialist at CAP

Abbreviation: CLMA, Clinical Laboratory Management Association.

COMMUNICATION

Multiple strategies for communicating the IQCP concept, its impact on laboratory medicine, and the resources are available to participating laboratories (**Table 3**). The CAP's monthly magazine, *CAP TODAY*, published 4 feature articles on risk-managed QC and IQCP between April 2014 and September 2015.[19–22] The college broadcasted a live, 1-hour webcast on the subject of laboratory compliance with the IQCP requirements for accreditation on August 19, 2015; that program is available for replay on demand on the CAP Web site. Seminars on accreditation of laboratories choosing the IQCP option were presented at national meetings of the CAP and of the Clinical Laboratory Management Association. CAP's social media product for college members, CAPcast, has an audio file on IQCP that is available for streaming on demand. The FAQ sheet on IQCP, discussed earlier, is frequently updated to communicate the most recent interpretations of the accreditation requirements. New information on IQCP and interim changes to the checklist are emailed to participants (e-Alerts). In addition, CAP operates a toll-free hotline during regular business hours that is staffed by technical specialists dedicated to the LAPs. In 2015, specialists answered thousands of calls, many of which concerned IQCPs.

SUMMARY

Recognition that accredited laboratories have the tools and expertise to individualize their QC strategies is a milestone in the history of the CAP accreditation program. The checklist requirements that frame the IQCP option were developed through the consensus of content experts and participants. Laboratory standards, no matter how well written, are insufficient to guarantee a successful accreditation program. The organization must commit resources to support the application of those standards. Inspectors and staff must be trained and educational tools developed. Participating laboratories need to know how to find the tools needed to implement a novel activity. The CAP helps with educational programs, Web site linkages to expert resources, and toll-free access to technical specialists on its staff. Customer feedback drives continuous improvement at the CAP. The future direction of the CAP's accreditation of laboratory QC will be driven by the needs of its participants.

ACKNOWLEDGMENTS

Hundreds of people contributed to the final set of accreditation requirements for IQCP and the systems that support them. Deborah A Perry MD, Sharon Geaghan

MD, Christopher Lehman MD, Denise K Driscoll MS, MT(ASCP)SBB, and Karen Peterson-Theis MT(HEW), MLT(ASCP) were key. The author particularly wishes to thank his colleague, Lyn Wielgos MT(ASCP), CAP Checklist Editor, for her tireless commitment.

REFERENCES

1. Centers for Medicare and Medicaid Services. Individualized quality control plan (IQCP): a new Quality Control (QC) Option. 2013. Memorandum S&C: 13-54-CLIA. Available at: https://www.cms.gov/Medicare/Provider-Enrollment-and-Certification/SurveyCertificationGenInfo/Downloads/Survey-and-Cert-Letter-13-54.pdf. Accessed March 13, 2016.
2. Code of Federal Regulations. Title 42, Part 493, §493.551. 2010.
3. Clinical and Laboratory Standards Institute. Quality management for unit-use testing; approved guideline. Wayne (PA): CLSI; 2002. CLSI document EP18-A.
4. Clinical and Laboratory Standards Institute. Risk management techniques to identify and control laboratory error sources; approved guideline—second edition. Wayne (PA): CLSI; 2009. CLSI document EP18–A2.
5. Clinical and Laboratory Standards Institute. Laboratory quality control based on risk management; approved guideline. Wayne (PA): CLSI; 2011. CLSI document EP23-A.
6. Centers for Medicare and Medicaid Services. CLIA Brochure #12, "Considerations when deciding to develop an IQCP" and brochure #13, "What is an IQCP?" Available at: http://www.cms.gov/Regulations-and-Guidance/Legislation/CLIA/CLIA_Brochures.html. Accessed March 13, 2016.
7. College of American Pathologists. Standards for laboratory accreditation. Northfield (IL): College of American Pathologists; 2013.
8. CLIA Final Rules, US Department of Health and Human Services. Medicare, Medicaid and CLIA programs: laboratory requirements relating to quality systems and certain personnel qualifications. Final rule. Fed Regist 2003;68:3640–714.
9. Centers for Medicare and Medicaid Services. Effect on microbiology laboratories due to the removal of references to the Clinical Laboratory Standards Institute (CLSI) and to CLSI Documents. 2015. Memorandum S&C: 15-07-CLIA. Available at: https://www.cms.gov/Medicare/Provider-Enrollment-and-Certification/SurveyCertificationGenInfo/Downloads/Survey-and-Cert-Letter-15-07.pdf. Accessed March 13, 2016.
10. Clinical and Laboratory Standards Institute. Performance standards for antimicrobial disk susceptibility tests; approved standard—twelfth edition. Wayne (PA): CLSI; 2015. CLSI document M02–A12.
11. Clinical and Laboratory Standards Institute. Methods for dilution antimicrobial susceptibility tests for bacteria that grow aerobically; approved standard—tenth edition. Wayne (PA): CLSI; 2015. CLSI document M07–A10.
12. National Committee for Clinical Laboratory Standards. Quality control for commercially prepared microbiological culture media; approved standard—third edition. Wayne (PA): NCCLS; 2004. NCCLS document M22–A3.
13. Clinical and Laboratory Standards Institute. Quality control for commercial microbial identification systems; approved guideline. Wayne (PA): CLSI; 2008. CLSI document M50-A.
14. Clinical and Laboratory Standards Institute. Verification of commercial microbial identification and antimicrobial susceptibility testing systems. 1st edition. Wayne (PA): CLSI; 2015. CLSI guideline M52.

15. Clinical and Laboratory Standards Institute. Performance standards for antimicrobial susceptibility testing. 25th edition. Wayne (PA): CLSI; 2015. CLSI supplement M100S.
16. Centers for Medicare and Medicaid Services. Interpretive guidelines for laboratories; Appendix C. Available at: https://www.cms.gov/Regulations-and-Guidance/Legislation/CLIA/Interpretive_Guidelines_for_Laboratories.html. Accessed March 13, 2016.
17. 2015 IQCP Requirements. CAP Web site. 2015. Available at: http://www.cap.org/ShowProperty?nodePath=/UCMCon/Contribution%20Folders/WebContent/pdf/iqcp-requirements.pdf. Accessed April 13, 2016.
18. American Society for Microbiology. IQCP. Available at: http://clinmicro.asm.org/index.php/lab-management/laboratory-management/445-iqcp-iqcp. Accessed March 14, 2016.
19. Paxton A. Risk management steps up labs' QC game under IQCP. College of American Pathologists: CAP TODAY Web site; 2014. Available at: http://www.captodayonline.com/risk-management-steps-up-labs-qc-game-under-iqcp/. Accessed April 13, 2016.
20. Paxton A. In lab QC, how much room for improvement? College of American Pathologists: CAP TODAY Web site; 2014. Available at. http://www.captodayonline.com/lab-qc-much-room-improvement/. Accessed April 13, 2016.
21. Paxton A. IQCP worries? Help with what ends and begins. College of American Pathologists: CAP TODAY Web site; 2015. Available at. http://www.captodayonline.com/iqcp-worries-help-ends-begins/. Accessed April 13, 2016.
22. Paxton A. Full-court collaboration in transition to IQCP. College of American Pathologists: CAP TODAY Web site; 2015. Available at. http://www.captodayonline.com/full-court-collaboration-transition-iqcp/. Accessed April 13, 2016.
23. Centers for Medicare and Medicaid Services (CMS). Individual Quality Control Plan (IQPC) for Clinical Laboratory Improvement Amendments (CLIA) laboratory nonwaived testing. Available at: http://www.cms.gov/Regulations-and-Guidance/Legislation/CLIA/Downloads/IQCP-announcement-letter-for-CLIA-CoC-and-PPM-labs.pdf. Accessed October 31, 2016.
24. Department of Health and Human Services, Centers for Medicare & Medicaid Services. Brochure #13. CLIA Individualized Quality Control Plan, What is an IQCP?. 2014. Available at: http://www.cms.gov/Regulations-and-Guidance/Legislation/CLIA/Downloads/CLIAbrochure13.pdf. Accessed October 31, 2016.
25. Nichols JH. Laboratory quality control based on risk management. Ann Saudi Med 2011;31:223–8.
26. Yundt-Pacheco J, Parvin CA. Validating the performance of QC procedures. Clin Lab Med 2013;33:75–88.

Sunway Medical Laboratory Quality Control Plans Based on Six Sigma, Risk Management and Uncertainty

CrossMark

Jamuna Jairaman, BSc, MPH*, Zarinah Sakiman, BSc, Lee Suan Li, BSc

KEYWORDS

- Analytical quality control • Six Sigma • Risk management • Uncertainty

KEY POINTS

- Measurement uncertainty, risk management, and Sigma metrics are often discussed as individual approaches, sometimes in conflict with each other. But in truth, these approaches can all be implemented together and provide complementary strength in assuring the quality of laboratory testing.
- Sustained effort and implementation of Sigma metrics result in continuous improvement of assay quality and reductions in costs and defective test results.
- Sigma metrics provide not only assistance in optimizing routine laboratory operation but also greatly assist in the selection of appropriate new instruments and methodology.
- Risk management allows laboratories to expand their quality assurance to cover the total testing process.
- Measurement uncertainty is an essential calculation for International Organization for Standardization 15189 certification, but often these figures are not routinely reported with patient test results and requires the greatest effort to educate laboratorians and clinicians about the meaningful use of these estimates.

INTRODUCTION

Any laboratory total testing process involves 3 major phases: the preanalytical, analytical, and postanalytical phases. All 3 areas can contribute to sources of errors resulting in poor patient care. Studies in the 1990s and 2000s led many to believe that about 80% of the errors are found in the preanalytical and postanalytical phases, whereas

Disclosures: None.
Pathology Laboratory Department, Sunway Medical Centre Sdn Bhd, No. 5 Jalan Lagoon Selatan, Bandar Sunway, Selangor 47500, Malaysia
* Corresponding author.
E-mail address: jamunaj@sunway.com.my

only 20% of the errors occur in the analytical phase. Thus, more support and improvements are focused on preanalysis and postanalysis, and less importance is given to analytical quality, which is assumed to be the least problematic area. Based on daily complaints from users, we noted preanalytical and postanalytical errors are obvious categories of errors, as they are easily detected by clinicians, in contrast to analytical errors in which clinicians depend totally on the laboratory for detection and correction of errors, unless the results are extremely divergent from clinical symptoms. If any test result has an error, the clinicians instruct the laboratory to perform repeat testing. Clinician voices are heard louder than any others, resulting in the perception that preanalytical and postanalytical errors are the bigger issues for laboratories. This finding leads to a misconception about which errors are bigger and need to be managed first. However, this triage might not be correct, as in a hospital laboratory all 3 phases carry equal weight and importance. If we can't get the patient specimen to the laboratory, if we can't perform the test correctly, and if we can't deliver the results back to the right patient, it leads to similar consequences of bad test results and poor patient care.

The core duty of a medical laboratory is to produce correct test results. Therefore, the interlinked 3 phases of the laboratory testing process need to be addressed concurrently and equally. Similar to US laboratories, Malaysian laboratories comply with regulatory requirements in implementation of quality control (QC) systems. Local standards, particularly Malaysian Standards (MS) International Organization for Standardization (ISO) 15189, have led medical laboratories to adopt uncertainty of measurement, "intended use" of clinical needs or requirements, and risk management to develop laboratory-specific quality control plans to reduce errors and enhance quality improvements and patient care. Similarly, international standards such as the Australian Council of Healthcare Standards (ACHS) and The Joint Commission International accreditations require health care sectors to adopt risk management in continuous quality improvement activities. QC is important in a health care setting to assure that a desirable quality standard is achieved. In a broad sense, QC is defined as processes, procedures, and techniques that are adopted to either prevent errors from occurring or to detect errors if they do occur.[1] Therefore, providing education, training, proper system in specimen collection, processing, analyzing correctly and reporting the test result to the right patient is part of the broad approach of QC. A more specific meaning of QC is statistical quality control (SQC), which focuses on monitoring and controlling the analytical phase of a laboratory testing process.[1] The biggest challenge faced by medical laboratories is to choose the right way of doing statistical QC and how much knowledge and skill the analyst has in applying the quality tools such as Six Sigma, measurement of uncertainty, and risk management to assure the quality of laboratory test results.

ANALYTICAL QUALITY CONTROL PLANS WITH SIX SIGMA QUALITY MANAGEMENT SYSTEM AT SUNWAY MEDICAL LABORATORY

In addition to assuring compliance with regulatory requirements, the goal of quality management is to satisfy stakeholders, such as doctors and patients, for reliable laboratory test results. Quality must meet the predetermined requirements to the satisfaction of the users for a particular substance or a service. Quality assurance is sum of all activities that are undertaken to ensure generation of reliable and accurate results or data.[2] An integral part of any analytical quality system is SQC.[1] QC in the medical laboratory is defined as a statistical process used to monitor and evaluate the analytical process that produces patient results.[3] It is essential and crucial for the medical laboratory to select the right QC procedures.

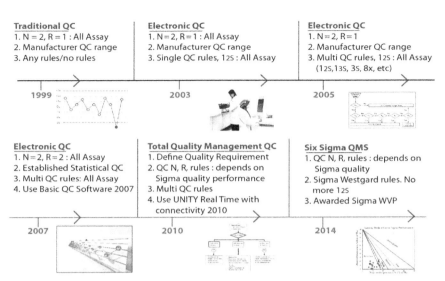

Traditional QC	Electronic QC	Electronic QC
1. N = 2, R = 1 : All Assay	1. N = 2, R = 1 : All Assay	1. N = 2, R = 1
2. Manufacturer QC range	2. Manufacturer QC range	2. Manufacturer QC range
3. Any rules/no rules	3. Single QC rules, 12S : All Assay	3. Multi QC rules, 12S : All Assay (12S,13S, 3S, 8x, etc)

1999   2003   2005

Electronic QC	Total Quality Management QC	Six Sigma QMS
1. N = 2, R = 2 : All Assay	1. Define Quality Requirement	1. QC N, R, rules : depends on Sigma quality
2. Established Statistical QC	2. QC N, R, rules : depends on Sigma quality performance	2. Sigma Westgard rules. No more 12S
3. Multi QC rules: All Assay	3. Multi QC rules	3. Awarded Sigma WVP
4. Use Basic QC Software 2007	4. Use UNITY Real Time with connectivity 2010	

2007   2010   2014

Fig. 1. SunMed journey on best QC practices.

For the last 2 decades, the QC practices of Malaysian medical laboratories have undergone constant evolution and change to provide the best practices and cost-effective monitoring of analytical processes. Traditional QC practices have been the heart of quality systems; however, now they have been expanded to develop a more comprehensive plan for managing analytical quality that will cover all the potential risks or errors and monitoring of the residual risks.[1]

Fig. 1 shows how the laboratory in one of the private hospitals in Malaysia, Sunway Medical Center (SunMed), evolved in their QC practices since the inception of the hospital in 1999.

Initially, SunMed adopted default QC of 2 levels once per day with no QC rules in place. We have been using electronic QC even as early as 2003. The manufacturer ranges were used instead of establishing our own mean and standard deviation. SunMed implemented a single "1:2s" rule for all assays and realized that this "one size fits all" QC rule was not enough for good error detection. Thus, in 2005, we further expanded to implement the multirule (Westgard Rules) for all assays. In 2007, statistical QC and basic QC software was used to monitor the QC performance. Eventually in 2010 the QC software was upgraded to a real-time quality data management system while also defining the quality requirement and running QC according to individual assay performance. SunMed laboratory realized that the use of electronic QC checks are not sufficient; therefore, the need for a quality system is essential to effectively monitor and control the error sources in the total testing process. While the laboratory was in the midst of being verified for a Sigma Verification Program, we implemented the Six Sigma Quality Management System (6σQMS), the new Westgard Sigma Rules, and selected QC runs and rules according to the respective assay performance. One of the reasons that triggered our turning point in QC plans in 2014 was the lack of QC knowledge and awareness among laboratory personnel. Without a sturdy understanding and knowledge about the total testing process and basic QC, it would have been a challenge to sustain good quality in the laboratory. The implementation of 6σQMS enabled us not only to look into the performance of our analyzers, but also take into account the preexamination steps on specimen collection, transportation, and sorting and the postexamination steps on test interpretation and transmission. This resulted in the need for preventive techniques and control mechanisms to prevent sources of errors and improve the current workflow to preserve the level of quality of laboratory test results. SunMed laboratory, while achieving status as a Sigma-verified laboratory, still felt that single QC procedures were not able to monitor all the sources of errors in the total testing process. QC plans and quality management systems (QMSs) were enhanced with additional tools and techniques, some of those are as mentioned below:

- Policies and procedures are in place to describe the standard operating procedures and processes for producing test results.
- Local MS ISO 15189 guidelines are used for essential requirements on best laboratory practices.
- International accreditation such as ACHS looks at overall processes in the hospital where cross-functional teams will be necessary to the preanalytical and postanalytical portion of the total testing processes to mitigate sources of errors and satisfy the needs of doctors and patients.
- Inspection is done by the hospital internal quality audit team and on accreditation assessment by the external assessors on the weak points in the total testing process that requires further improvements.
- External monitoring is done of the analytical performances by comparison and participation in proficiency testing and external quality assessment.
- Quality indicators such as critical value reporting, turnaround time, and specimen rejection rates, give quantitative performance of the testing processes.
- SQC is established for monitoring the analytical performances of the laboratory testing process. The 2 important aspects related to statistical QC are quality planning and quality goals. Quality planning results in the selection and validation of new methods or instruments, whereas quality goals fulfill the ISO standard requirement on the phrase *intended use*. The need to define tolerance limits or total allowable errors is an essential part of 6σQMS. Sigma metrics enable us to quantify the performance of individual assays and indicate if the instruments are performing well in terms of measurable quantitative data. They also provide a benchmark to select QC protocols and target assay improvement.
- Analytical QC plans take into account the statistical (which is the SQC) and the nonstatistical elements of the procedures to mitigate potential risks or errors. The approach to the analytical QC plan began with the definition of the goal for intended use that complies with ISO 15189 regulatory requirements; total allowable error (TEa) from Clinical Laboratory Improvement Amendments were used. The calculation of Sigma metric takes into account the measurement procedure by assessing the precision (coefficient of variation) and inaccuracy (bias); these lead to validation of the QC design. The appropriate statistical QC procedure is designed by establishing the required control rules, total number of control measurements, and the frequency. Once the appropriate QC procedure is designed, strategies are developed by incorporating risk analysis and recommendations from the manufactures as part of the procedures.

SOME OF THE POSITIVE IMPACTS OF ANALYTICAL QUALITY CONTROL PLANS WITH THE SIX SIGMA QUALITY MANAGEMENT SYSTEM

1. Via the 6σQMS, we were able to quantify individual assay performances and compare them with those of previous years. With the QMS in place, not only did we manage to improve the Sigma quality of individual assays from preverification and postverification (2014 to 2015), we managed to reduce the number of assays

with ≤3σ and 4σ and increase number of assays with 5σ and ≥6σ (**Figs. 2–4**). We found more than 70% of the assays maintained a world class performance of Six

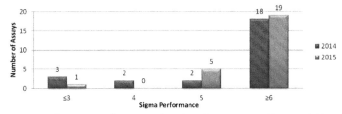

Fig. 2. Comparison of Sigma performance for chemistry assays—2014 and 2015 (level 1).

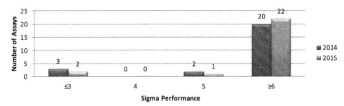

Fig. 3. Comparison of Sigma performance for chemistry assays—2014 and 2015 (level 2).

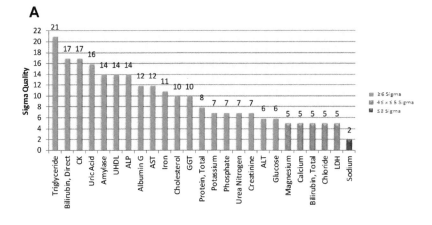

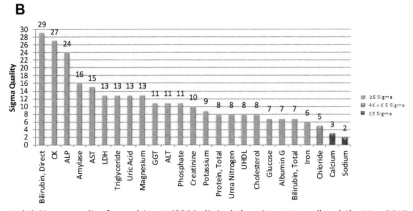

Fig. 4. (*A*) Sigma quality for architect ci8200 clinical chemistry assays (level 1)—Nov 2015. (*B*) Sigma quality for architect ci8200 clinical chemistry assays (level 2)—Nov 2015.

Table 1
Comparison of Sigma metric obtained by manual calculation using the Sigma metric equation for the 4 assays on 4 different analyzers

Assay	Analyzer	TEa from Ricos Database	QC Mean	Coefficient of Variation, %	Bias, %	Sigma Metric
Sodium	EPOC blood	± 4 mmol/L	139.6	0.2	0.7	10.7
Potassium	gas	±0.5 mmol/L	4.1	0.5	2.5	19.4
Glucose	analyzer	± 6 mg/dL or ± 10% (greater)	5.5	1.0	10.0	<3
Hemoglobin		± 7%	10.9	0.4	10.0	<3
Sodium	I-STAT blood	± 4 mmol/L	141.4	0.2	1.4	14.2
Potassium	gas analyzer	±0.5 mmol/L	4.5	0.5	2.2	17.8
Hemoglobin		± 7%	10.2	0.4	7.5	<3
Sodium	Architect ci	± 4 mmol/L	141.6	0.8	0.7	<3
Potassium	8200	±0.5 mmol/L	3.9	0.8	0.1	15.5
Glucose		± 6 mg/dL or ± 10% (greater)	4.8	1.1	0.3	6.0
Hemoglobin	CD Sapphire	± 7%	12.2	1.8	1.6	3.0

Sigma. We investigated the 3 Sigma metric performing assays; looked into the pre-analytical issues on sample collection, transportation, and processing; ensured staff is aware of the available policies and procedures; and ensured training and education were performed to enhance staff knowledge on how to review the QC. Furthermore, the frequency of control testing is based on the recommendation and application of the Westgard Sigma Rules. Close monitoring of the assays has resulted improvement in the performances.

Medical laboratories can use the Sigma metric to make decisions about method quality when a new analytical system is in place. In addition, we are able to monitor the method quality throughout the lifetime of the system.[4] When purchasing new equipment and instruments, it is a requirement to verify those instruments against current method using correlation, impression study, and linearity (**Table 1**). By only looking at correlation and impression studies, we cannot truly determine whether assays are providing world class performance. However, by converting the data into Sigma metrics, it is practical to determine if the instruments are performing well. At SunMed, we aimed to verify and select an acceptable blood gas analyzer based on precision data, correlation coefficient of selected assays, and Sigma performance of the assays carried out in 2 portable blood gas analyzers, EPOC and I-Stat, in the intensive care unit, against the laboratory analyzers, Architect ci8200 and CD Sapphire. EPOC and I-Stat showed excellent precision for all parameters except for Pco_2 in EPOC. As for the slope of regression, sodium, potassium, glucose, and hemoglobin showed a correlation coefficient of more than 0.900. The 3 analyzers showed variable Sigma performances, and not all assays met the minimum performance goal of 3.0 Sigma. This study enabled us to select the acceptable method based on precision, correlation coefficient, and sigma performance and at the same time establish a proper QC plan for poor performing assays.

2. With a good QMS in place, patients and doctors have confidence in the test results. Accurate and reliable results are vital to assist doctors in providing the best

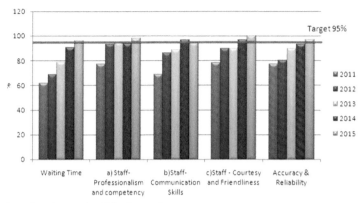

Fig. 5. Internal customers' satisfaction rate.

diagnosis and treatment to the patients. The application of Westgard Sigma Rules has helped reduce QC rework and costs caused by reduction in false rejection. These rules also improved the turnaround time of the test allowing us to provide timely and quality laboratory results to doctors and patients while also improving customer satisfaction toward our services (**Fig. 5**).

3. Initially, when we started our Six Sigma journey, our aim was reducing operational costs. It was discovered that the Sigma metric helps significantly in reducing the cost of QC materials and cost of failures annually with improved performance characteristics on most assays. Thus, patient safety is not compromised. We have been monitoring analytical performance based on Sigma metrics, and the QC procedures vary according to assays, resulting in a reduction in cost (**Fig. 6**).

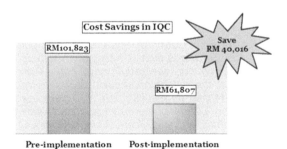

Fig. 6. Cost savings in IQC.

4. Internal failure costs from the rework of QC (simply rerunning or repeating QCs) are reduced. With unnecessary rework reduced, we can realize tangible cost savings. External failures are related to nonconformance or complaints from customers caused by error rates, inaccuracy, or turnaround time. And because we have a proper approach in monitoring quality by the Six Sigma process management system, customer complaints have been reduced. And despite the increase in

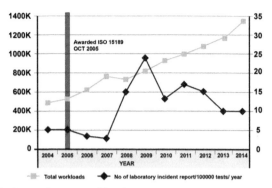

Fig. 7. Total incident report over workload per year.

workload, the laboratory error rate was reduced and has remained stable for the last several years (**Fig. 7**).

5. The 6σQMS also takes into account the competency and capability of the laboratory personnel, which is also crucial. Findings from our previous external audit by accreditation team showed that nonconformance related to staff competency decreased tremendously because staff are educated about the overall testing process from the specimen collection to the release of result. Additionally, the staff is able to handle QC-related issues and is more competent since the implementation of the 6σQMS. Thus, the implementation of a good QMS has given rise to a department with professional and well-trained personnel.

6. An independent verification by an external third party program such as a Sigma Verification Program enabled our laboratory to be assessed and validated, providing a strong incentive and motivation to continuously improve on Sigma metric performance and understand each assay's specific performance.

7. The implemented quality planning and goals are established as policies and procedures and are documented in the quality manual and reviewed yearly or as required.

8. The Sigma metric can be used as a predictor of risk, according to researcher Woodworth and colleagues (2014)[5]:

A risk assessment can be performed to determine if the current QC practice is adequate or requires revision. Currently, there is minimal guidance available regarding how laboratories may quantitatively estimate risk to optimize analytical QC criteria appropriate for an Individualized Quality Control Plan (IQCP). For the laboratory, risk is related to the chance of producing and reporting unreliable patient results, which are defined as results containing measurement errors that exceed a TEa specification. Evaluation of analytical performance characteristics, assay requirements, σ metrics, and statistical QC plans is one way to estimate risk during the analytical phase of testing.

A low Sigma metric results in high defect rates resulting in high number of unreliable results; thus, there is need to for close monitoring of such assays with frequent runs of control.

RISK MANAGEMENT WITH ANALYTICAL QUALITY CONTROL PLAN

Many international guidelines such as ACHS and The Joint Commission International, regulatory standards and accreditation requirements have made manufacturers implement and take responsibility for risk management of measuring systems and reagents. But today great emphasis is placed on medical laboratories to adopt risk management and develop laboratory specific QC plans.

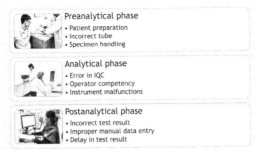

Fig. 8. Risk in the laboratory.

At SunMed, in 2014 we further adopted a risk management approach to develop a customized QC plan (QCP) based on Clinical Laboratory Improvement Amendments–approved guidelines on EP23-A Laboratory QC Based on Risk Management. This QC plan ensures addressing proactively any potential risk before wrong or unreliable results are released (**Fig. 8**).

Some of the steps taken in risk analysis and establishing the QCP include:

1. Hazard Identification through process map, followed by potential failure modes for each step in the diagram are plotted in a Fishbone cause and effect diagram (**Figs. 9** and **10**).

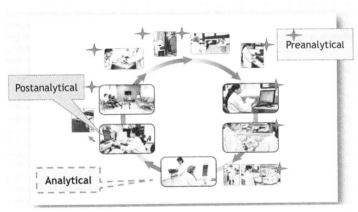

Fig. 9. Step 1a: process map. Risk in the laboratory: from blood requesting to the releasing of the report.

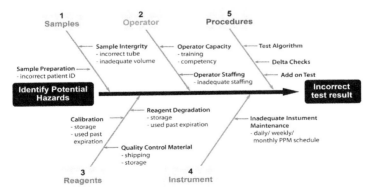

Fig. 10. Step 1 b: hazard identification.

2. Risk estimation and evaluation based on the ISO 14971 risk acceptability matrix. A Pareto chart is often plotted to show the highest failure modes with highest risk priority numbers (**Figs. 11** and **12**).

	Targeted failure mode	Cause of Hazard	S (Severity of Harm)	P (Probability of harm)	D (Detectability)	Hazard score	Risk acceptability
1	**Samples**	1. Incorrect tube	1	4	3	12	A
		2. Inadequate volume	1	4	2	12	A
		3. Incorrect patient ID	4	3	2	24	U
2	**Operator**	1. Lack of Training & Competency	3	4	3	36	U
		2. Incorrect and inadequate staffing	1	4	3	12	A
3	**Reagent**	1. Reagent and control degradation	2	4	2	16	A
		2. QC material	2	3	3	18	A
4	**Instrument**	1. IQC	3	5	3	45	U
		2. Instrument failure	1	3	1	3	A
		3. Inadequate instrument	3	3	1	9	A
5	**Procedure**	1. Test algorithm	2	4	3	24	U
		2. Delta check	2	5	1	10	A

Fig. 11. Steps 2 and 3: risk estimation and evaluation.

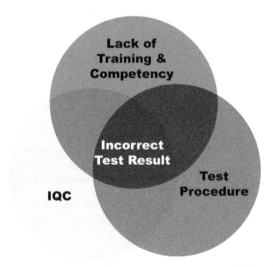

Fig. 12. Three major contributing factors to incorrect test result based on risk priority number.

3. Risk controls are implemented to ensure the whole testing process is addressed. This process is integrated with the careful design of SQC procedures (**Table 2**).

Table 2
Steps 4 and 5: risk control and implementation

Hazard	Cause of Hazard	Control Plan	Measurand
1. Operator	Lack of training & competency	1. Gap analysis 2. Individual internal & external training plan 3. Training policy	1. CME hours 2. Competency scoring 3. Incident report 4. External audit compliance 5. Internal customers' satisfaction
2. Instrument	IQC (chemistry)	1. AQC Strategy	1. Sigma metric 2. External quality assessment performance
3. Procedure	Test algorithm (HIV)	1. Revised test algorithm 2. Reflex test for positive case	Incorrect reported HIV test result

Abbreviations: AQC, analytical quality control; CME, continuing medical education; HIV, human immunodeficiency virus.

The above risk management concept led to tremendous benefits in terms of personnel, procedures and policies, compliances to accreditation, satisfaction of consumers, and improvement in SQC design. These established steps provide a safety net that enables us to detect errors as early as possible and prevent harm to patients. The implemented QCP enables our laboratory to mitigate, sustain, and assist in preventing possible hazards or risks that may occur before incorrect results are reported to health care providers. SunMed QCP planning is an ongoing process that requires constant planning and review.

UNCERTAINTY OF MEASUREMENTS

In SunMed, besides the implementation of quality tools and techniques such as Six Sigma and risk management, we also measure uncertainty of measurement (MU) as one of our quality tools. MU is a mandated requirement of ISO 15189.
MU as defined by MS ISO 15189: 2014 in Section 5.5.1.4:

The laboratory shall determine measurement uncertainty for each measurement procedure in the examination phases used to report measured quantity values on patients' samples. The laboratory shall define the performance requirements for the measurement uncertainty of each measurement procedure and regularly review estimates of measurement uncertainty.

To determine the true value of a measured quantity is an important asset for good laboratory practice in every area of measurement. Determining the random and systematic errors along the processing of samples provides us information on total error and creates a doubt (uncertainty) about the true value of the measured quantity. The so called uncertainty of measurement (MU) has become an important issue in

---

Box 1
Why measurement of uncertainty is important

- ISO 15189:2012; page 6 Clause 8.3

- When using an empirical method, care is required in defining the measurand to ensure that all uncertainty components are identified and accounted for including the use of different analysers in the laboratory.

- Laboratories are responsible to ensure test outputs are fit for clinical purposes by:
  - Defining what an analytical method measures
  - Meeting a defined analytical goal
  - Indicating the confidence that can be placed in a test result
  - Contributing to defining, monitoring, and indicating where a test procedure may be improved

---

clinical practice, and its importance has been increasingly realized by clinical laboratories.[6]

MU parameters involve variable sources that potentially contribute to dispersion of the values that could be finally attributed to the measurand. All possible variable sources that can contribute to MU must be taken into account, and several possible sources of uncertainty are listed below[7]:

- The measuring instruments can suffer from errors including bias, changes caused by aging or other kinds of drift, poor readability, and noise from electrical instruments
- The measurement process—preanalytical, analytical, and postanalytical
- Imported uncertainty—calibrator, control
- Operator skill and changes
- The environment

Thus, in every result, the value will contain the actual result given by the instruments and uncertainty measurement from variable sources gained along the processes.

At SunMed, MU is calculated at the analytical process, and bias is ignored and not assessed. Even though MU from preanalytical and postanalytical phases cannot be determined, MU still plays an important role in defining a good quality result. The importance of MU is simplified in **Box 1**.

In the beginning stage of adopting this tool, we were unfamiliar, and we stumbled in the calculation process of MU. Despite having 2 consecutive observations from the auditors during external assessment by an accreditation team, we were still uncertain about the procedure and the importance; nevertheless, we ensured the calculated value was always there for assessment purposes. Only procedures for which we are able to include all the sources of variables will give the total true estimate of MU, which we at SunMed were unable to do. However, in 2012, calculation of MU became mandatory by MS ISO15189 and with the guidance of Guideline Uncertainty Measurement article,[8] we started to calculate the MU following the top-down approach. We also updated it in our Quality Control Manual and is now calculated on yearly basis.

Some of the benefits gained after many years of calculating measurements of uncertainty include:

1. Adherence and compliance to the mandated requirement of the accreditation standard MS ISO15189:2014
2. For improvement of the sample testing process, the numerical value given also indicates the magnitude of doubt about that certain result. This doubt or standard

deviation will include systematic and random error. The total error from biological variation provides quantitative estimates of the level of confidence that a laboratory has in its analytical precision of test results. The value of uncertainty helps improve quality of services of clinical chemistry either to the diagnosis or monitoring effects of the treatment of patients.

3. MU is an essential parameter of the reliability of measurement results. MU provides quantitative evidence that measurement results meet clinical requirements for reliability.[9,10] We are in the progress of setting rules in middleware for auto verification. If there is any repeat run needed, the acceptance on repeat rerun will rely on the MU value of the analytes.

4. MU is useful in alleviating concern from clinicians. MU will determine the variation between two results are acceptable or not, therefore the value of MU shall be available for Clinicians if requested to clear their doubt on variation of test results.

Limitation of MU through SunMed experience.

1. Variable sources: There are many sources and contributing factors to MU. We are unable to determine all variable sources. Not only by precision and calibrator but other factors will also contribute variances, for example, sample matrix, instrument noise, operator, or preparation of QC.

2. Standardization: Multiple analyzers will have slightly different MU. The laboratory needs to be certain which patient samples are running on which analyzers. No standardization on calculating MU is possible if we have more than 1 instrument.

3. Standardization of calibrators: Major sources of calibrator error include differences in analysis methods used by different laboratory instruments, lot-to-lot variance in calibration materials, and lack of traceability between secondary reference material and primary standards. Some of the commercial suppliers provide the uncertainty estimates of assigned value, but there are still some manufacturers who do not provide information.[6] Of course, the former is preferable by clinical laboratory practitioners.

4. MU values for calibrators are from vendors: If information on restandardization of calibrator values or levels is not disseminated in a timely manner to the end user, delays for data collection or MU review will occur.

5. Limited MU range: If we use intermediate-term precision from controls as our approach to estimate MU, then our estimates depend on the QC range. Beyond this range we can only assume the percentage of the MU.

6. Awareness: Initially, MU needs to be reported with patient results on a routine basis. But practically there is a need for ongoing education and training to create awareness, both for laboratories and requesting doctors to understand its benefit and limitation of MU concepts. With more stable and modern instruments, the margin of doubt is smaller, but less technical training is being provided on MU, making it more challenging for increasing clinician awareness.

MU with its benefits and limitation is still crucial for the clinical laboratory, especially to know test performance, even if currently the value is not reported with the patient's results. As Albert Einstein famously said," Every number has its value but not all value has numbers."

SUMMARY

Quality is a priority if we wish to gain and sustain the confidence of our customers, both clinicians and patients, and satisfy their evolving needs. In order to provide our continuous commitment toward enhancing the overall quality of test results in line with our vision as leading medical center in ASEAN region and our mission to achieve world standard in quality services, safe facilities and increase consumers either patients or doctors satisfaction, thus the use of appropriate tools and techniques is crucial as well as essential. We feel that the tools adopted such as TEa and MU help the laboratory in ensuring reliability of test results, each from a different perspective. However, tools for establishing the statistical QC alone are not sufficient to ensure the quality of service that we provide to our customers. A good QMS with an excellent analytical QC plans is essential to provide the bigger picture, which will not only give confidence in our analytical performance but span to provide assurance across the total testing process, workflow, and staff competency. It's not an easy task to achieve good quality, but with a proper QMS in place, it is definitely within our grasp.

REFERENCES

1. Westgard JO. Six sigma risk analysis-designing analytical QC plans for the medical laboratory. Madison, WI: Westgard QC; 2011.
2. Gami B, Patel DS, Chauhan K. Sigma metrics as a quality marker for analyzing electrolytes in laboratory. Int J Adv Res (Indore) 2013;1(7):197–201.
3. Cooper G. Bio-Rad LaboratoriesQC Education: Basic Lessons in LaboratoryQuality-Control. 2008. Available at: http://www.qcnet.com/Portals/50/PDFs/QCWorkbook 2008_Jun08.pdf. Quality control is essential for two reasons: to detect error and avoid false rejections. Accessed January 6, 2016.
4. Westgard JO, Stein B. An automated process for selecting statistical QCprocedures to assure clinical and analytical quality requirements. Clin Chem 1997; 43:400–3.
5. Woodworth A, Korpi-Steiner N, Miller JJ, et al. Utilization of assay performance characteristics to estimate Hemoglobin A1c result reliability. Clin Chem 2014; 60:1073–9.
6. Demirel GY, Tamer S, Topbas F. Measurement uncertainty in clinical laboratories: implementation to daily practise. Turkey: Centro Laboratuvarlari; 2007.
7. Linko S, Ornemark U, Kessel R. Evaluation of measurement uncertainty in clinical chemistry. Belgium: IRMM European Commission-JRC; 2001.
8. Guide to, the expression of uncertainty in measurement. Geneva (Switzerland): JCGM/WG 1; 1993.
9. Graham White, The hitch-hiker's guide to measurement uncertainty (MU) in clinical laboratories, 2012. Available at: https://www.westgard.com/hitchhike-mu. htm. Accessed November 25, 2016.
10. Westgard JO. Basic QC practices-training in statistical quality control for medical laboratories. 3rd edition. Madison, WI: Westgard QC; 2010.

Applying Sigma Metrics to Reduce Outliers

Joseph Litten, PhD

KEYWORDS

- Six sigma • Sigma metrics • Instrumentation assessment • Quality control
- Laboratory standardization • QC rules failure rates

KEY POINTS

- Sigma metrics can be used to aid in the evaluation and selection of clinical laboratory instrumentation.
- A Six Sigma–designed quality control (QC) program can be used in monitoring the performance of assays, resulting in cost savings in reagents, supplies, and labor, especially if most of the assays are of 5 sigma or better.
- QC rules failure rates increase dramatically as the sigma metric of the method decreases.
- Reproducibility of results between laboratories is much better with methods of 5-sigma or 6-sigma metrics.

Over the last several decades, laboratory testing results have improved in both accuracy and precision. This improvement has mostly been caused by changing technology of instrumentation and the quality of the assays developed with that instrumentation. With this improved assay quality, the following questions need to be asked: how does this quality relate to acceptable quality goals set forth by the laboratory, what accuracy and precision are required by the method to achieve these quality goals, and how is this determined? It is necessary to answer these questions to assess the quality of the laboratory results being generated by the laboratory. Without this knowledge, the laboratory cannot accurately determine whether or not their results are within allowable clinical error.

ASSESSMENT OF NEW INSTRUMENTATION

When evaluating new instrumentation, there are numerous factors to consider; most of these factors are related to costs. These factors include, but are not limited to:

- Cost of instrumentation, including automation, middleware, and service costs
- Cost of reagents and supplies

Disclosure: The author has nothing to disclose.
Laboratory, Valley Health, 1840 Amherst Street, Winchester, VA 22601, USA
E-mail address: jlitten@valleyhealthlink.com

Clin Lab Med 37 (2017) 177–186
http://dx.doi.org/10.1016/j.cll.2016.09.014   labmed.theclinics.com
0272-2712/17/© 2016 Elsevier Inc. All rights reserved.

- Reliability of the instruments
- Ease of use
- Instrument throughput
- Specimen requirements
- Test menu (consolidation of workstations)
- Middleware capabilities
- Turnaround times
- Vendor support

All of these factors affect the overall cost of the operation of the instrumentation. However, one important factor that is too often overlooked is assay quality. Quality measures such as accuracy and reproducibility affect physician decisions, which in turn can affect patient outcomes. Assay quality also affects the laboratory. Poor assay quality can affect the efficiency of the QC program used to monitor the assays, and this can translate into time and cost and may also affect proficiency testing.

SIGMA-METRIC ANALYSIS

In our laboratory, we conducted a quality comparison of the different vendor instruments, performing a sigma-metric analysis for each instrument. The Six Sigma approach is a universal benchmark that describes the number of defects per million of a process or system. For laboratory assays, a defect is defined as an event that is outside the tolerance limits of an assay. The sigma metric is measured on a scale of 0 to 6, with 6 being world class (3.4 defects per million) and 3 being the minimum level of performance for a system (about 66,800 defects per million). It uses basic laboratory quality measures, bias and imprecision, and can be used to compare assay quality across multiple instrument systems, or to evaluate the assay performance of a given instrument system and to set the appropriate QC rules required to effectively monitor the assays.[1] The sigma metric is calculated using the following equation:

Sigma metric = (TEa − Bias$_{observed}$)/CV(coefficient of variation)$_{observed}$

where TEa is total allowable error. For the purposes of comparing estimated sigma metrics for different vendor systems during the instrument assessment phase, bias and imprecision values are available from several sources, such as external proficiency testing programs, quality control (QC) programs, information from the vendor, and literature sources. TEa can be taken from several different analytical or clinical benchmarks, such as proficiency testing criteria, external quality assessment standards, RiliBAK guidelines (Guidelines for Quality Assurance of Medical Laboratory Examinations of the German Medical Association), desirable biological variation database,[2] and ISO (International Standards Organization) 15189.

Once the instrumentation is in place, the same quality measures can be used to evaluate the true assay performance and to set the appropriate QC rules required to effectively monitor an assay. Imprecision data from the laboratory replication study and the measured bias against a reference method or peer group can be used along with the TEa to generate a sigma metric. These values can also be correlated with Westgard Sigma Rules to set the QC procedures. Five-sigma and 6-sigma methods only require a simple QC rule to monitor the method with fewer controls per run. Three-sigma and 4-sigma methods require multiple QC rules to monitor the method with a higher number of controls per run. Methods with a sigma metric of less than 3 are difficult to monitor even with multiple QC rules and many controls per run; these methods should be avoided.

To aid in the vendor decision process, our laboratory used sigma metrics to predict the quality of clinical chemistry assays from 6 different instruments. Sigma metrics were estimated for 30 chemistry tests across each of the 6 vendor's instruments (**Box 1**).

Box 1
Chemistry tests evaluated for sigma metrics

- Albumin
- Alkaline phosphatase
- ALT
- Amylase
- AST
- Bilirubin, direct
- Bilirubin, total
- Calcium
- Chloride
- Cholesterol
- CK
- CO_2
- Creatinine
- GGT
- Glucose
- HDL
- Iron
- LDH
- LDL cholesterol
- Lipase
- Magnesium
- Phosphorus
- Potassium
- Prealbumin
- Protein, total
- Sodium
- Transferrin
- Triglycerides
- BUN
- Uric acid

Abbreviations: ALT, alanine transaminase; AST, aspartate transaminase; BUN, blood urea nitrogen; CK, creatinine kinase; HDL, high-density lipoprotein; LDH, lactate dehydrogenase; LDL, low-density lipoprotein; GGT, gamma-glutamyl transferase.

There are several sources of bias and imprecision data that can be used during the instrument assessment phase to help predict the sigma performance. These sources include proficiency testing results, information from the vendor, literature sources, and QC programs. In this study, data were obtained from the College of American Pathologists (CAP) proficiency surveys. Clinical Laboratory Improvement Amendments (CLIA) and CAP performance standards were used for the TEa. For CO_2, because the CLIA standard is ±3 standard deviations (SDs), the average SD for all instruments was used (**Table 1**). Because the total error may vary across the analytical range, the total error at the critical medical decision level was used to determine the sigma metric for each assay.

The sigma-metric performance of the 6 vendor instruments was calculated for each assay using only the CV for each instrument because there was no reference method to refer to for the accuracy of each analyte. Each assay was categorized by sigma

Table 1 Total allowable error for chemistry tests	
Albumin	±10%
Alkaline phosphatase	±30%
ALT	±20%
Amylase	±30%
AST	±20%
Bilirubin, direct	±0.4 mg/dL or 20%
Bilirubin, total	±0.4 mg/dL or 20%
Calcium	±1.0 mg/dL
Chloride	±5%
Cholesterol	±10%
CK	±30%
CO_2	±3 SD (±25%)
Creatinine	±0.3 mg/dL or 15%
GGT	±20%
Glucose	±6.0 mg/dL or 10%
HDL	±30%
Iron	±20%
LDH	±20%
LDL cholesterol	±30%
Lipase	±30%
Magnesium	±25%
Phosphorus	±0.3 mg/dL or 10.7%
Potassium	±0.5 mmol/L
Prealbumin	±5.0 mg/dL or 25%
Protein, total	±10%
Sodium	±4.0 mmol/L
Transferrin	±20%
Triglycerides	±25%
BUN	±2.0 mg/dL or 9%
Uric acid	±17%

metric from less than 3 to 6 and the total number of assays in sigma-metric categories for an instrument was determined (**Table 2**). One vendor instrument was substantially better than the others, with 73% of the assays at the medical decision levels at 5 or 6 sigma. The next best vendor had 60.7% of the medical decision points at 5 or 6 sigma, followed by 57.1%, 53.6%, 48.2%, and 44.7%. Because assays with a sigma metric of less than 3 are very hard to control regardless of how many controls are run or how many QC rules are used, they should be avoided. Instrument 1 had no methods with a sigma metric of less than 3; all the other instruments had at least 1 assay with a sigma metric less than 3. Instruments 4 and 6 had more than 10% of the medical decision points with sigma metrics less than 3 (**Fig. 1**).

ASSESSMENT OF SIGMA METRICS IN THE LABORATORY

After an analysis of all the factors being considered by our search committee for chemistry and immunoassay instrumentation, the vendor of instrument 1 was selected for our health system. After the instrumentation had been in operation for approximately 9 months, the laboratory QC data were used to generate real-world sigma performance metrics on the 30 tests originally evaluated. Twenty-eight of the 30 chemistry assays were 5 sigma or better; 1 assay was 4 sigma, and 1 was 3 sigma. None of the assays were less than 3 sigma (**Table 3**). The in-house data showed the tests to be as good as estimated or better. **Fig. 2** shows how the estimated sigma metric compared with the actual sigma metric.

SIX SIGMA QUALITY CONTROL PROGRAM

Traditional QC programs are based on the imprecision and bias of the methods used in the laboratory. The imprecision of the methods is determined by the day-to-day SD of QC material. Means and limits are established and the methods are monitored by the use of common Westgard Rules, especially the 1:2s and 1:3s rules. Whether or not these limits are clinically relevant is too often not taken into consideration.

A Six Sigma QC program takes into account the clinically relevant error for each test method.[1] In a Six Sigma QC–designed program, the TEa is determined for each analyte. TEa is an expression of how much error can be tolerated in the test result without negatively affecting patient care based on interpretation of that result.

Sigma-metric analysis provides information on the proper number of control measurements required per run and which Westgard Rules are needed to adequately monitor the performance of a test. The higher the sigma metric of a method, the better the method will deliver results within the total allowable limits. Once the sigma metric has been calculated, Westgard Rules appropriate for the quality of the method are

Table 2					
Percentage of tests by sigma metric for each instrument					
Instrument	6 Sigma (%)	5 Sigma (%)	4 Sigma (%)	3 Sigma (%)	<3 Sigma (%)
Instrument 1	58.9	14.3	19.6	7.1	0
Instrument 2	50.0	10.7	16.1	17.9	5.4
Instrument 3	37.5	19.6	14.3	23.2	5.4
Instrument 4	37.5	16.1	14.3	16.1	16.1
Instrument 5	33.9	14.3	32.1	17.9	1.8
Instrument 6	26.8	17.9	17.9	23.2	14.3

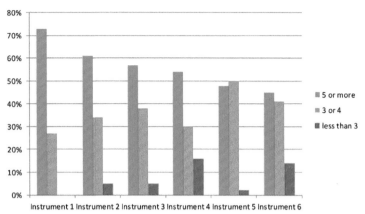

Fig. 1. Summary of 30 chemistry assays. Percentage of assays at 5 sigma or greater, 3 to 4 sigma, and less than 3 sigma.

selected to monitor its performance. The higher the sigma metric, the fewer controls are required per run and the simpler the Westgard Rules required. The goal is to have the QC program detect at least 90% of clinically significant errors and have few (<5%) false rejections of QC rules. Too high a percentage of false rejections of a QC rule leads to unnecessary investigations. The Westgard Rules needed for 5 sigma and higher assays are less demanding than those required for 3-sigma or 4-sigma methods. Therefore, the more methods an instrument can deliver at a 5-sigma metric or better, the simpler the QC program required to monitor the performance of the assays.

Table 3
Sigma metric of chemistry tests

6 Sigma	5 Sigma	4 Sigma	3 Sigma	<3 Sigma
Albumin	BUN	Sodium	CO_2	—
ALT	Chloride			
Alkaline phosphatase	LDL			
Amylase	Phosphorus			
AST	Total bilirubin			
Calcium				
Cholesterol				
CK				
Creatinine				
Direct bilirubin				
GGT				
Glucose				
HDL				
Iron				
LD				
Lipase				
Magnesium				
Potassium				
Prealbumin				
Total protein				
Transferrin				
Triglycerides				
Uric acid				

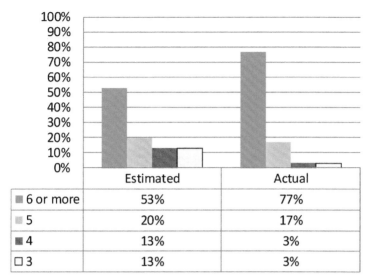

	Estimated	Actual
■ 6 or more	53%	77%
■ 5	20%	17%
■ 4	13%	3%
□ 3	13%	3%

Fig. 2. Comparison of the estimated sigma metric with the actual sigma metric. Percentages of assays at 5 sigma or greater (excellent), 4 sigma (good), 3 sigma (marginal), and less than 3 sigma (poor).

A Six Sigma–designed QC program was instituted in our laboratory for these instruments. It was decided to run 3 to 4 QC controls each day with at least 1 control every 12 hours for the high-volume testing. The rules used to monitor the tests by Sigma metric are listed in **Table 4**.[1]

The Six Sigma QC program was run in the background for 3 months. During that time, a traditional QC program was still being used to monitor the assays. An analysis of the data showed that there were 53% fewer QC rules failures using the Six Sigma program versus the traditional QC program, which would have resulted in fewer unnecessary repeats of controls, fewer recalibrations of assays, and less time investigating QC rules failures. It was also noted that no clinically significant errors were missed using the Six Sigma QC program during that time period.

The Six Sigma QC program was next applied to all quantitative methods performed on both the chemistry and immunoassay instruments. Implementing a Six Sigma QC program resulted in:

- Fewer controls per run
- Simpler Westgard Rules used to monitor method performance
- Fewer false rejections

Table 4	
Quality control rules used for sigma metric of method	
Sigma Metric	**QC Rules Used**
6 Sigma	1-3.5s
5 Sigma	1-3s
4 Sigma	1-3s, R4s, 2 of 2-2s, and 2 of 3-2s
3 Sigma	1-3s, R4s, 2 of 2-2s, 2 of 3-2s, 4-1s and 12x

The implementation of the Six Sigma QC program led to increased savings across multiple areas of the laboratory. There was a 45% saving on reagents and supplies that would have been consumed while running controls.

- $8000 savings for the chemistry instrument
- $55,000 savings for cardiac markers in the immunoassay instrument

There was also a 45% saving in control material, resulting in another $10,000 in annual savings. Additional labor savings of 1.5 to 2.0 hours per day were realized in running QC and investigating QC rules failure (**Fig. 3**).

QUALITY CONTROL FAILURE RATES BY SIGMA METRIC OF METHOD

A study was performed to determine the rate of QC rules violations for a method depending on its sigma metric. QC values were reviewed for 70 different chemistry, TDM (therapeutic drug monitoring), and immunoassay methods over a 3-month period. Methods were grouped as follows:

- Six sigma
- Five sigma
- Four sigma or less

More than 45,000 QC points were collected over a 3-month period. The failure rate by sigma metric is shown in **Table 5**.

The failure rate of the 3-sigma and 4-sigma tests was more than 20 times higher than that of the 6-sigma methods and 7 times higher than the 5-sigma methods. A third of the failures for the 5-sigma and 6-sigma methods were caused by the wrong controls being run, which would reduce the QC failure rate for 6-sigma methods from 0.7% to 0.5% and of the 5-sigma methods to 1.4%. In addition, by eliminating the need for the 1-2s rule for 5-sigma and 6-sigma methods, another 6% of QC failures were avoided. Therefore, the combination of high-quality methods with optimized QC design resulted in significant resource and labor efficiencies, ensuring quality while providing needed savings in both labor and reagents and supplies.

INTERNAL PROFICIENCY TESTING PROGRAM FOR HEALTH SYSTEM

Standardization of the hospital laboratories within the health system was a major objective for the vendor selection. In order to achieve standardized testing within

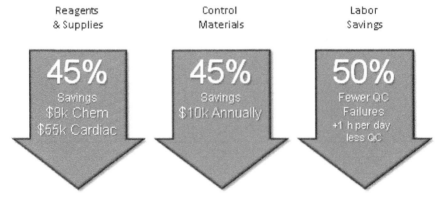

Fig. 3. Summary of Six Sigma QC program savings. Chem, chemistry.

Table 5
Quality control failures by sigma metric of method

Sigma Metric	QC Performed	QC Rule Failure	QC Failure Rate (%)
6 Sigma	30,044	209	0.7
5 Sigma	10,875	224	2.1
3 and 4 Sigma	5572	818	14.7

the health system with excellent correlation between sites, the instrumentation must have assays with high-sigma metrics. To ensure compliance between the different laboratories, 29 common methods were tested each month by assaying pooled patient specimens and control materials. Acceptable limits were established for each

Table 6
Tolerance limits for interlaboratory correlation studies

Test	Limits
Albumin	±0.3 g/dL
Alkaline phosphatase	±10 U/L or 12%
ALT	±5 U/L or 10%
Amylase	±5 U/L or 14.6%
AST	±3 U/L or 16.7%
Bilirubin, direct	±0.2 mg/dL or 10%
Bilirubin, total	±0.2 mg/dL or 10%
BUN	±2 mg/dL or 9%
Calcium	±0.4 mg/dL
Chloride	±2.5%
Cholesterol	±3%
CK	±10 U/L or 10%
CO_2	±2 mmol/L or 12%
Creatinine	±0.2 mg/dL or 8.9%
Glucose	±4 mg/dL or 6.9%
HDL	±4 mg/dL or 11.6%
LD	±11.4%
Lipase	±5 U/L or 15%
Magnesium	±0.3 mg/dL or 4.8%
Phosphorus	±0.2 mg/dL or 10.1%
Potassium	±5.6%
Sodium	±3 mmol/L
Total protein	±0.2 mg/dL or 4%
Triglycerides	±5 mg/dL or 10%
Uric acid	±12%
Troponin I	±0.04 ng/mL or 10%
Free T4	±15%
HCG	±2 mIU/mL or 15%
TSH	±12%

Abbreviations: HCG, human chorionic gonadotropin; TSH, thyroid-stimulating hormone.

method using Ricos and colleagues'[2] Desirable Biological Variation Database with optimal TEa, CLIA limits, and internal TEa limits (**Table 6**).

Data are analyzed using EP Evaluator multi-instrument comparison. All failures are investigated immediately. Most of the failures are corrected by recalibration, but some require instrument maintenance and further troubleshooting. The high quality of the assay methods allows tight control over test results to be maintained from one hospital to another. Many of the hospitals are feeder hospitals to our flagship hospital. Because tight limits are kept on the assays, patients coming from one hospital to another do not have to be rebaselined and the results can be trended.

SUMMARY

Sigma metrics can be used to predict the quality of an instrument's assay. Sigma-metric analysis allows easy comparison of instrument quality and can predict which tests will require minimal QC rules to monitor the performance of the method. A Six Sigma QC program can result in fewer controls and fewer QC rules failures for methods with a sigma metric of 5 or better. The higher the number of methods with a sigma metric of 5 or better, the lower the costs for reagents, supplies, and control material required to monitor the performance of the methods. This outcome also translates into less labor required to run QC and troubleshoot QC rules failures. Methods that are 4 sigma or lower have 20 times higher QC rules failures than 6-sigma methods, which requires follow-up investigation by the staff. Standardization throughout a health system is much easier with better reproducibility of results when the methods are of a high-sigma metric. Tight standards for results from one laboratory to another allow better trending of values and provide better patient history. Having methods with high-sigma metrics helps to improve patient care and should be an important factor when selecting instrumentation for the clinical laboratory.

REFERENCES

1. Westgard JO. Six sigma quality design and control: desirable precision and requisite QC for laboratory measurement processes. Madison (WI): Westgard QC; 2001.
2. Ricos C, Alvarez V, Cava F, et al. Current databases on biological variation: pros, cons and progress. Scand J Clin Lab Invest 1999;59:491–500.

Quality Indicators for the Total Testing Process

Mario Plebani, MD*, Laura Sciacovelli, Biol Sci, Ada Aita, Biol Sci

KEYWORDS

- Errors in laboratory medicine • Quality indicators • Extra-analytical phases
- Quality specifications • External quality assurance program

KEY POINTS

- In laboratory medicine the extra-analytical phases have the highest error rates.
- ISO 15189:2012 requires the establishment of quality indicators to monitor and evaluate laboratory performance throughout critical aspects of pre-examination, examination, and postexamination processes.
- The use of quality indicators that meet requirements for effectiveness and harmonization is an important quality improvement tool.
- The participation in External Quality Assurance Program managed by the working group Laboratory Errors and Patient Safety of IFCC (www.ifcc-mqi.com) allows a laboratory to compare its performance with that of other participants.

INTRODUCTION

The increasingly dominant role of laboratory medicine in clinical decision making and the pressure on cost containment have led to a more careful evaluation of the effectiveness of, and improvement in, clinical outcomes. Because laboratory tests play an extremely important role in diagnosing, monitoring, and evaluating patient outcomes, evidence-based evaluation of laboratory performances is crucial to ensuring that patients receive safe, efficient, and effective care.

Efforts to reduce errors and enhance patient safety in medicine must focus on risk procedures and processes with a high likelihood of error generation. Analytical activities must be improved in the effort to achieve consistently higher levels of quality in laboratory medicine. Yet, in the last few decades, performance measurements have focused mainly on analytical processes with a view to meeting the quality specifications of precision and trueness.[1,2] Clinical laboratories can measure, monitor, and improve their analytical performances over time thanks to internal quality control

The authors have nothing to disclose.
Department of Laboratory Medicine, University Hospital of Padova, via Giustiniani, 2, 35128 Padova, Italy
* Corresponding author.
E-mail address: mario.plebani@unipd.it

Clin Lab Med 37 (2017) 187–205
http://dx.doi.org/10.1016/j.cll.2016.09.015   labmed.theclinics.com
0272-2712/17/© 2016 Elsevier Inc. All rights reserved.

(IQC) rules, objective analytical quality specifications, and proficiency testing/external quality assessment (EQA) programs, which have provided clinical laboratories with a valuable benchmark based on objective data. IQC procedures and EQA programs have significantly improved the intra-analytical quality of laboratory testing. However, studies on errors in laboratory medicine confirm that most errors occur in the preanalytical and postanalytical phases of testing.[3–6] The implementation of performance measurements to evaluate the preanalytical and postanalytical stages of the total testing process (TTP) is therefore needed to maximize the overall testing cycle and the quality of patient care. In addition, recent regulation and accreditation guidelines require laboratories to focus improvement efforts not only on the intra-analytical phase, but also on all steps of the TTP.[7]

ERRORS IN THE EXTRA-ANALYTICAL PHASES

Although the frequency of laboratory errors varies greatly depending on the study design and steps of the TTP investigated, a series of papers have drawn the attention of laboratory professionals to the preanalytical and postanalytical phases, which have been demonstrated to be more vulnerable to errors than the analytical phase; the pre-analytical phase has the highest error rates, accounting for up to 70% of all mistakes in laboratory diagnostics.[3–6,8–10] Several technological, informatics, and computer science advances introduced in the preanalytical phase have the potential to decrease the risk of errors. The complexity of the process, and the variety of owners and mutual responsibilities at the interfaces of several steps calls for adequate governance based on reliable measures. Indeed, the development of preanalytical robotic workstations and their employment in clinical practice have significantly reduced errors in the conventional preanalytical steps involved in making a sample suitable for analysis (centrifugation, aliquoting, diluting, and sorting specimens into batches for their introduction into automated analyzers).[11–13] The preanalytical phase consists of a pre-preanalytical phase and "true" preanalytical phase. The pre-preanalytical phase involves selecting and ordering appropriate tests, and collecting, identifying, labeling, handling, and transporting biologic samples. These processes are neither performed by, nor usually under the control of, laboratory staff. Evidence collected demonstrates that the staff in clinical wards is at a significantly higher risk of error than those in the laboratory.[14–16] In the preanalytical phase, the laboratory accepts samples, centrifuging, aliquoting, diluting, and sorting the biologic samples. This categorization is not only of "taxonomic" value, but also underpins the responsibilities and duties of nonlaboratory personnel, most of the processes being performed by other health care operators (eg, nurses and physicians).[9]

An important factor affecting quality in the postanalytical phase is poor communication between laboratory professionals and clinicians, in particular in relation to timeliness of reporting, notification of significantly abnormal test results, and presentation of relevant information through reports and interpretative comments. Breakdowns in communication lead to errors that compromise patient safety, and lead to the inefficient and ineffective use of resources.

Clinicians are interested in service quality, which encompasses total testing error (imprecision and trueness), availability, cost, relevance, and timeliness. However, because the quality of a laboratory is often judged on timeliness, many laboratories may be ready to sacrifice analytical quality for a faster turnaround time (TAT). Timeliness is measured by monitoring the TAT of some specific tests, and the time required for notification of critical results. The automation of various steps in the analytical phase, the increased use of electronic results reporting, and the development of automatic electronic alerting systems for critical values have contributed to reducing the time required for results reporting. Prompt reporting of test results can improve efficiency in patient care and enhance clinician and patient satisfaction, even when it does not affect health outcomes.[8,17]

The correct monitoring of TAT calls for knowledge of the different measurement approaches used by laboratories, such as test typology, need for priority reporting (eg, urgent or routine), patient typology (eg, inpatients, outpatients, urgent cases), and the activities incurred (eg, interval of measurement). Another important aspect is the procedure used for notifying critical values; this plays a key role in safe and effective patient care. Yet there is still a lack of consensus on the choice of analytes and critical ranges, and notification times vary depending on patient typology (inpatients or outpatients). Likewise, mistakes in the content and completeness of laboratory reports and misunderstanding by the treating physician as to the significance of the information in the report, among other factors, can delay the treatment of a serious disease and alter outcomes. Specific report content issues can include any of the following: noninterpretable information, incorrect reference interval data, inaccurate personal patient details, and/or incorrect reporting of measurements. Moreover, different types of error can occur during report formatting. Reports lacking units of measurement or using inappropriate units of measurement can lead to harmful misinterpretation of results and/or underestimation of vital information. The correct interpretation of results is crucial to patient outcome yet, wishing to avoid giving inappropriate advice, many laboratories fail to provide interpretative comments in the absence of complete clinical information. Studies conducted have revealed that although most comments provided in laboratory reports are acceptable, some are inappropriate or misleading and, in a few cases, dangerous, leading to inaccurate assumptions by staff, particularly if the available clinical information is insufficient or the expertise in a clinical chemistry subspecialty area (eg, toxicology, endocrinology, and tumor markers) is inadequate.[18] The aim of interpretative comments on laboratory reports is to help clinicians interpret complex data provided, particularly when dynamic or rare test results are reported, when significant abnormalities are present, and/or when analytical or preanalytical factors might compromise the interpretation. Although several authors have described this process and indicated its value, there is little evidence that it has improved patient outcomes, mainly because of difficulties involved in collecting data.[19–22]

IMPROVEMENT PROCESS

Quality improvement initiatives, in compliance with systematic criteria and organization, are key elements in ensuring an effective quality management system and favorable outcomes by reducing errors. That which is not measured cannot be improved on. Improvement actions in laboratory activities are as many and varied as the relationships and interactions between multiple processes and activities are complex. Success depends on leadership committed to improving quality as its modus operandi, organizational culture that calls for efforts from all employees involved in improvement activities, integrated and well-defined processes and procedures that define how the improvement can be implemented and how shared responsibility is to be achieved, and application by management and staff of knowledge and skills for continuous improvement and tools.[23]

The identification of improvement opportunities in clinical laboratories must include all TTP activities, especially those in the extra-analytical phases; this calls for proactive and reactive methods, not only concerning the processes but also, and above all, regarding the risks related to patient safety.[4,5,24,25] Improvement opportunities are based on information arising from a robust and integrated quality management system that provides a wide variety of information sources, generated from symptomatic (eg, incident reporting) or asymptomatic (eg, analysis of the strengths, weaknesses, opportunities) events, and managed within processes pertaining to evaluation, monitoring, and improvement.[23] In particular, results of quality indicators (QIs), performances obtained in EQA programs, reports of external audits for accreditation and/or certification, and management of undesirable events (errors, complaints, adverse events, nonconformities).

Other important sources of information are activities focusing on users outside (eg, citizens, patients, clinicians) and within (laboratory staff) the organization. Surveys on user satisfaction and the analysis of users' needs provide data for the definition of organizational and quality goals, and values and intervention priorities. The reliability of information on opportunities for improvement reflects the criteria to be used, and the way the information itself is to be collected and handled.

QUALITY INDICATORS

The need to reduce the error rate has highlighted, especially in preanalytical and postanalytical phases, the difficulty involved in identifying adverse events and complying with the International Standard for Accreditation of Clinical Laboratories, ISO 15189:2012, thus prompting laboratory professionals to develop and implement QIs.[26–30] As stated by the ISO 15189:2012, "The laboratory shall establish QIs to monitor and evaluate performance throughout critical aspects of pre-examination, examination and post examination processes"; and "The process of monitoring QIs shall be planned, which includes establishing the objectives, methodology, interpretation, limits, action plan and duration of measurement."[7]

In recent years, different QIs have been developed to monitor critical processes and identify errors and mistakes in laboratories based on their particular characteristics and organization. This monitoring is based on the laboratories' different health care contexts, purposes and goals, patient number and typology, activity typology, and sensitivity and training of staff.

Many laboratories have introduced QIs based on different criteria and methods and, in the last decade, interesting programs for indicators of the extra-analytical phases have been developed in some countries and regions, such as Australia and New Zealand, Brazil, and Catalonia, and other surveys and programs have been promoted in the UK, China, and Croatia.[31–36]

The different experiences worldwide in the use of QIs have made it difficult to establish a reliable state-of-the art because data reported are not comparable.[37–40] Because of differences in methods used for data collection processing and analysis of results this incomparability underlines the need for international consensus on the adoption of universal QIs and common terminology. Because laboratory results have such an important impact on patient safety, activities related to evaluation, monitoring, and quality improvement within the TTP, it is clearly of crucial importance for laboratory professionals to focus their attention on harmonization of the management of QIs. The harmonization process must hinge on the recognition, understanding, and explanation of the differences between criteria used and procedures used to overcome the differences and achieve uniformity in compliance with organizational and management peculiarities. The first step must therefore be designed with an awareness of the differences, and the recognition that a common model must be used to assess appropriateness, identify strengths and weaknesses, and define uniform criteria and procedures.[41]

Because various QIs and terminologies are currently used in laboratory medicine, the path toward harmonization should be based on sound criteria. Consensus has been achieved regarding the main characteristics of QIs, which should be (1) patient-centered to promote total quality and patient safety; (2) consistent with the definition of "laboratory error " specified in the ISO/TS 22367: 2008[42] and conducive to addressing all TTP stages, from initial pre-preanalytical (test request and patient/sample identification) to post-postanalytical (acknowledgment of data communication, appropriate result interpretation, and use) steps; and (3) consistent with ISO 15189: 2012[7] requirements. In addition, essential prerequisites of QIs, as measurable and objective tools, are (1) importance and applicability to a wide range of clinical laboratories worldwide, (2) scientific robustness with a focus on areas of great importance for quality in laboratory medicine, (3) the definition of evidence-based thresholds for acceptable performance, and (4) timeliness and possible use as a measure of laboratory improvement.

The revision issued in 2012 of ISO 15189 focuses on the definition of QIs and the rationale for their use, and calls for establishment of QIs concerning the preanalytical, intra-analytical, and postanalytical phase; definition of goals, method, interpretation, limits, action plans, and measurement times to ensure a monitoring process; and appropriateness continued through periodic reviews enabling the systematic monitoring and evaluation of the laboratory's contribution to patient care.

In the harmonization process, a model QI (MQI) is defined as an indicator where identification of indicator and reporting system is well designed; is of strategic importance in comparing the results of different laboratories, identifying the true state-of-the-art, and defining quality specifications for each indicator; and contributes to reducing errors and maximizing patient safety. An accurate definition of each indicator helps staff to understand the following:

- What they must measure
- The performance standard expected of them
- The TTP phase involved
- The reason for the importance of the previous points
- The way in which events under control have to be measured and what the measurement problems are
- The information to be transmitted

Likewise, it is of great importance to implement a reporting system that specifies the

- Individual who is to collect or analyze data and identify the corrective actions
- Frequency of data collection
- Way in which data are to be analyzed
- Approach required for evaluating quality improvement

Moreover, to be effective, the management of QIs must be designed as part of a coherent and integrated system in quality improvement strategies,[43] and based on an internal assessment evaluation system and participation in an interlaboratory program.

The internal assessment system includes the definition of a list of QIs to be used in different laboratory areas, both technical and managerial; a form for each indicator that defines the specifications (what has to be measured, how to collect data, acceptability limits for results, laboratory areas where they are to be carried out, responsibilities); and instructions describing operational arrangement for managing the QIs system.

The effectiveness of QIs is closely related to the complete understanding of all staff involved as to the importance of using the specific indicator, the method for data collection and processing, and result evaluation. The definition of a form for each indicator that describes the rationale, the activities/processes involved, and any necessary information regarding the collection and analysis of data is conducive to achieving full staff awareness (**Table 1**). The form not only formalizes statements, but also obliges staff to assume full responsibility by signing it.

Likewise, it is important to issue an operating instruction to describe the operational procedures to be followed and to ensure uniform behavior so that goals can be achieved. The operating instructions must describe all activities involved in the QIs management system and, in particular, the criteria and procedures for the following:

- Identification and definition of indicator
- Design of QIs system
- Method for data collection and analysis of results and related frequency
- Method for reviewing the system
- Responsibilities for each step, including system testing, putting into practice, implementing improvement actions

Employment of QIs calls for a data collection system that guarantees:

- Accuracy, so that all events to be measured are effectively collected
- Traceability, which raises staff awareness of their responsibilities in recording information to provide evidence of procedures used and to simplify investigation into causes of error

Table 1
Quality indicator form

Identification code
Purpose/rationale
Process/activity involved
Method of data collection
Times for data collection
Method for data processing
Results presentation
Goal for corrective action
Goal for improvement action
Person appointed for data collection
Person in charge of data collection
Person in charge of periodic data analysis
Problems of the measurement

Classification

☐ Efficiency	☐ Structure	☐ Preanalytical phase
☐ Effectiveness	☐ Activity/process	☐ Intra-analytical phase
☐ Timeliness	☐ Results	☐ Postanalytical phase
☐ Safety of the staff	☐ Outcome	☐ Support processes
☐ Competence		

Laboratory area where the indicator has to be used

Note

- Standardization, so that data collected in different periods of time are comparable
- Efficiency, making data analysis easier and timelier for the implementation of improvement actions

It is therefore advisable to use software to guarantee standardized data collection independently of operator, the measure of all events that must be recorded, reduced recording and processing times, ease of procedures, and improved staff satisfaction.

A well-designed and managed internal assessment system enables the laboratory to assess QIs results over time but does not provide information on its performance with respect to other laboratories, at either a national or international level. The participation in an interlaboratory program, proposed and approved by the scientific community, is therefore indispensable in improving on process and reducing error, and in monitoring the appropriateness of the internal assessment system used.

To promote the harmonized use of QIs, since 2008 the Working Group on Laboratory Errors and Patient Safety (WG-LEPS) of the International Federation of Clinical Chemistry and Laboratory Medicine (IFCC) has implemented a project aiming to develop an MQI for use in clinical laboratories throughout the world.[44,45] It is designed, above all, to identify a list of QIs that can be applied in all laboratories worldwide, define the procedures for data collection, and provide quality specifications for evaluating laboratory results.

Three different MQIs have followed in succession because during the project's experimental phase it emerged that there was a need to improve aspects, such as wording, the number of indicators, and the information included in the periodic and confidential report.

The MQI, discussed and approved in the Consensus Conference held in Padova (Italy) in 2013, has been tested since 2014 through an external quality assurance program (EQAP). A dedicated Web site (www.ifcc-mqi.com) has been implemented to manage uniform data collection and centralized data processing, and to provide a report for each participant. Participation is free and confidentiality is ensured. A criterion to define the performance specifications for each indicator has been proposed. MQI includes 53 QIs of which, concerning the key processes, 28 indicators were defined for the preanalytical phase, six for the intra-analytical phase, and 11 for the postanalytical phase. Moreover, five indicators were defined to monitor the support processes (two for staff competence, two users' satisfaction, one efficiency of laboratory information system) and three the outcome measures (**Tables 2–4**).

To facilitate the introduction into practice for each indicator, an order of priority has been assigned based on the importance of the specific indicator and the difficulty of data collection (one the highest priority, four the lowest). The QIs with priority one, which are mandatory, are to be put into practice first.

In many cases in the MQI, different measures have been defined to keep a single event under control to make data from laboratories comparable. In fact, in cases of different laboratories (ie, for context or user typology) it is important to split the collected data to guarantee that, for the same QI, the data collected have the same origin.

Regarding the identification of common QIs, mounting evidence underscores the importance of a standardized reporting system as an essential step toward harmonization. First and foremost, the standardization of the system for data collection and reporting plays a key role in ensuring the comparability of data collected by different

Table 2
Quality indicators of key processes

Code	Quality Indicator	Priority Order
Preanalytical Phase		
Misidentification errors		
Pre-MisR	Percentage of number of misidentified requests/ total number of requests	1
Pre-MisS	Percentage of number of misidentified samples/ total number of samples	1
Pre-Iden	Percentage of number of samples with fewer than two identifiers initially supplied/total number of samples	1
Pre-UnlS	Percentage of number of unlabeled samples/ total number of samples	1
Inappropriate test requests		
Pre-Quest	Percentage of number of requests without clinical question (outpatients)/total number of requests (outpatients)	2
Pre-OutReq	Percentage of number of inappropriate requests, with respect to clinical question (outpatients)/number of requests reporting clinical question (outpatients)	4
Pre-InReq	Percentage of number of inappropriate requests, with respect to clinical question (inpatients)/number of requests reporting clinical question (inpatients)	4
Test transcription errors		
Pre-OutpTN	Percentage of number of outpatients requests with erroneous data entry (test name)/total number of outpatients requests	1
Pre-OutpMT	Percentage of number of outpatients requests with erroneous data entry (missed test)/total number of outpatients requests	1
Pre-OutpAT	Percentage of number of outpatients requests with erroneous data entry (added test)/total number of outpatients requests	1
Pre-InpTN	Percentage of number of inpatients requests with erroneous data entry (test name)/total number of inpatients requests	1
Pre-InpMT	Percentage of number of inpatients requests with erroneous data entry (missed test)/total number of inpatients requests	1
Pre-InpAT	Percentage of number of inpatients requests with erroneous data entry (added test)/total number of inpatients requests	1
Unintelligible requests		
Pre-OutUn	Percentage of number of unintelligible outpatients requests/total number of outpatients requests	3

(continued on next page)

Table 2
(continued)

Code	Quality Indicator	Priority Order
Pre-InpUn	Percentage of number of unintelligible inpatients requests/total number of inpatients requests	3
Incorrect sample type		
Pre-WroTy	Percentage of number of samples of wrong or inappropriate type (ie, whole blood instead of plasma)/total number of samples	1
Pre-WroCo	Percentage of number of samples collected in wrong container/total number of samples	1
Incorrect fill level		
Pre-InsV	Percentage of number of samples with insufficient sample volume/total number of samples	1
Pre-SaAnt	Percentage of number of samples with inappropriate sample-anticoagulant volume ratio/total number of samples with anticoagulant	1
Unsuitable samples for transportation and storage problems		
Pre-NotRec	Percentage of number of samples not received/total number of samples	1
Pre-NotSt	Percentage of number of samples not properly stored before analysis/total number of samples	1
Pre-DamS	Percentage of number of samples damaged during transportation/total number of samples	1
Pre-InTem	Percentage of number of samples transported at inappropriate temperature/total number of samples	1
Pre-ExcTim	Percentage of number of samples with excessive transportation time/total number of samples	1
Contaminated samples		
Pre-MicCon	Percentage of number of contaminated samples rejected/total number of microbiologic samples	1
Sample hemolysed		
Pre-Hem	Percentage of number of samples with free Hb >0.5 g/L (clinical chemistry)/total number of samples (clinical chemistry)[a]	1
Samples clotted		
Pre-Clot	Percentage of number of samples clotted/total number of samples with an anticoagulant	1
Inappropriate time in sample collection		
Pre-InTime	Percentage of number of samples collected at inappropriate time of sample collection/total number of samples	2

(continued on next page)

Table 2 (continued)		
Code	**Quality Indicator**	**Priority Order**
Intra-analytical Phase		
Test with inappropriate ICQ performances		
Intra-Var	Percentage of number of tests with CV% higher than selected target, per year/total number of tests with CV% known for at least • Glucose • Creatinine • Potassium • C-reactive protein • Troponin I or troponin T • TSH • CEA • PT (INR) • Hb	1
Test uncovered by an EQA-PT control		
Intra-EQA	Percentage of number of tests without EQA-PT control/total number of tests in the menu	1
Unacceptable performances in EQA-PT schemes		
Intra-Unac	Percentage of number of unacceptable performances in EQAS-PT schemes, per year/total number of performances in EQA schemes, per year	1
Intra-PPP	Percentage of number of unacceptable performances in EQAS-PT schemes per year occurring to previously treated cause/total number of unacceptable performances	3
Data transcription errors		
Intra-ErrTran	Percentage of number of incorrect results for erroneous manual transcription/total number of results that need manual transcription	1
Intra-FailLIS	Percentage of number of incorrect results for information system problems-failures/total number of results	1
Postanalytical Phase		
Inappropriate turnaround times		
Post-OutTime	Percentage of number of reports delivered outside the specified time/total number of reports	1
Post-PotTAT	Turnaround time (minutes) of potassium (K) at 90th percentile (STAT)	1
Post-INRTAT	Turnaround time (minutes) of INR value at 90th percentile (STAT)	1
Post-WBCTAT	Turnaround time (minutes) of WBC at 90th percentile (STAT)	1
Post-TnTAT	Turnaround time (minutes) of troponin I or troponin T at 90th percentile (STAT)	1

(continued on next page)

Table 2 (continued)		
Code	Quality Indicator	Priority Order
Incorrect laboratory reports		
Post-IncRep	Percentage of number of incorrect reports issued by the laboratory/total number of reports issued by the laboratory	1
Notification of critical values		
Post-InpCV	Percentage of number of critical values of inpatients notified after a consensually agreed time (from result validation to result communication to the clinician)/total number of critical values of inpatients to communicate	1
Post-OutCV	Percentage of number of critical values of outpatients notified after a consensually agreed time (from result validation to result communication to the clinician)/total number of critical values of outpatients to communicate	1
Results notification (TAT)		
Post-InCVT	Time (from result validation to result communication to the clinician) to communicate critical values of inpatients (minutes)	4
Post-OutCVT	Time (from result validation to result communication to the clinician) to communicate critical values of outpatient (minutes)	4
Interpretative comments		
Post-Comm	Percentage of number of reports with interpretative comments, provided in medical report, impacting positively on patient's outcome/total number of reports with interpretative comments	4

Abbreviations: CEA, arcinoembryonic antigen; CV, coefficient of variation; Hb, hemoglobin; INR, international normalized ratio; IQC, Internal Quality Control; PT, prothrombin time; TSH, thyroid-stimulating hormone; WBC, white blood cell count.
[a] Clinical chemistry: all samples that are analyzed on the chemistry analyzer, which is used for detection of HIL indices. If laboratories are detecting hemolysis visually, they count all samples with visible hemolysis. We suggest that a color chart is provided for this purpose.

laboratories worldwide. This aspect prompted us to split some QIs into different groups to facilitate the understanding and collection of data:

a. Four measures are included in MQI for misidentification errors: misidentified requests, misidentified samples, samples with fewer than two identifiers initially supplied, and unlabeled samples

b. Six measures for the test transcription errors: the errors concerning the missed test, the added test, the misnamed test, split into outpatients and inpatients

c. Seven measures for unsuitable samples: samples of wrong or inappropriate type; samples collected in wrong container; samples with insufficient sample volume; samples with inappropriate sample-anticoagulant volume ratio; and hemolyzed, clotted, and/or contaminated samples

Table 3
Quality indicators of support processes

Code	Quality Indicator	Priority Order
Employee competence		
Supp-Train	Number of training events organized for all staff, per year	2
Supp-Cred	Percentage of number of credits obtained by employee, per year/total number of credits to be obtained, per year	2
Client relationships		
Supp-Phys	Percentage of sum of point given in the enquiry to the question of global satisfaction of the physician/ multiplication of the maximum point defined in the enquiries by the number of enquiries	2
Supp-Pat	Percentage of sum of point given in the enquiry to the question of global satisfaction of the patient/ multiplication of the maximum point defined in the enquiries by the number of enquiries	2
Efficiency of laboratory information system		
Supp-FailLIS	Number of Laboratory Information System downtime episodes, per year	3

d. Five measures for unsuitable samples caused by transportation and storage problems: samples not received, not properly stored before analysis, excessive transportation time, transported at inappropriate temperature, and/or damaged during transport

e. Seven measures to evaluate the appropriateness of time to release results: number of reports delivered outside the specified time, TAT (minutes) at 90th percentile (STAT) (potassium, international normalized ratio, white blood cell count, troponin I or troponin T), number of critical values notified after a mutually agreed time (from result validation to result communication to the clinician for inpatients and outpatients)

f. One measure for incorrect laboratory report

Data from participating laboratories are collected and processed, and a report is-sued by the WG-LEPS contact person. In the report the laboratory results are described in relation to a specific period of time and the corresponding Sigma value

Table 4
Quality indicators of outcome measures

Code	Quality Indicator	Priority Order
Sample recollection		
Out-RecOutp	Percentage of number of outpatients with recollected samples for laboratory errors/total number of outpatients	1
Out-RecInp	Percentage of number of inpatients with recollected samples for laboratory errors/total number of inpatients	1
Inaccurate results		
Out-InacR	Percentage of number of inaccurate results released/total number of results released	1

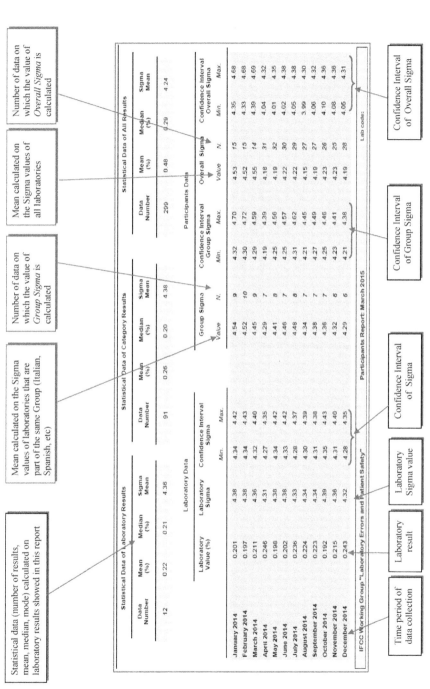

Fig. 1. Report concerning quality indicator results and Sigma values of participating laboratory.

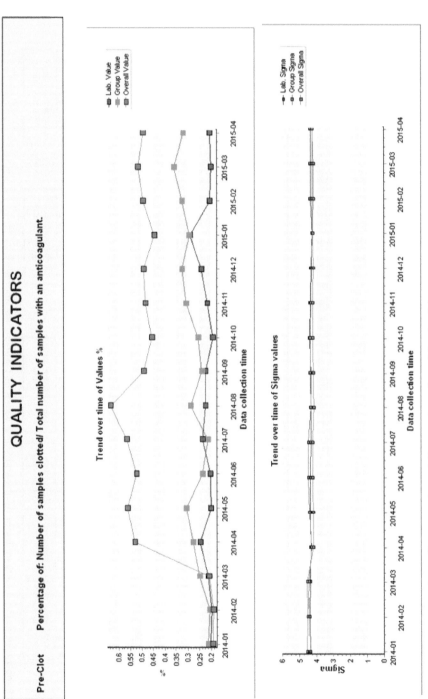

Fig. 2. Trend concerning quality indicator results and Sigma values of participating laboratory.

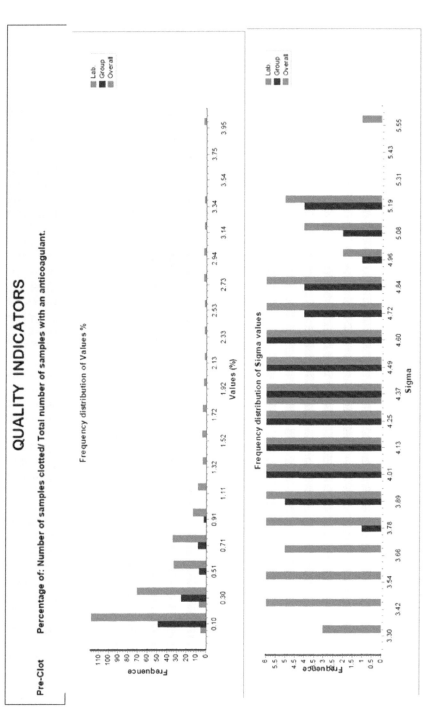

Fig. 3. Frequency distribution of quality indicator results and Sigma values of participating laboratory.

with confidence range is specified. The laboratory can compare its performance with that of other participants on the basis of the mean calculated on the Sigma values of laboratories from the same country and all participating laboratories. Laboratories are provided with the results and Sigma value trends in a graph, and the frequency distribution (**Figs. 1–3**).

QUALITY SPECIFICATIONS IN THE EXTRA-ANALYTICAL PHASES

A significant decrease in error rates in the analytical phase has been achieved in the last three decades thanks to automation; standardization and optimization of reagents; improved training of the laboratory staff; and above all to the development and implementation of valuable analytical quality specifications and their use in setting objective goals in routine practice, and in measuring, recording, and improving laboratory performances in IQC and EQAPs.[4] The hierarchy of models to establish analytical quality specifications defined in the Stockholm Conference was the fruit of years of work, publications, and scientific debate, whereas only a few preliminary proposals are available for the extra-analytical phases.

The definition of performance specifications for each indicator facilitates the interpretation of QIs results and the identification of action priorities. This criterion is based on the results of participating laboratories. The definition of three different performance goals allows laboratories to compare their performance with that of other laboratories, and to ascertain whether improvement actions are possible and feasible: the lower percentiles represent the better, and the higher percentiles, the worse performance. The use of the 75th percentile as a lower limit seems to be the most practical possible approach, because no more than 25% of laboratories are considered to have a poor performance.

The proposal for performance specifications is based on data collected in the last year by IFCC WG-LEPS to provide a reliable picture of the current state-of-the-art. However, because the ideal performance criteria should be "zero defects," we made a preliminary definition of the following three levels: high, medium, and low. Although for analytical performance criteria the levels are defined with respect to biologic variation, for preanalytical and postanalytical issues, errors and defects are linked specifically to the quality of the procedures and, at least in theory, the final goal is zero tolerance. This approach allows laboratories not only to ascertain whether their performance lies within an acceptable range, but also to identify any negative trend when their performance shifts from a high, to a medium or low level.

The quality specifications defined represent a starting point for activating the improvement process. In fact, the system cannot be effective without the proper analysis and identification of error sources and the implementation of appropriate corrective actions. Also, the continuous exchange of experience between laboratory professionals is a further key element conferring added value to the system.

SUMMARY

The identification of a management system of QIs that meets requirements for effectiveness and harmonization may have important implications in many aspects of the laboratory. The implementation and management of a QI system that includes internal assessment and participation in interlaboratory comparison, a suitable tool for supporting the management decisions for quality, should be considered one of the fundamental components of a continuous quality improvement system.

Because different QIs and terminologies are currently used, there is the need to pursue a harmonization process involving the identification of common QIs and a standardized reporting system. Although the identification of harmonized, universal QIs seems to be the mainstay, the standardization of data collection and reporting systems are critical steps in effective harmonization initiatives. The IFCC project WG-LEPS applies to all laboratories nationally and worldwide, thus effectively coordinating opinions and contributions, and promoting quality improvement in laboratory medicine.[45,46]

REFERENCES

1. Kallner A, McQueen M, Heuck C. Foreword. The Stockholm Consensus on quality specifications in laboratory medicine 25-26 April 1999. Scand J Clin Lab Invest 1999;59:475–6.
2. Sandberg S, Fraser CG, Horvath AR, et al. Defining analytical performance specifications: consensus statement from the 1st strategic conference of the European Federation of Clinical Chemistry and Laboratory Medicine. Clin Chem Lab Med 2015;53:833–5.
3. Bonini P, Plebani M, Ceriotti F, et al. Errors in laboratory medicine. Clin Chem 2002;48:691–8.
4. Plebani M. The detection and prevention of errors in laboratory medicine. Ann Clin Biochem 2010;47:101–10.
5. Plebani M, Carraro P. Mistakes in a stat laboratory: types and frequency. Clin Chem 1997;43:1348–51.
6. Carraro P, Plebani M. Errors in a stat laboratory: types and frequencies 10 years later. Clin Chem 2007;53:1338–42.
7. UNI EN ISO 15189. Medical laboratories: requirements for quality and competence. Geneva (Switzerland): International Organization for Standardization; 2013.
8. Sciacovelli L, Aita A, Padoan A, et al. Performance criteria and quality indicators for the post-analytical phase. Clin Chem Lab Med 2016;54:1169–76.
9. Plebani M, Sciacovelli L, Aita A, et al. Performance criteria and quality indicators for the pre-analytical phase. Clin Chem Lab Med 2015;53:943–8.
10. Plebani M. Errors in clinical laboratories or errors in laboratory medicine? Clin Chem Lab Med 2006;44:750–9.
11. Lippi G, Becan-McBride K, Behúlová D, et al. Preanalytical quality improvement: in quality we trust. Clin Chem Lab Med 2013;51:229–41.
12. Holman JW, Mifflin TE, Felder RA, et al. Evaluation of an automated preanalytical robotic workstation at two academic health centers. Clin Chem 2002;48:540–8.
13. Da Rin G. Pre-analytical workstations: a tool for reducing laboratory errors. Clin Chim Acta 2009;404:68–74.
14. Wallin O, Söderberg J, Van Guelpen B, et al. Preanalytical venous blood sampling practices demand improvement: a survey of test-request management, test-tube labelling and information search procedures. Clin Chim Acta 2008; 391:91–7.
15. Söderberg J, Brulin C, Grankvist K, et al. Preanalytical errors in primary healthcare: a questionnaire study of information search procedures, test request management and test tube labelling. Clin Chem Lab Med 2009;47:195–201.
16. Kemp GM, Bird CE, Barth JH. Short-term interventions on wards fail to reduce preanalytical errors: results of two prospective controlled trials. Ann Clin Biochem 2012;49:166–9.
17. Valestein P. Laboratory turnaround time. Am J Clin Pathol 1996;105:676–88.
18. Lim EM, Sikaris KA, Gill J, et al. Quality assessment of interpretative commenting in clinical chemistry. Clin Chem 2004;50:632–7.

19. Dighe AS, Sodeberg BI, Laposata M. Narrative interpretation for clinical laboratory interpretations. Am J Clin Pathol 2001;116:S123–8.
20. Macmillian DH, Sodeberg BI, Laposata M. Regulations regarding reflexive testing and narrative interpretations in laboratory medicine. Am J Clin Pathol 2001;116: S129–32.
21. Kratz A, Sodeberg BI. The generation of narrative interpretations in laboratory medicine. Am J Clin Pathol 2001;116:S133–40.
22. Plebani M. Interpretative commenting: a tool for improving the laboratory-clinical interface. Clin Chim Acta 2009;404:46–51.
23. Clinical and Laboratory Standards and Institute. Quality management system: continual improved. Approved Guideline – Third Edition. QMS06–A3, 2011.
24. Plebani M. Harmonization in laboratory medicine: requests, samples, measurements and reports. Crit Rev Clin Lab Sci 2016;53(3):184–96.
25. Carraro P, Zago T, Plebani M. Exploring the initial steps of the testing process: frequency and nature of pre-preanalytic errors. Clin Chem 2012;58:638–42.
26. Plebani M. Quality indicators to detect pre-analytical errors in laboratory testing. Clin Biochem Rev 2012;33:85–8.
27. Wagar EA, Tamashiro L, Yasin B, et al. Patient safety in the clinical laboratory: a longitudinal analysis of specimen identification errors. Arch Pathol Lab Med 2006; 130:1662–8.
28. Lippi G, Blanckaert N, Bonini P, et al. Causes, consequences, detection, and prevention of identification errors in laboratory diagnostics. Clin Chem Lab Med 2009;47:143–53.
29. Plebani M, Sciacovelli L, Aita A, et al. Quality Indicators to detect pre-analytical errors in laboratory testing. Clin Chim Acta 2014;432:44–8.
30. Plebani M, Sciacovelli L, Marinova M, et al. Quality indicators in laboratory medicine: a fundamental tool for quality and patient safety. Clin Biochem 2013;46: 1170–4.
31. Khoury M, Burnett L, Mackay M. Error rate in Australian chemical pathology laboratories. Med J Aust 1996;165:128–30.
32. Shcolnik W, de Oliveira CA, de São José AS, et al. Brazilian laboratory indicators program. Clin Chem Lab Med 2012;50:1923–34.
33. Kirchner MJ, Funes VA, Adzet CB, et al. Quality indicators and specifications for key processes in clinical laboratories: a preliminary experience. Clin Chem Lab Med 2007;45:672–7.
34. Barth JH. Selecting clinical quality indicators for laboratory medicine. Ann Clin Biochem 2012;49:257–61.
35. Barth JH. Clinical quality indicators in laboratory medicine. Ann Clin Biochem 2012;49:9–16.
36. Simundic AM, Topic E. Quality indicators. Biochem Med 2008;18:311–9.
37. Llopis MA, Trujillo G, Llovet MI, et al. Quality indicators and specifications for key, analytical–extranalytical processes in the clinical laboratory: five years' experience using the six sigma concept. Clin Chem Lab Med 2011;49:463–70.
38. Barth JH. Clinical quality indicators in laboratory medicine: a survey of current practice in the UK. Ann Clin Biochem 2011;48:238–40.
39. Sciacovelli L, Sonntag O, Padoan A, et al. Monitoring quality indicators in laboratory medicine does not automatically result in quality improvement. Clin Chem Lab Med 2011;50:463–9.
40. Sciacovelli L, O'Kane M, Skaik YA, et al. Quality indicators in laboratory medicine: from theory to practice. Preliminary data from the IFCC working group project "laboratory errors and patient safety". Clin Chem Lab Med 2011;49:835–44.

41. Plebani M. Harmonization in laboratory medicine: the complete picture. Clin Chem Lab Med 2013;51:741–51.
42. ISO/PDTS 22367. Medical laboratories: reducing error through risk management and continual improvement. Geneva (Switzerland): International Organization for Standardization; 2008.
43. Clinical and Laboratory Standards and Institute (CLSI). Development and use of quality indicators for process improvement and monitoring of laboratory quality. Approved Guideline. QMS12–A3, 2010.
44. Sciacovelli L, Plebani M. The IFCC Working Group on laboratory errors and patient safety. Clin Chim Acta 2009;404(1):79–85.
45. Plebani M, Astion ML, Barth JH, et al. Harmonization of quality indicators in laboratory medicine. A preliminary consensus. Clin Chem Lab Med 2014;52:951–8.
46. Plebani M, Chiozza ML, Sciacovelli L. Towards harmonization of quality indicators in laboratory medicine. Clin Chem Lab Med 2013;51:187–95.

Using Sigma Quality Control to Verify and Monitor Performance in a Multi-Instrument, Multisite Integrated Health Care Network

Harold H. Harrison, MD, PhD, FACB, FCAP[a],*, Jay B. Jones, PhD, D(ABCC), FACB[b]

KEYWORDS

- Sigma metrics • Multisite instrument system • Clinical chemistry • Coagulation
- Hematology • Networked QC management

KEY POINTS

- Develop a multisite integrated instrument network with ongoing Sigma-driven quality control (QC) rules management.
- Establish baseline Sigma performance for several instrument-method types in each discipline of chemistry, coagulation, and hematology based on laboratory size and scope.
- Evaluate monthly and annual variation in Sigma performance metrics for ongoing justification of change in rules, for example, 1-2s to 1-3s rejection, or retention of standard Westgard rule sets.
- Measure run rejection rates and evaluate the operational gains resulting from decreased run rejections.
- Show stability in performance over time and changes in lots of QC materials for core methods on Roche chemistry and immunochemistry instruments, Diagnostica Stago coagulation instruments, and Sysmex hematology instruments.

INTRODUCTION

The Sigma-metric statistical approach to clinical instrument and method evaluation developed by Professor James Westgard and colleagues[1–3] provides a powerful technique for characterizing the performance of specific instrument-method combinations in the context of precision and total allowable error (TEa). The inclusion of both analytical and clinically acceptable variation into a TEa allows the derivation of power

[a] Laboratory Medicine, Geisinger Health System, 100 North Academy Avenue, Danville, PA 17822, USA; [b] Clinical Chemistry, Geisinger Regional Laboratories, 100 North Academy Avenue, Danville, PA 17822, USA
* Corresponding author.
E-mail address: hharrison@geisinger.edu

Clin Lab Med 37 (2017) 207–241
http://dx.doi.org/10.1016/j.cll.2016.10.001
0272-2712/17/© 2016 Elsevier Inc. All rights reserved.

labmed.theclinics.com

functions and OpSpecs charts that define the number and frequency of control materials and control rule limits necessary to adequately monitor quantitative process performance for individual instrument and method combinations. This customization of quality control (QC) rules brings a contextual dimension that melds analytical and clinical quality goals into a single indicator.

This new Sigma QC approach has been transformational to quantitative analytical process management by providing rules for minimizing false run rejections and maximizing true error detection as needed for specific analyte-instrument combinations.

Generally the application of Sigma analysis has been a cross-sectional analytical event with calculations based on data collected for a relatively brief period, commonly 1 month or less, using QC materials or a group average of results for a common sample event, such as proficiency testing. This usage yields a powerful and useful moment-in-time result for comparing QC number and frequency requirements across methods and instrument families. The Sigma-driven QC design process results in a laboratory monitoring approach whereby one is no longer limited to the same one-size-fits-all classic set of QC rules and responses of first-generation Westgard rules and Shewhart/Levey-Jennings charts. The Sigma-metric approach empowers the laboratory to customize rule sets to the specific precision and operational specification for each method-instrument combination. As the authors sought to incorporate this type of QC approach into daily operations and system-wide QC management, they identified it as the Advanced Analytical QC (AAQC) program to distinguish it from the more traditional QC rule approaches engrained in medical technology education and instrument-dwelling or manufacturer-supplied QC software. This article describes the authors' use of Sigma-metrics on a system level and its growth and extension in disciplinary scope and number of sites. As noted earlier, the Sigma values reported in the literature have generally been developed as single window-in-time calculations, yet for ongoing management in a networked regional laboratory system, some understanding of stability and variation were needed to determine applicability. Therefore, the authors set out to evaluate the Sigma-metric approach over time with chemistry and extension to other core assays in coagulation and hematology. Some of these data have been presented in preliminary form as AACC annual meeting posters.[4–6]

History

The Geisinger Medical Laboratory (GML) system is a large and growing integrated laboratory system that is highly focused on standardization and operational efficiency. It covers an area of 25,000 square miles in north central Pennsylvania that has an encompassed population of 3 million. At the start of the AAQC program in 2010 the system included 2 hospitals and 7 regional clinic laboratories. Since the beginning of the program, the authors' system has grown substantially, principally by acquisition and merger. As of the summer of 2016, the GML incorporates 7 hospitals ranging from 50 to 500 beds, 10 large regional multispecialty clinics with nonwaived, instrumented laboratories, a stand-alone outpatient reference laboratory, and approximately 75 waived testing physician offices and small clinics (**Fig. 1**).

Information technology

The laboratory information technology (IT) network includes Epic EHR (Epic Systems Corporation, Verona, WI) for ordering and reporting, Sunquest for the common laboratory information system (LIS), and Copath for pathology and interpretive reporting. CareEvolve is also included for reporting to physician offices.

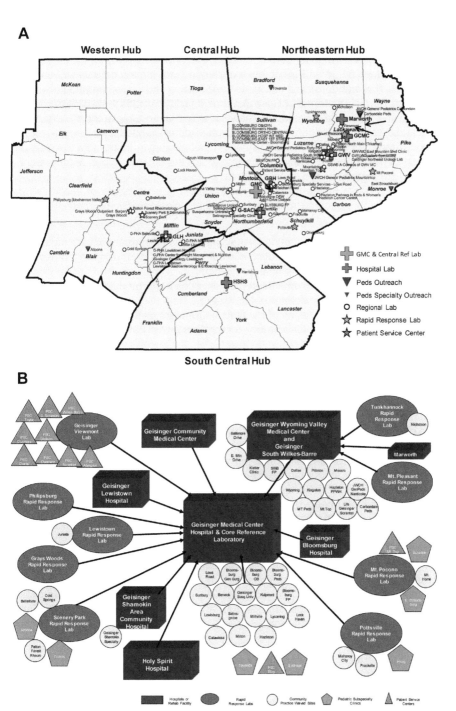

Fig. 1. (*A*) GML in Central Pennsylvania. (*B*) GML interlaboratory referral relationships. Lab, laboratory; PSC, patient service centers.

Harmonization and standardization

The authors' goal is to use similar manufacturers and methods across the system to provide uniformity of results, common reference ranges as patients move from site to site for various centers of treatment excellence, and primary care versus specialty care needs. This standardization requires the adoption and implementation of not only system standard IT platforms but also instruments and methods that validate common analytical and reference ranges at the new sites. To that end, the authors' current system standard sources for core analytics include Roche Diagnostics (chemistry), Diagnostica Stago (coagulation), and Sysmex (hematology). Instrument models are selected to match the workload needs of each of the different types of laboratories. These instruments are cited explicitly later.

Given the system needs for standardization and harmonization of analytical processes, the authors became interested in using the Westgard Sigma-metric approach for several purposes:

1. To verify that the initially obtained values for Sigma performance were measurable and maintained in ongoing, routine clinical instrument performance (not just optimized data reported for one time publication)
2. To demonstrate that instruments at different sites performed acceptably on installation and continuously during routine usage
3. To evaluate the performance of multiple instruments as a group by model type as well as detect individual laboratory outliers performing at lower or higher Sigma levels than the others
4. To identify specific analytes where high Sigma values (consistently in excess of 4.0) allow for more relaxed QC limits, for example, 1-3s versus 1-2s as initial warning and, thereby, fewer QC out-of-control events
5. To quantify the improved operational impact of the decreased false rejections occurring with Sigma-derived QC rules selection
6. To demonstrate to the technical staff the value of Sigma-derived changes in warning limits and build confidence in the new approach to QC rule determination
7. To measure and monitor month-to-month and year-to-year variations and trends in Sigma values for instrument performance over long production run time intervals expected of typical instrument usage
8. To compare instruments that have the same reagents but different mechanics, fluidics, and computerization for baseline and stability levels of Sigma values

Organization

To organize efforts for multiple sites, the authors established an oversight committee for AAQC, which included operations, technical, and medical scientific leadership. This program has been rolled out progressively over the past 5 years, during which time the authors have also added 5 hospitals and incorporated unanticipated variation in instrumentation and QC methods, policies, and procedures. The AAQC committee functioned to

1. Select the supplier and materials for standardization of the analytical QC materials: For chemistry, unassayed Bio-Rad Liquichek controls (Bio-Rad Laboratories, Inc, Hercules, CA) were used; for coagulation, Diagnostica Stago N and ABN controls (Diagnostica Stago Inc, Parsippany, NJ) were used; and for hematology, Sysmex level 1, 2, and 3 controls (Sysmex Corporation, Kobe, Japan) were used. Each of these companies now produces a report that contains peer group means (Unity, Clarity, and Insight, respectively, for Bio-Rad, Stago, and Sysmex). These reports were used for monthly assessment of bias. Arrangements were made with each

company to produce, sequester, and ship satisfactory amounts of identical lot control materials to all of the GML sites.

2. Create commonly accessible online file folders to maintain the data files, calculation spreadsheets, and trend graphs, which is maintained on a virtual disk drive that is accessible from all sites in the GML-wide area Intranet system

3. Develop discipline-related subteams and technical leaders to collate the mean, standard deviation, and bias and calculate and record the Sigma value for each area monthly

4. Standardize the use of comment codes in response to out-of-control alerts, necessitating reducing the number of codes in use from approximately 40 to 10: Before this standardization, the choice of comment code was up to the individual technologist to select from a long list that contained conceptual redundancies. (This is a most important area of education as new institutions join the system.)

5. Manage ongoing activities and challenges to the AAQC program for
   - Educating staff to understand the concepts and calculation of Sigma values
   - Create standard templates for access and use by multiple sites
   - Standardize control material types, production lots, and inventory
   - Incorporate new institutions and colleagues as added to the GML system
   - Time to implement in each site and scientific area: 5 years since the start in 2010, now there are 5 more hospitals than the two with which the authors started and 3 added regional laboratories, with progression from chemistry to coagulation to hematology
   - Instruments with control cutoffs that are hard coded or difficult to alter by method
   - Maintaining momentum during periods of merger transitions, technical leadership turnover, and instrumentation changes.
   - Accommodating software version changes and maintenance of compatibility among the onboard instrument software, middleware, and LIS systems

6. Report on achievements of the project at scientific meetings (AACC, American Society for Clinical Pathologists, College of American Pathologists [CAP], and so forth) and in publications

METHODS

Sigma values were calculated based on QC sample data. Chemistry QC materials were sourced from Bio-Rad (Liquichek level 1 and 2), coagulation QC was from Diagnostica Stago (STA normal and abnormal), and hematology QC (3 levels) was from Sysmex.

Sigma values were calculated using the following equation: Sigma = [(TEa − bias)/ SD], where SD is standard deviation and TEa was determined by Clinical Laboratory Improvement Amendments requirement or CAP Scientific Committee Consensus (from proficiency testing participant summaries). Bias was determined from the difference of the measured mean value and a peer group mean. The standard deviation or coefficient of variation (CV) was determined for each group of QC measurements, typically 1 month for chemistry and coagulation and one period (4–6 weeks) for hematology. These results were then recorded into spreadsheets accessible to staff from all sites. For assessment of bias, where possible, lot-specific peer means were obtained online or in printed reports from Bio-Rad (Unity) and Sysmex (Insight). For coagulation testing (prothrombin time [PT] and partial thromboplastin time [PTT]), a self-generated, local peer group of 11 instruments was used to determine a group mean for calculation of bias. Recently the authors have begun to use the new Stago Clarity statistical report as more participants join to provide a broader participant peer group.

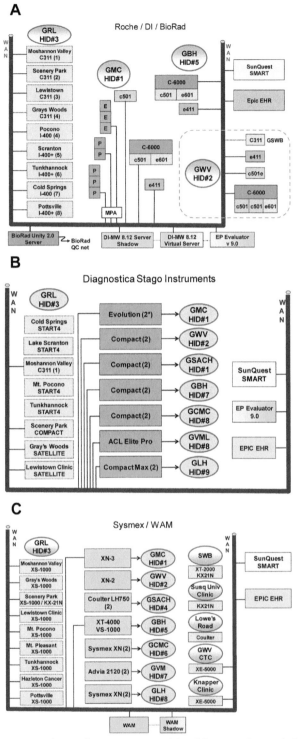

Fig. 2. (*A*) Enterprise analytics: chemistry connectivity. (*B*) Enterprise analytics: coagulation connectivity. (*C*) Enterprise analytics: hematology connectivity. DI, data innovations; WAN, wide area network.

System-wide computer connectivity has been key to centralizing data gathering and analysis. The system connections for the chemistry, coagulation, and hematology instrument platforms are shown in **Fig. 2**. Chemistry instruments on the network included the modular E and P units, c501, Integra, and c311 models. Chemistry QC data were transmitted through Roche-Data Innovations Middleware to a wide area network (WAN) that also communicated with Bio-Rad Unity Real Time. Coagulation instruments included the Stago Evolution, Compact, Satellite, and STart4. Coagulation data were collected in a central Excel spreadsheet database for monthly Sigma calculations as shown in **Table 1** and **Fig. 3**. The Satellite and STart4 were not interfaced, but the WAN was used for the interfaced Compact and Evolution models. Hematology data were interfaced through the same WAN and Sunquest but also through the Sysmex WAM interface.

Chemistry Sigmas were calculated by a combination of networked Excel spreadsheets and the online BioRad Westgard Advisor module. However, as a final common pathway for all data, they were manually entered into the spreadsheets to generate dashboard (trend) plots. As the program has progressed, the number and proportion of online laboratories has increased. Monthly Sigmas were plotted from each instrument cited on a trend plot (dashboard) or Sigma scatterplot as shown in **Figs. 3** and **4**. To avoid some of the visual confusion created with the large number of interwoven representations in the trend plot, the authors created another graph that they refer to as a Sigma scatterplot to allow distinction of performance of each individual instrument grouped by model.

Preparations for implementing the Sigma approach at each site included (1) purchase of sufficient QC material to use the same lot number on all instruments for the longest possible period of time based on stability and availability. For chemistry and coagulation, this was typically 9 to 12 months and 2 to 3 months for hematology cell-based controls. (2) The program also necessitated advance operational planning and cooperation from the suppliers to sequester enough designated lots and inventory to provide the specified QC material supply throughout the GML multisite system. (3) When changing production lots of QC, an overlap baseline period for at least 1 month was used for chemistry and coagulation and 2 weeks for hematology.

Frequency of QC performance varied based on the site. For hospitals, QC was run at least once per shift and every 2 to 4 hours at the central medical center laboratory for chemistry. Coagulation and hematology QC was run once per shift. The hospital laboratories are all around-the-clock operations. For the clinic sites, QC was run twice or 3 times per day of operation, which was generally weekdays only.

Table 1
Average Sigmas for selected chemistry analytes on Roche analytics

Test	H1	H2	RL1	RL2	RL3	RL4	RL5	RL6	RL7
Alkaline phosphatase	8.9	12.8	9.4	11.5	10.3	11.9	7.4	7.3	6.4
	12.9	15.1	21.5	26.5	15.5	20.0	17.6	11.1	9.0
Glucose	3.7	6.7	6.3	9.1	7.6	8.9	6.0	4.5	5.1
	4.7	7.9	7.9	11.1	5.8	9.2	8.1	5.2	6.4
Potassium	8.0	7.4	13.2	12.2	15.2	10.9	9.1	8.0	6.4
	7.0	7.4	8.0	9.2	8.7	8.5	7.2	5.3	5.3
Sodium	3.8	2.8	1.8	2.8	3.5	3.7	3.4	1.9	2.4
	3.8	3.1	2.7	1.5	3.6	3.4	3.0	1.7	2.3

Upper row for each analyte: Bio-Rad level 1; lower row for each analyte: Bio-Rad level 2.
Analytical platforms: hospital site 1 (H1) = Modular P; H2 = c501; regional clinical laboratory (RL) 1 to 4 = Integra 400; RL5 to 7 = c311.
Abbreviations: H, hospital site; RL, regional clinical laboratory.

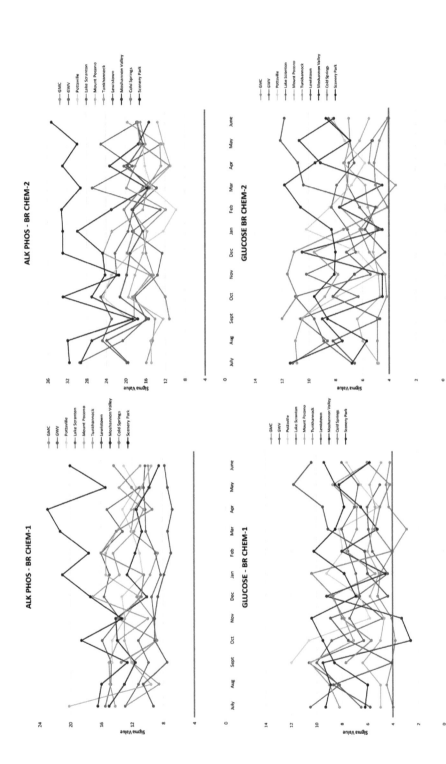

Fig. 3. Monthly Sigma trend plots (dashboards) for selected chemistries (CHEM) on Roche analytical platforms. ALK PHOS, alkaline phosphatase.

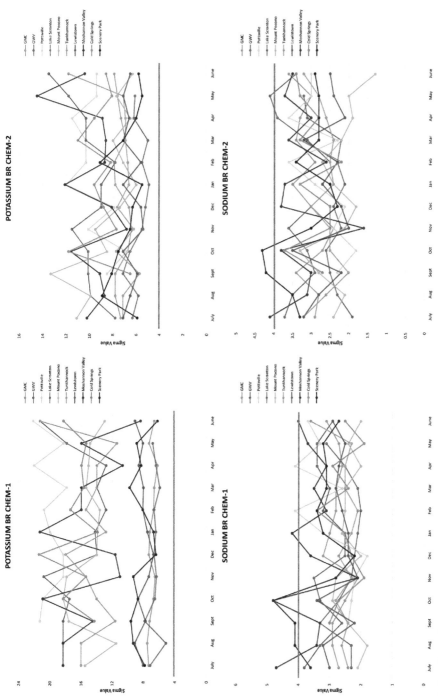

Fig. 3. (continued).

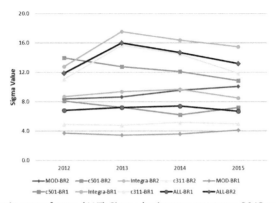

Fig. 4. Alanine aminotransferase (ALT) Sigma by instrument type: 2012 to 2015.

RESULTS AND DISCUSSION
Chemistry

Sigma variation by method-instrument combination
The evaluation of method-instrument combinations shows clear variation among chemical analytes and instruments. **Table 1** and **Fig. 3** show an early selected sub-group of methods and variation between instruments for 4 representative analytes. There were consistently low and high Sigma analytes. In this selection, alkaline phosphatase, glucose, and potassium gave relatively high Sigma values, whereas sodium was much lower at all sites and instruments. Potassium and sodium determinations both use ion selective electrode methodology, yet potassium performs at much higher Sigma level. Thus, one cannot generalize Sigma performance by method type. However, note the detail of the Sigma values for glucose determination at hospital site 1 (H1) relative to hospital 2 (H2) and the regional clinical laboratories (RL3 through RL7). The H1 Sigma is clearly lower for the modular instrument compared with the c501, Integras, and c311s. Compiled chemistry data by analyte are shown in **Table 2** with comments as to which method-instrument combinations had low Sigma performance (<4.0) for months or years of data. It is important to point out that for most of the analytes with low Sigma performance, it was, like the glucose example, usually on a limited number of platforms. In those cases, the authors modified QC rules on a site-by-site basis with each site keeping a logbook of specific changes made. Thus, these results show that it is key to evaluate method-instrument combinations overall, combination by combination rather than by analyte- or instrument-alone generalizations. And this represents the incorporation of the additional features of imprecision and allowable error.

Impact of Sigma-based rules revision
For the chemistry methods with Sigma values consistently more than 4.0 had the QC rejection rule changed from 1-2s to 1-3s. The impact of this is summarized in **Table 3**, which shows the high-performing subgroup from **Table 2**. Over the 3-month tracking interval, there was a 76.9% reduction in rejection events without apparent diminution in patient result quality and CAP proficiency scores at or near 100%. This reduction in rejection events yielded fewer production line stoppages, fewer unnecessary QC repeats, and elimination of waste labor associated with the troubleshooting and QC record-keeping processes. As a consequence of these improvements, the authors

Table 2					
Average chemistry Sigma values (4-year cumulative)					
Analyte	TEa	BR-1	BR-2	Any <4.0, Which?	
Albumin	10%	4.8	6.2		
Alkaline phosphatase	30%	13.8	19.3		
ALT	20%	6.8	13.2	Yes	Modular
Amylase	30%	26.2	30.2		
AST	20%	9.2	21.2		
Bilirubin, direct	0.4 or 20%	39.6	13.1	Yes	c501
Bilirubin, total	0.4 or 20%	11.7	9.2		
BUN	2 or 9%	5.3	4.3	Yes	All but c311
Calcium	1.0 mg/dL	6.6	5.0	Yes	Integra
Chloride	5%	3.7	4.4	Yes	All
Cholesterol, HDL	30%	7.8	8.4		
Cholesterol, LDL	30%	12.8	12.6		
Cholesterol, total	10%	5.2	6.1		
Carbon dioxide	3 SD	2.8	2.9	Yes	All
Creatine kinase	30%	19.9	25.1		
Creatinine	0.3 or 15%	15.5	10.3		
Digoxin	0.2 or 20%	3.6	9.5	Yes	Modular
GGTP	3 SD	4.4	8.1	Yes	c311
Glucose	6 or 10%	6.9	7.0		
Iron	20%	7.1	13.0		
LDH	20%	12.7	16.5		
Lipase	30%	14.6	15.6		
Magnesium	25%	12.4	17.2		
Phenobarbital	20%	3.3	5.7	Yes	Modular
Phenytoin	25%	5.8	4.2	Yes	Mod + c311
Phosphorus	0.3 or 10%	5.2	7.7	Yes	Modular
Potassium	0.5 mmol/L	12.1	7.8		
Protein, total	10%	5.8	7.0		
Sodium	4 mmol/L	3.1	2.9	Yes	All
Triglycerides	25%	9.1	13.5		
UIBC	3 SD	5.5	8.5		
Uric acid	17%	11.9	13.7		
Valproic acid	25%	4.1	5.1	Yes	Modular

Abbreviations: ALT, alanine transaminase; AST, aspartate transaminase; BR, Bio-Rad; BUN, blood urea nitrogen; GGTP, gamma glutamyl transpeptidase; HDL, high-density lipoprotein; LDH, lactate dehydrogenase; LDL, low-density lipoprotein; TEa, total allowable error; UIBC, unsaturated iron binding capacity.

moved forward with extending the AAQC to more chemistry analytes and to coagulation and hematology assays.

Immunochemistry analytes

Table 4 shows the Sigma values obtained for 1 year's performance of immunoassays on Roche Modular E and Elecsys systems (Indianapolis, IN). The Sigma performance of these immunoassays is relatively high for most analytes except therapeutic drug

Table 3 Reduced rejection rate with Sigma quality control						
Test Name (Abbr)	Pre–Sigma QC Rejects	Total QC Points	Pre–Sigma QC Reject (%)	Post–Sigma QC Rejects	Total QC Points	Post–Sigma QC Reject (%)
ALKP	108	2372	4.55	2	2599	0.08
K	47	4589	1.02	17	3058	0.56
AMY	31	1107	2.80	11	1613	0.68
HDL	25	1358	1.84	10	1211	0.83
LDL	36	482	7.47	4	543	0.74
CK	80	1332	6.01	38	1741	2.18
LIPA	17	950	1.79	6	1341	0.45
AST	73	2588	2.82	17	2821	0.60
TBILI	36	1468	2.45	2	1399	0.14
LDH	2	409	0.49	2	714	0.28
TRIG	120	1411	8.50	3	1202	0.25
URIC	2	409	0.49	0	654	0.00
GLU	70	706	9.92	5	694	0.72
Total	455	16,655	2.73	105	14,927	0.70

Overall rejection reduction: 76.9%.
Abbreviations: ALKP, alkaline phosphatase; AMY, amylase; AST, aspartate transaminase; CK, creatine kinase; GLU, glucose; HDL, high-density lipoprotein; K, potassium; LIPA, lipase; LDH, lactate dehydrogenase LDL, low-density lipoprotein; TBILI, total bilirubin; TRIG, triglycerides; URIC, uric acid.

monitoring. Partly this has to do with allowable error tolerances, which are tighter for the drugs than for most of the other analytes shown. The Sigma values for digoxin, phenytoin, phenobarbital, and valproic acid were also measured on the c311 platform and showed somewhat better performance than the central laboratory's Modular units (**Table 5**).

Performance over time
Monthly Month-to-month intrinsic variation in Sigma values for 9 individual instruments that represent 4 model types of Roche chemistry instruments is shown in **Table 5**. These data, from one single 12-month period, show both the site-to-site variation and the month-to-month statistical variation in calculated Sigma values by analyte for 2 levels of controls. These data were mostly from single lots of QC materials. Sigma values are frequently reported without any specification of variation, yet they are not invariant, as that is an intrinsic component of any process that involves measurement. The analysis presented in **Table 5** provides an overall specification of the month-to-month variation in Sigma on an instrument-by-instrument basis. The average value of all of the CVs was 23%. There are a few methods that have very low CVs, but these characteristics occur because of control materials and method combinations with relatively invariant results at low values.

This intrinsic month-to-month Sigma variation suggests that for an average Sigma of 5.0 one should not be alarmed by excursions in the 1.0 range. However, for a Sigma that averages at or near the 4.0 threshold and includes values that dip less than 4.0, there may be wisdom in retaining the 1-2s warning rule set. The statistical variations in Sigma values can also be used as a criterion to evaluate apparent drifts or trends in a Sigma value. Yet, although the authors have seen occasional trends in the data

Table 4
Sigma values for Roche immunoassays

| | Control Material | | |
Analyte	IAP-1	IAP-2	IAP-3
Digoxin	2.1	3.6	5.5
Phenobarbital	2.9	4.3	5.6
Phenytoin	3.6	5.3	6.0
Salicylates	7.7	10.6	10.0
Theophylline	4.3	6.1	6.6
Valproate	2.9	3.4	3.2
Total T4	5.5	5.5	5.4
PSA	13.0	14.4	13.6
Ferritin	7.6	7.9	12.9
Prolactin	10.2	11.3	10.6
CEA	6.7	7.2	7.0
Insulin	16.2	16.2	17.8
SHBG	16.0	15.0	17.3

| | Control Material | |
Analyte	IM-1	IM-3
CRP	46.8	26.7
C4	10.2	14.0
Haptoglobin	13.0	14.4
Prealbumin	6.4	8.4
A1AT	4.8	5.4
C3	6.2	5.7
IgA	4.0	4.6
IgG	10.5	13.2

Sigma value average for 12 consecutive months.
Abbreviations: A1AT, alpha-1-antitrypsin; C3, complement factor 3; C4, complement factor 4; CEA, carcinoembryonic antigen; CRP, C-reactive protein; IAP, inhibitor of apoptosis protein; IgA, immunoglobulin A; IgG, immunoglobulin G; PSA, prostate specific antigen; SHBG, sex hormone binding globulin.

plots, these usually occur in a range of Sigmas that is very high and of limited clinical relevance. In practicality when there are large Sigma swings between months, there is usually a nonmethodologic explanation related to skewed outlier data, clerical error, or bad spreadsheet cell references. The baseline trend plots and Sigma scatterplots provide a good visual representation for assessment of Sigma stability.

Annually Year-to-year variation for 4 years of compiled chemistry Sigma data are shown in **Table 6** and the alanine aminotransferase (ALT) yearly trend graph in **Fig. 4**. **Table 6** shows compiled sigma data for each analyte and QC material over the period 2012 to 2015. The analytes are organized by analyte type (enzymes, electrolytes, TDM (Therapeutic Drug Monitoring), and so forth) During this 4-year period, there were multiple lots of QC material in use. All lots were Bio-Rad unassayed liquid controls, but the year-to-year Sigma comparison includes this variable of QC lot number. As can be seen from the example graph in **Fig. 4** for ALT, there is good year-to-year stability. **Fig. 4** also shows a method that consistently performs

Table 5
Month-to-month variation in Sigma values

Analyte	Instrument	Sigma (X̄)	SD	CV (%)
Analyses Performed on 4 Roche Instrument Types				
Albumin BR-1	Mod-1	3.94	0.81	21
	c501–2	3.32	0.53	16
	Integra-3	4.97	1.81	32
	Integra-4	5.6	1.12	20
	Integra-5	4.54	1.25	27
	Integra-9	4.61	0.97	21
	c311–7	4.94	0.91	19
	c311–8	4.17	1.52	36
	c311–10	4.74	1.02	21
Albumin BR-2	Mod-1	5.81	1.6	28
	c501–2	5.44	1.99	37
	Integra-3	5.74	1.72	30
	Integra-4	6.61	1.17	18
	Integra-5	4.95	1.47	30
	Integra-9	5.02	1.83	36
	c311–7	7.03	1.55	22
	c311–8	5.54	2.26	41
	c311–10	6.68	1.21	18
Alk Phos BR-1	Mod-1	10.41	1.51	15
	c501–2	14.58	1.48	10
	Integra-3	11.87	3.92	33
	Integra-4	10.21	1.21	12
	Integra-5	4.95	1.47	30
	Integra-9	5.02	1.83	36
	c311–7	7.03	1.55	22
	c311–8	5.54	2.26	41
	c311–10	6.68	1.21	18
Alk Phos BR-2	Mod-1	16.08	2.18	14
	c501–2	20.14	4.0	20
	Integra-3	17.31	4.5	26
	Integra-4	19.18	5.48	29
	Integra-5	13.87	4.19	30
	Integra-9	15.22	4.77	31
	c311–7	18.81	2.51	13
	c311–8	22.84	5.21	23
	c311–10	30.21	5.02	17
ALT BR-1	Mod-1	3.71	0.86	23
	c501–2	8.12	1.88	23
	Integra-3	7.38	1.09	15
	Integra-4	11.34	4.55	40
	Integra-5	8.83	1.83	21
	Integra-9	7.38	1.93	26
	c311–7	6.65	1.43	22
	c311–8	2.58	0.52	20
	c311–10	5.38	0.99	18
ALT BR-2	Mod-1	8.41	1.15	14
	c501–2	13.98	5.46	39
	Integra-3	11.98	2.07	17
	Integra-4	14.28	3.21	22
	Integra-5	14.04	4.6	33
	Integra-9	10.86	3.08	28
	c311–7	10.8	4.14	38
	c311–8	8.2	2.14	26
	c311–10	14.4	3.51	24

(continued on next page)

Table 5
(continued)

Analyte	Instrument	Sigma ($\overline{X}$)	SD	CV (%)
AST BR Chem-1	Mod-1	4.28	0.71	17
	c501–2	6.14	2.15	35
	Integra-3	12.44	2.04	16
	Integra-4	12.31	2.43	20
	Integra-5	9.75	2.29	23
	Integra-9	12.28	4.08	33
	c311–7	7.88	1.93	24
	c311–8	6.33	6.26	99
	c311–10	7.07	1.47	21
AST BR Chem-2	Mod-1	14.48	2.5	17
	c501–2	14.49	6.99	48
	Integra-3	18.23	4.87	27
	Integra-4	23.89	9.38	39
	Integra-5	17.23	5.36	31
	Integra-9	21.12	4.71	22
	c311–7	21.51	9.16	43
	c311–8	18.82	4.86	26
	c311–10	32.32	5.14	16
Amylase BR-1	Mod-1	16.36	4.62	28
	c501–2	25.35	3.82	15
	Integra-3	26.98	6.7	25
	Integra-4	32.48	7.77	24
	Integra-5	21.06	4.28	20
	Integra-9	25.48	8.29	33
	c311–7	29.6	9.15	31
	c311–8	33.58	6.84	20
	c311–10	30.48	4.96	16
Amylase BR-2	Mod-1	24.71	5.92	24
	c501–2	27.95	4.95	18
	Integra-3	26.89	5.11	19
	Integra-4	31.13	5.41	17
	Integra-5	19.88	2.4	12
	Integra-9	26.84	4.35	16
	c311–7	36.28	12.16	34
	c311–8	41.18	11.98	29
	c311–10	39.52	2.7	7
Lipase BR Chem-1	Mod-1	8.14	2.24	28
	c501–2	14.81	2.63	18
	Integra-3	16.96	4.09	24
	Integra-4	18.53	6.55	35
	Integra-5	12.79	2.14	17
	c311–10	11.5	1.25	11
Lipase BR Chem-2	Mod-1	9.62	2.64	27
	c501–2	19.5	6.14	31
	Integra-3	16.65	3.71	22
	Integra-4	20.08	6.99	35
	Integra-5	12.31	3.48	28
	c311–10	14.6	2.96	20

(continued on next page)

Table 5
(continued)

Analyte	Instrument	Sigma ($\overline{X}$)	SD	CV (%)
Chloride BR Chem-1	Mod-1	3.98	0.40	10
	c501–2	2.88	0.47	16
	Integra-3	3.14	0.66	21
	Integra-4	2.63	0.81	31
	Integra-5	2.58	0.81	31
	Integra-9	2.64	0.99	38
	c311–7	3.08	0.57	19
	c311–8	4.57	1.46	32
	c311–10	4.65	1.2	26
Chloride BR Chem-2	Mod-1	5.51	0.49	9
	c501–2	4.36	0.52	12
	Integra-3	3.81	1.13	30
	Integra-4	3.69	1.02	28
	Integra-5	3.03	1.25	41
	Integra-9	5.12	1.14	22
	c311–7	3.94	0.79	20
	c311–8	6.14	1.62	26
	c311–10	5.92	1.48	25
CO_2 BR Chem-1	Mod-1	2.98	0.22	7
	c501–2	3.69	0.39	11
	Integra-3	2.67	0.23	9
	Integra-4	2.67	0.24	9
	Integra-5	2.98	1.1	37
	Integra-9	2.63	0.69	26
	c311–7	2.53	0.39	15
	c311–8	2.68	0.4	15
	c311–10	4.01	1.16	29
CO_2 BR Chem-2	Mod-1	3.33	0.56	17
	c501–2	4.35	0.69	16
	Integra-3	2.6	0.31	12
	Integra-4	2.64	0.27	10
	Integra-5	2.66	0.25	9
	Integra-9	3.05	0.84	28
	c311–7	2.83	0.53	19
	c311–8	3.62	0.95	26
	c311–10	5.19	1.76	34
Creatine Kinase BR Chem-1	Mod-1	21.98	3.93	18
	c501–2	23.71	6.61	28
	Integra-3	16.58	3.19	19
	Integra-4	20.45	5.41	26
	Integra-5	13.64	4.36	32
	Integra-9	14.11	4.19	30
	c311–7	18.56	7.0	38
	c311–8	17.89	4.57	26
	c311–10	27.38	8.28	30
Creatine Kinase BR Chem-2	Mod-1	26.11	5.42	21
	c501–2	26.89	7.39	27
	Integra-3	21.21	5.83	27
	Integra-4	25.84	5.4	21
	Integra-5	17.93	5.56	31
	Integra-9	20.83	4.31	21
	c311–7	22.19	9.65	43
	c311–8	23.44	8.05	34
	c311–10	32.44	8.9	27

(continued on next page)

Table 5
(continued)

Analyte	Instrument	Sigma (X̄)	SD	CV (%)
LDH BR Chem-1	Mod-1	9.63	1.65	17
	c501–2	13.45	4.01	30
	Integra-3	11.32	2.2	19
	Integra-9	11.2	3.16	28
	c311–10	17.21	4.74	28
LDH BR Chem-2	Mod-1	12.16	2.73	22
	c501–2	16.57	3.98	24
	Integra-3	13.63	2.38	17
	Integra-9	13.35	3.76	28
	c311–10	24.94	5.79	23
BUN BR Chem-1	Mod-1	3.43	0.57	17
	c501–2	—	—	—
	Integra-3	3.46	0.62	18
	Integra-4	4.37	0.7	16
	Integra-5	3.83	0.7	18
	Integra-9	4.23	1.26	30
	c311–7	7.01	1.7	24
	c311–8	7.05	2.71	38
	c311–10	7.08	2.79	39
BUN BR Chem-2	Mod-1	3.74	0.57	15
	c501–2	3.43	1.49	43
	Integra-3	2.59	0.63	24
	Integra-4	3.25	0.37	11
	Integra-5	3.41	0.77	23
	Integra-9	3.73	0.86	23
	c311–7	5.73	0.98	17
	c311–8	5.63	1.05	19
	c311–10	6.68	1.26	19
Creatinine BR Chem-1	Mod-1	23.80	9.06	38
	c501–2	10.20	—	—
	Integra-3	12.48	3.79	30
	Integra-4	13.32	4.28	32
	Integra-5	13.18	2.8	21
	Integra-9	9.81	2.15	22
	c311–7	9.3	—	—
	c311–8	21.4	—	—
	c311–10	—	—	—
Creatinine BR Chem-2	Mod-1	10.94	1.77	16
	c501–2	10.3	2.59	25
	Integra-3	9.35	3.4	36
	Integra-4	10.78	2.62	24
	Integra-5	6.35	1.74	27
	Integra-9	7.15	2.33	33
	c311–7	13.15	2.28	17
	c311–8	12.01	1.98	16
	c311–10	12.81	1.42	11
Calcium BR Chem-1	Mod-1	4.55	0.32	7
	c501–2	6.97	0.73	10
	Integra-3	4.68	0.67	14
	Integra-4	4.33	1.00	23
	Integra-5	5.85	1.25	21
	Integra-9	4.09	0.66	16
	c311–7	8.27	1.42	17
	c311–8	7.97	1.82	23
	c311–10	8.58	2.25	26

(continued on next page)

Table 5
(continued)

Analyte	Instrument	Sigma (X̄)	SD	CV (%)
Calcium BR Chem-2	Mod-1	3.58	0.25	7
	c501–2	5.02	0.67	13
	Integra-3	3.16	0.37	12
	Integra-4	2.72	0.59	22
	Integra-5	3.91	0.85	22
	Integra-9	3.23	0.95	29
	c311–7	6.25	1.39	22
	c311–8	5.48	1.51	28
	c311–10	5.94	1.4	24
Magnesium BR Chem-1	Mod-1	8.04	2.85	35
	c501–2	11.10	1.56	14
	Integra-5	10.06	1.6	16
	c311–7	15.24	7.94	52
	c311–8	11.83	5.13	43
Magnesium BR Chem-2	Mod-1	11.64	4.45	38
	c501–2	17.77	6.21	35
	Integra-5	11.66	2.41	21
	c311–7	29.18	13.26	45
	c311–8	16.05	2.54	16
	c311–10	21.34	6.38	30
Phosphorus BR Chem-1	Mod-1	2.96	0.71	24
	c501–2	3.13	1.24	40
	Integra-3	6.09	2.4	39
	Integra-4	5.41	0.95	18
	Integra-9	5.11	2.01	39
	c311–7	4.78	0.65	14
	c311–8	5.07	1.53	30
	c311–10	5.03	1.47	29
Phosphorus BR Chem-2	Mod-1	5.39	1.07	20
	c501–2	4.95	3.5	71
	Integra-3	7.7	1.84	24
	Integra-4	9.21	1.59	17
	Integra-9	8.34	2.46	29
	c311–7	8.15	1.3	16
	c311–8	7.51	2.23	30
	c311–10	6.85	2.65	39
Uric Acid BR Chem-1	Mod-1	9.12	1.80	20
	c501–2	8.97	1.19	13
	Integra-3	13.81	3.07	22
	Integra-5	11.28	2.06	18
	Integra-9	13.08	5.15	39
	c311–8	11.53	3.17	27
	c311–10	13.21	3.65	28
Uric Acid BR Chem-2	Mod-1	10.51	2.72	26
	c501–2	10.25	1.56	15
	Integra-3	14.71	4.31	29
	Integra-5	11.99	3.51	29
	Integra-9	15.62	6.22	40
	c311–8	13.43	4.12	31
	c311–10	18.03	4.8	27

(continued on next page)

Table 5
(continued)

Analyte	Instrument	Sigma ($\overline{X}$)	SD	CV (%)
Potassium BR Chem-1	Mod-1	6.93	0.42	6
	c501–2	6.50	0.67	10
	Integra-3	21.26	3.24	15
	Integra-4	16.68	3.0	18
	Integra-5	15.06	2.06	14
	Integra-9	16.61	2.28	14
	c311–7	8.08	0.72	9
	c311–8	15.13	4.3	28
	c311–10	8.26	1.25	15
Potassium BR Chem-2	Mod-1	7.33	0.55	8
	c501–2	5.83	0.68	12
	Integra-3	9.62	1.59	17
	Integra-4	10.09	1.64	16
	Integra-5	8.44	2.17	26
	Integra-9	8.99	1.57	17
	c311–7	6.47	0.67	10
	c311–8	9.6	2.5	26
	c311–10	6.85	1.28	19
Sodium BR Chem-1	Mod-1	2.78	0.29	10
	c501–2	2.45	0.42	17
	Integra-3	2.97	0.82	28
	Integra-4	3.12	0.42	13
	Integra-5	2.29	0.42	18
	Integra-9	2.55	0.47	18
	c311–7	2.68	0.4	15
	c311–8	3.63	0.74	20
	c311–10	3.36	0.71	21
Sodium Chem-2	Mod-1	3.08	0.36	12
	c501–2	2.44	0.4	16
	Integra-3	2.7	0.62	23
	Integra-4	3.27	0.53	16
	Integra-5	2.25	0.52	23
	Integra-9	2.97	0.49	16
	c311–7	2.59	0.49	19
	c311–8	3.42	0.83	24
	c311–10	3.23	0.8	25
Protein, Total BR Chem-1	Mod-1	5.72	1.09	19
	c501–2	7.00	1.10	16
	Integra-3	6.49	2.46	38
	Integra-4	7.49	1.64	22
	Integra-5	3.75	0.63	17
	Integra-9	4.89	1.49	30
	c311–7	7.8	1.0	13
	c311–8	5.19	1.67	32
	c311–10	8.29	2.0	24
Protein, Total BR Chem-2	Mod-1	7.13	1.41	20
	c501–2	8.52	1.47	17
	Integra-3	6.64	2.61	39
	Integra-4	7.66	1.63	21
	Integra-5	4.93	1.13	23
	Integra-9	5.63	1.68	30
	c311–7	9.93	1.71	17
	c311–8	6.31	2.19	35
	c311–10	9.81	1.44	15

(continued on next page)

Table 5
(continued)

Analyte	Instrument	Sigma ($\bar{X}$)	SD	CV (%)
Glucose BR Chem-1	Mod-1	4.22	0.59	14
	c501–2	6.55	1.78	27
	Integra-3	7.95	2.16	27
	Integra-4	7.81	1.41	18
	Integra-5	5.39	0.52	10
	Integra-9	6.52	2.09	32
	c311–7	7.7	2.42	31
	c311–8	7.08	2.54	36
	c311–10	7.99	1.56	20
Glucose BR Chem-2	Mod-1	4.85	0.74	15
	c501–2	7.2	1.93	27
	Integra-3	7.65	1.84	24
	Integra-4	8.23	1.68	20
	Integra-5	5.62	0.8	14
	Integra-9	7.32	3.68	50
	c311–7	8.04	3.11	39
	c311–8	7.38	3.05	41
	c311–10	8.55	1.69	20
Analyses Performed on Limited Instrument Types				
Cholesterol, HDL BR Chem-1	Mod-1	5.88	1.98	34
Cholesterol, HDL BR Chem-2	Mod-1	5.88	1.98	34
Cholesterol, LDL BR Chem-1	Mod-1	12.61	3.51	28
Cholesterol, LDL BR Chem-2	Mod-1	12.62	3.61	29
Cholesterol, Total BR Chem-1	Mod-1	4.70	0.72	15
	c501–2	4.46	0.96	22
	Integra-3	6.62	1.59	24
	Integra-4	6.98	1.6	23
Cholesterol, Total BR Chem-2	Mod-1	5.68	0.8	14
	c501–2	5.68	1.46	26
	Integra-3	6.89	1.75	25
	Integra-4	7.78	1.92	25
Triglycerides BR Chem-1	Mod-1	7.29	1.13	16
	c501–2	12.49	1.80	14
	—	—	Mean CV:	15
Triglycerides Chem-2	Mod-1	10.29	1.43	14
	c501–2	18.65	4.2	23
	—	—	Mean CV:	18
GGTP Chem-1	Mod-1	5.62	1.66	30
	c501–2	9.25	5.25	57
	Integra-9	7.69	2.97	39
	c311–7	7.78	3.77	48
	c311–10	7.03	3.66	52
GGTP Chem-2	Mod-1	8.43	4.92	58
	c501–2	13.47	10.68	79
	Integra-9	9.2	4.52	49
	c311–7	12.04	6.22	52
	c311–10	10.65	5.86	55

(continued on next page)

Table 5
(continued)

Analyte	Instrument	Sigma (X̄)	SD	CV (%)
Bilirubin, Total BR Chem-1	Mod-1	8.74	1.54	18
	c501–2	—	—	—
	Integra-3	15.16	2.54	17
	Integra-4	13.06	5.07	39
	Integra-5	10.93	2.43	22
	Integra-9	11.76	4.72	40
	c311–7	10.83	3.57	33
	c311–8	13.85	5.31	38
	c311–10	13.08	2.52	19
Bilirubin, Total BR Chem-2	Mod-1	8.67	1.08	12
	c501–2	7.76	2.00	26
	Integra-3	11.47	1.81	16
	Integra-4	9.45	2.71	29
	Integra-5	7.98	1.39	17
	Integra-9	13.87	19.97	144
	c311–7	4.86	1.36	28
	c311–8	7.43	2.26	30
	c311–10	9.99	1.83	18
Bilirubin, Direct BR Chem-1	Mod-1	—	—	—
	c501–2	—	—	—
	Integra-3	69.41	5.66	8
	Integra-4	64.75	17.1	26
	Integra-5	65.74	11.35	17
	Integra-9	52.7	11.39	22
	c311–7	7.33	1.22	17
	c311–8	10.07	2.47	25
	c311–10	10.66	3.43	32
Bilirubin, Direct BR Chem-2	Mod-1	8.9	4.28	48
	c501–2	7.36	4.14	56
	Integra-3	18.71	1.45	8
	Integra-4	19.72	2.44	12
	Integra-5	17.45	2.96	17
	Integra-9	14.03	3.2	23
	c311–7	5.03	1.19	24
	c311–8	7.88	2.45	31
Digoxin BR Chem-1	Mod-1	2.39	0.43	18
	c311–7	3.93	0.95	24
	c311–8	4.36	1.11	25
	c311–10	3.8	1.48	39
Digoxin BR Chem-2	Mod-1	5.17	1.11	21
	c311–7	11.34	2.89	25
	c311–8	8.27	1.74	21
	c311–10	10.3	3.48	34
Phenobarbital BR Chem-1	Mod-1	2.15	0.79	37
	c311–10	6.23	2.67	43
Phenobarbital BR Chem-2	Mod-1	3.0	1.06	35
	c311–10	10.61	2.98	28
Phenytoin BR Chem-1	Mod-1	3.38	0.80	24
	c311–7	8.06	3.3	41
	c311–8	5.94	1.92	32
	c311–10	6.7	2.29	34

(continued on next page)

Table 5 (continued)				
Analyte	Instrument	Sigma (X̄)	SD	CV (%)
Phenytoin BR Chem-2	Mod-1	5.48	1.19	22
	c311–7	2.83	0.92	33
	c311–8	4.47	1.06	24
	c311–10	4.78	0.85	18
Valproate BR Chem-1	Mod-1	2.81	0.46	16
	c311–10	5.78	1.53	26
Valproate BR Chem-2	Mod-1	3.43	0.64	19
	c311–10	7.53	3.1	41
Iron BR Chem-1	Mod-1	11.79	2.13	18
	c501–2	4.81	0.92	19
Iron BR Chem-2	Mod-1	17.28	3.19	18
	c501–2	11.9	1.51	13
UIBC BR Chem-1	Mod-1	5.85	0.57	10
UIBC BR Chem-2	Mod-1	9.64	1.1	11

Abbreviations: Alk Phos, alkaline phosphatase; ALT, alanine transaminase; AST, aspartate transaminase; BR, Bio-Rad; BR-1,Bio-Rad Level 1; BR-2, Bio-Rad Level 2; BR Chem-1, Bio-Rad chemistry Level 1; BUN, blood urea nitrogen; Chem, chemistry; CO2, carbon dioxide; GGTP, gamma glutamyl transpeptidase; HDL, high-density lipoprotein; LDL, lowdensity lipoprotein; LDH, lactate dehydrogenase; UIBC, unsaturated iron binding capacity.

less than the 4.0 threshold (Bio-Rad level 1 on the Modular) and the rest that are all in excess of this threshold. Several of the high-level Sigmas show a progressive decline over 2013 to 2015, but these are at a level of Sigma that is greater than 10 and of no clinical impact.

Coagulation

In 2012 the authors extended the Sigma QC program to PT measurements. The background incorporated standardizing system reference ranges and obtaining QC material for all sites. The system of instruments included Evolutions, Compacts, Satellite, and STart4. **Table 7** shows the Sigma values generated in 2012 to 2013 for PT QC. **Table 8** shows the spreadsheet that was used to calculate the monthly Sigma values. This spreadsheet was identical to the spreadsheet used to calculate the chemistry Sigma values. **Fig. 5** shows this first year's dashboard/trend plot, which is every bit as complex and visually confusing as the chemistry dashboards.

Fig. 6 shows a representation of contemporary PT and activated PTT data that contains the standard trend plot on the left and a Sigma scatterplot on the right. The coagulation group shown here contains, in comparison with **Fig. 5**, additional instruments from the hospitals and clinics added during 2012 to 2015. The trend plot shows the usual Sigma by month by instrument. The scatterplot on the right shows the monthly Sigma values for each instrument plotted in one vertical location. These values are then grouped by instrument type as Compacts, Evolutions, STart4s, and Satellites (left to right). The time axis is eliminated but the Sigma scatter distribution is evident, and (1) biases between instrument types and (2) performance relative to the 4.0 threshold line are cleanly represented. Most of the instruments performed consistently at world-class levels with the exception of the Satellites, which were generally lower in Sigma performance. These data are consistent with other published reports of coagulation test performance.[7,8]

Table 6
Year-to-year variation

Enzymes

Alk Phos BR-1 & 2	2012	2013	2014	2015	Amylase BR-1 & 2	2012	2013	2014	2015
Modular	10.41	12.69	10.41	13.20	Modular	16.36	17.28	20.08	19.85
	16.08	16.19	15.30	18.20		24.71	25.57	24.73	21.98
c501	*14.58*	*14.64*	*14.76*	*12.50*	c501	25.35	22.41	22.23	25.25
	20.14	17.18	16.87	16.00		27.95	25.53	26.63	26.08
Integra Group	11.80	14.03	12.42	14.90	Integra Group	26.50	22.60	22.68	24.30
	16.39	17.35	17.90	20.00		26.18	22.50	28.57	25.91
c311 Group	12.60	15.47	15.15	17.20	c311 Group	31.22	29.70	32.09	36.71
	23.89	21.76	21.75	24.40		38.99	35.94	40.36	41.49
All Instruments	12.22	14.39	13.27	15.20	All Instruments	26.82	24.18	25.48	28.52
	19.27	18.54	18.69	20.83		30.48	27.14	31.86	31.29
ALT BR-1 & 2	**2012**	**2013**	**2014**	**2015**	**Lipase BR-1 & 2**	**2012**	**2013**	**2014**	**2015**
Modular	3.71	3.42	3.60	4.10	Modular	8.14	8.96	10.24	8.45
	8.41	8.68	9.60	10.10		9.62	11.53	11.97	10.23
c501	8.12	7.23	6.20	7.20	c501	14.81	15.88	15.97	19.00
	13.98	12.78	12.10	10.90		19.50	17.97	18.13	23.42
Integra Group	8.70	9.40	9.70	8.50	Integra Group	16.09	14.16	15.17	17.88
	12.80	17.60	16.40	15.50		16.35	15.21	16.01	15.79
c311 Group	4.90	4.80	5.20	5.00	c311 Group	—	—	—	—
	11.10	16.70	14.50	11.90		—	—	—	—
All Instruments	7.06	7.47	5.73	7.09	All Instruments	14.25	13.46	14.34	16.22
	12.23	17.34	10.45	12.87		15.63	15.03	15.63	16.20
AST BR-1 & 2	**2012**	**2013**	**2014**	**2015**	**Creatine kinase BR-1 & 2**	**2012**	**2013**	**2014**	**2015**
Modular	4.28	4.88	5.34	5.29	Modular	21.98	22.04	21.22	18.73
	14.48	11.83	16.17	15.93		26.11	25.88	25.59	21.52
c501	6.14	6.45	5.98	5.56	c501	23.71	22.21	22.15	20.92
	14.49	15.47	14.29	19.37		26.89	26.03	24.56	23.82
Integra Group	11.70	12.25	11.42	11.37	Integra Group	16.19	16.17	17.90	18.09
	20.12	19.97	19.78	18.39		21.45	22.06	22.89	23.48
c311 Group	7.10	7.14	7.44	10.05	c311 Group	21.28	23.29	25.05	22.77
	24.22	27.19	29.00	30.42		26.02	27.97	33.36	29.51
All Instruments	8.72	9.40	9.07	9.61	All Instruments	19.37	19.50	20.80	20.04
	20.23	20.87	21.63	22.24		24.10	24.61	26.47	25.31
GGTP BR-1 & 2	**2012**	**2013**	**2014**	**2015**	**LDH BR-1 & 2**	**2012**	**2013**	**2014**	**2015**
Modular	5.62	4.11	6.09	5.83	Modular	9.63	10.74	9.75	11.93
	8.43	6.07	10.12	12.30		12.16	13.71	12.69	14.48
c501	9.25	7.93	—	—	c501	13.45	13.55	13.04	14.33
	13.47	8.58	8.89	27.38		16.57	16.33	14.20	15.48
Integra Group	6.54	—	—	—	Integra Group	11.26	13.36	13.10	—
	10.40	—	—	—		13.49	15.89	18.50	—
c311 Group	7.40	2.79	1.85	1.28	c311 Group	17.21	10.69	15.79	12.75
	11.35	2.75	2.15	1.24		24.94	13.22	21.06	25.30
All Instruments	7.13	4.41	3.26	2.79	All Instruments	12.56	12.34	12.92	13.00
	10.90	5.04	5.83	10.54		16.13	15.01	16.61	18.42

Lipids & Liver Function Tests

Cholesterol, Total BR-1 & 2	2012	2013	2014	2015	D Bilirubin BR-1 & 2	2012	2013	2014	2015
Modular	4.70	4.53	5.35	4.27	Modular	—	15.89	—	—
	5.68	5.63	6.35	5.18		8.90	8.08	6.77	7.56

(continued on next page)

Table 6
(continued)

Lipids & Liver Function Tests								
c501	4.46	5.21	4.42	4.75	c501	0.40	1.00	3.61	3.68
	5.68	6.36	5.34	5.84		7.36	5.30	13.69	6.95
Integra Group	8.67	5.02	3.65	—	Integra Group	63.15	58.51	66.64	71.04
	9.49	5.23	4.35	—		17.48	19.04	17.74	19.09
c311 Group	—	—	—	—	c311 Group	9.35	18.37	17.93	19.29
	—	—	—	—		6.45	8.64	8.51	8.49
All Instruments	7.03	4.94	4.47	4.51	All Instruments	35.13	36.46	43.40	43.22
	7.96	5.61	5.34	5.51		12.38	13.45	13.47	12.93

Triglycerides	2012	2013	2014	2015	T Bilirubin BR-1 & 2	2012	2013	2014	2015
BR-1 & 2									
Modular	7.29	6.56	7.39	5.64	Modular	8.74	7.65	7.72	7.89
	10.29	9.17	15.37	8.30		8.67	7.85	8.14	7.88
c501	12.49	10.98	11.53	10.83	c501	—	10.24	8.94	12.33
	18.65	14.79	16.93	14.88		7.76	9.14	10.30	11.31
Integra Group	—	—	—	—	Integra Group	12.73	12.28	10.98	14.83
	—	—	—	—		10.69	8.47	8.33	9.55
c311 Group	—	—	—	—	c311 Group	12.59	16.66	10.10	7.98
	—	—	—	—		7.43	9.38	9.53	11.81
All Instruments	9.89	8.77	9.46	8.23	All Instruments	12.18	12.93	10.18	11.50
	14.47	11.98	16.15	11.59		9.05	8.75	8.87	10.31

Cholesterol, HDL	2012	2013	2014	2015	Cholesterol, LDL	2012	2013	2014	2015
BR-1 & 2					*BR-1 & 2*				
Modular	5.88	8.08	8.77	8.46	Modular	12.61	12.94	12.85	12.91
	5.88	8.48	10.18	9.00		12.62	14.04	12.55	11.17
All Instruments	—	—	—	—	All Instruments	—	—	—	—
	—	—	—	—		—	—	—	—

Albumin BR-1 & 2	2012	2013	2014	2015	T Protein BR-1 & 2	2012	2013	2014	2015
Modular	3.94	3.67	3.97	4.05	Modular	5.72	5.84	7.05	4.10
	5.81	5.81	5.32	5.69		7.13	7.03	7.51	7.27
c501	3.32	3.30	3.12	3.54	c501	7.00	5.70	5.40	3.50
	5.44	5.37	4.53	5.69		8.52	6.86	6.15	6.26
Integra Group	4.93	5.08	5.55	5.73	Integra Group	5.66	5.21	6.50	5.73
	5.58	5.94	6.30	6.62		6.22	6.12	6.98	7.41
c311 Group	4.62	4.59	4.73	5.19	c311 Group	7.09	6.62	5.39	5.20
	6.41	6.96	6.76	6.99		8.70	7.57	6.29	7.46
All Instruments	4.54	4.61	4.90	5.12	All Instruments	6.29	5.74	6.11	5.12
	5.87	6.17	6.16	6.57		7.40	6.72	6.74	7.28

Electrolytes and Basic Chemistry								
Calcium BR-1 & 2	2012	2013	2014	2015	Sodium BR-1 & 2	2012	2013	2014	2015
Modular	4.55	5.18	5.59	5.75	Modular	2.78	2.71	2.58	2.42
	3.58	4.09	4.21	4.08		3.08	3.00	2.95	2.88
c501	6.97	6.50	8.69	9.57	c501	2.45	2.49	2.97	3.18
	5.02	4.95	6.48	7.18		2.44	2.50	3.04	3.50
Integra Group	4.74	5.68	7.16	6.75	Integra Group	2.73	3.20	3.54	3.27
	3.25	3.88	4.50	5.28		2.80	2.92	2.99	2.67

(continued on next page)

Table 6
(continued)

Electrolytes and Basic Chemistry								
c311 Group	8.26	7.50	7.93	5.64	c311 Group	3.22	3.07	3.91	3.08
	5.89	5.33	6.11	6.78		3.08	2.82	3.59	2.56
All Instruments	6.14	6.26	7.39	6.58	All Instruments	2.87	3.04	3.50	3.10
	4.36	4.44	5.15	5.86		2.88	2.86	3.17	2.75
Magnesium BR-1 & 2	**2012**	**2013**	**2014**	**2015**	**Potassium BR-1 & 2**	**2012**	**2013**	**2014**	**2015**
Modular	8.04	7.12	7.78	8.40	Modular	6.93	7.09	7.33	7.53
	11.64	11.96	12.04	11.37		7.33	6.66	6.50	6.90
c501	11.10	22.20	12.75	11.85	c501	6.50	6.27	6.54	5.67
	17.77	15.95	13.16	12.77		5.83	5.46	5.98	5.56
Integra Group	10.06	11.37	11.89	10.88	Integra Group	17.40	15.55	14.74	14.51
	11.66	14.29	14.96	15.22		9.29	9.09	8.40	7.88
c311 Group	13.54	11.89	15.21	16.64	c311 Group	10.49	9.65	10.81	11.65
	22.19	18.03	19.55	26.91		7.64	7.31	8.30	7.37
All Instruments	11.26	12.53	12.85	12.85	All Instruments	12.72	12.01	12.00	11.80
	17.94	15.80	16.25	18.81		8.14	7.95	7.94	7.34
Phosphorus BR-1 & 2	**2012**	**2013**	**2014**	**2015**	**Chloride BR-1 & 2**	**2012**	**2013**	**2014**	**2015**
Modular	2.96	3.48	4.28	4.00	Modular	3.98	3.68	3.63	3.03
	5.39	5.33	6.75	6.99		5.51	5.17	4.68	4.13
c501	3.13	5.12	7.44	6.81	c501	2.88	2.86	2.97	3.62
	4.95	6.99	10.67	9.31		4.36	4.21	5.29	5.98
Integra Group	5.54	5.28	5.65	5.57	Integra Group	2.75	4.38	3.50	3.20
	8.42	7.23	8.29	7.32		3.91	3.70	2.95	2.51
c311 Group	4.96	5.26	5.25	5.56	c311 Group	4.10	4.04	4.61	3.77
	7.50	7.69	9.36	7.93		5.33	5.48	6.37	5.83
All Instruments	4.70	5.08	5.57	5.53	All Instruments	3.35	4.06	3.79	3.42
	7.26	7.16	8.69	7.71		4.61	4.43	4.38	4.18
Uric Acid BR-1 & 2	**2012**	**2013**	**2014**	**2015**	**CO_2 BR-1 & 2**	**2012**	**2013**	**2014**	**2015**
Modular	9.12	8.81	10.26	10.49	Modular	2.98	3.02	3.05	2.98
	10.51	10.50	11.45	11.18		3.33	3.58	3.81	3.55
c501	8.97	9.07	9.00	10.34	c501	3.69	3.68	3.36	3.60
	10.25	10.98	10.19	10.53		4.35	3.75	3.48	3.47
Integra Group	12.72	13.58	12.54	12.68	Integra Group	2.74	2.56	2.97	2.44
	14.11	14.46	14.10	13.80		2.74	2.59	2.53	2.41
c311 Group	12.37	11.93	12.25	12.46	c311 Group	3.07	2.48	2.34	2.43
	15.73	13.97	15.04	16.96		3.88	2.62	2.43	2.24
All Instruments	11.57	12.00	11.74	12.10	All Instruments	2.98	2.69	2.82	2.62
	13.50	13.41	13.51	14.20		3.36	2.82	2.72	2.60
Therapeutic Drugs, Basic Metabolites, & Iron/UIBC									
Digoxin BR-1 & 2	**2012**	**2013**	**2014**	**2015**	**Phenobarbital**	**2012**	**2013**	**2014**	**2015**
					BR-1 & 2				
Modular	2.39	2.07	2.16	2.59	Modular	2.15	2.95	3.61	2.57
	5.17	3.47	4.04	6.80		3.00	4.22	5.00	3.83
c311 Group	4.03	—	5.57	4.61	c311 Group	6.23	—	—	—
	9.97	—	21.30	9.31		10.61	10.00	—	—
All Instruments	3.62	2.07	4.72	4.10	All Instruments	4.19	2.95	3.61	2.57
	8.77	3.47	16.98	8.68		6.80	7.11	5.00	3.83

(continued on next page)

Table 6
(continued)

Therapeutic Drugs, Basic Metabolites, & Iron/UIBC

Phenytoin BR-1 & 2	2012	2013	2014	2015	Valproic Acid BR-1 & 2	2012	2013	2014	2015
Modular	3.38	3.60	3.21	3.59	Modular	2.81	2.90	2.97	3.05
	5.48	5.35	5.01	5.07		3.43	3.32	3.82	3.62
c311 Group	6.90	5.56	5.91	7.89	c311 Group	5.78	4.35	3.59	6.95
	4.02	3.49	4.11	4.24		7.53	5.63	5.39	8.07
All Instruments	6.02	5.07	5.23	6.82	All Instruments	4.30	3.63	3.28	5.00
	4.39	3.96	4.34	—		5.48	4.47	4.60	5.84

Iron BR-1 & 2	2012	2013	2014	2015	UIBC BR-1 & 2	2012	2013	2014	2015
Modular	11.79	10.58	7.65	8.84	Modular	5.85	6.09	4.50	5.11
	17.28	15.17	12.75	12.96		9.64	9.28	7.22	7.43
c501	4.81	5.38	4.85	5.34	c501	—	—	6.06	6.43
	11.90	12.34	12.11	12.72		—	—	9.98	9.38
All Instruments	—	7.98	6.25	7.09	All Instruments	—	—	5.28	5.77
	—	13.76	12.43	12.84		—	—	8.60	8.40

BUN BR-1 & 2	2012	2013	2014	2015	Creatinine BR-1 & 2	2012	2013	2014	2015
Modular	3.43	3.31	3.20	3.62	Modular	23.80	15.21	17.00	15.92
	3.74	3.78	3.38	4.03		10.94	9.83	10.24	9.42
c501	—	4.82	15.02	—	c501	10.20	6.11	5.94	6.33
	3.43	4.48	4.83	4.92		10.30	9.21	8.29	9.65
Integra Group	3.97	3.89	3.63	3.78	Integra Group	12.20	13.98	17.25	16.32
	3.24	3.41	3.31	3.42		8.41	8.38	11.07	10.08
c311 Group	7.05	11.74	6.62	4.82	c311 Group	—	19.33	17.90	20.96
	6.01	6.13	6.24	4.85		12.66	11.54	10.59	12.70
All Instruments	5.06	6.28	5.62	4.15	All Instruments	14.19	14.92	16.29	16.71
	4.24	4.37	4.35	4.13		10.32	9.55	10.57	10.83

Glucose BR-1 & 2	2012	2013	2014	2015
Modular	4.22	4.19	5.27	4.68
	4.85	4.08	5.41	4.98
c501	6.55	5.76	6.26	6.97
	7.20	6.40	6.49	7.38
Integra Group	6.92	6.61	7.45	7.58
	7.20	6.66	7.78	7.81
c311 Group	7.59	6.99	8.47	7.18
	7.99	7.96	6.20	6.63
All Instruments	6.80	6.40	7.42	7.06
	7.20	6.76	6.94	7.05

Abbreviations: Alk Phos, alkaline phosphatase; ALT, alanine transaminase; AST, aspartate transaminase; BR, Bio-Rad; BUN, blood urea nitrogen; CO_2, carbon dioxide; D Bilirubin, Direct bilirubin; GGTP, gamma glutamyl transpeptidase; HDL, high-density lipoprotein; LDL, low-density lipoprotein; LDH, lactate dehydrogenase; T Bilirubin, Total bilirubin; UIBC, unsaturated iron binding capacity.

Hematology

GML implemented new analytical hematology instrumentation during the first 3 years of the AAQC program and now has Sysmex installed at all sites. As with the Roche and Stago instrumentation, there is a spectrum of Sysmex models depending on the size

Table 7
Example of monthly Sigma calculation spreadsheet for prothrombin time

Laboratory Site	Device	Control	TEa (%)	Site Mean	Site CV	Peer Mean	Bias	Bias (ABS)	Bias (%)	TEa/CV	Sigma (TEa-%Bias)/CV
Lake Scranton	STart4	COAGN	15	12.3	1.14	13.0	-0.7	0.7	5.38	13.2	8.4
		COAG ABN	15	34.9	2.41	36.6	-1.7	1.7	4.64	6.2	4.3
Lewistown	Satellite	COAGN	15	13.3	1.28	13.0	0.3	0.3	2.31	11.7	9.9
		COAG ABN	15	32.8	1.04	36.6	-3.8	3.8	10.38	14.5	4.5
Moshannon Valley	STart4	COAGN	15	12.6	1.67	13.0	-0.4	0.4	3.08	9.0	7.2
		COAG ABN	15	37.9	2.16	36.6	1.3	1.3	3.55	6.9	5.3
Mount Pocono	STart4	COAGN	15	12.9	1.78	13.0	-0.1	0.1	0.77	8.4	8.0
		COAG ABN	15	37.0	1.65	36.6	0.4	0.4	1.09	9.1	8.4
Scenery Park	Compact	COAGN	15	12.9	1.71	13.0	-0.1	0.1	0.77	8.8	8.3
		COAG ABN	15	36.2	1.57	36.6	-0.4	0.4	1.09	9.5	8.8
Tunkhannock	STart4	COAGN	15	12.2	0.90	13.0	-0.8	0.8	6.15	16.6	9.8
		COAG ABN	15	34.9	1.46	36.6	-1.7	1.7	4.64	10.3	7.1
GMC-7062537	Evolution	COAGN	15	13.4	1.64	13.0	0.4	0.4	3.08	9.1	7.3
		COAG ABN	15	37.7	1.70	36.6	1.1	1.1	3.01	8.8	7.1
GMC-7092615	Evolution	COAGN	15	13.3	1.50	13.0	0.3	0.3	2.31	10.0	8.4
		COAG ABN	15	37.5	1.63	36.6	0.9	0.9	2.46	9.2	7.7
GWV-0082250	Compact	COAGN	15	13.0	1.85	13.0	0	0	0.00	8.1	8.1
		COAG ABN	15	36.8	1.55	36.6	0.2	0.2	0.55	9.7	9.3
GWV-7116671	Compact	COAGN	15	13.0	1.46	13.0	0	0	0.00	10.3	10.3
		COAG ABN	15	36.5	2.82	36.6	-0.1	0.1	0.27	5.3	5.2
Shamokin	Compact	COAGN	15	12.8	1.64	13.0	-0.2	0.2	1.54	9.1	8.2
		COAG ABN	15	36.6	1.83	36.6	0	0	0.00	8.2	8.2
	AVG COAGN:	8.5		AVG COAG ABN:		6.9	—			—	—

Abbreviations: Abs, absolute; Avg, average; COAGN, Roche trade name for normal range control material; COAGABN, Roche trade name for abnormal range control material; GMC, Geisinger Medical Center; GWC, Geisinger Wyoming Valley.

Table 8
Monthly Sigma values for prothrombin time quality control

	RL1	RL2	RL6	RL4	RL3	RL7	RL5	H1A	H1B	H2A	H2B	H4	Mean
					COAG Normal								
Oct	—	—	7.5	8.6	9.5	7.0	8.4	7.7	8.8	6.6	5.6	—	7.7
Nov	—	10.0	12.6	10.2	8.5	8.2	7.9	8.4	5.0	7.0	7.8	7.5	8.5
Dec	—	8.4	9.9	7.2	8.0	8.3	9.8	7.3	8.4	8.1	10.3	8.2	8.5
Jan	—	9.9	9.1	11.8	13.3	10.8	14.1	11.3	9.4	10.8	11.8	8.8	11.0
Feb	10.3	13.8	10.7	10.8	12.4	11.8	10.5	9.9	13.1	12.4	12.6	8.6	11.4
Mar	10.4	10.5	10.7	9.8	9.6	12.9	13.7	11.2	12.3	9.6	12.5	12.3	11.3
Apr	9.1	8.9	9.9	7.8	10.8	9.9	9.9	10.7	11.2	10.3	11.3	11.3	10.1
May	13.6	11.8	12.0	7.3	10.0	8.5	13.7	10.2	12.3	10.3	12.3	10.3	11.0
Jun	12.4	12.4	12.4	12.4	12.4	12.4	12.4	12.4	12.4	12.4	12.4	12.4	12.4
Site Avg:	11.2	10.7	10.5	9.5	10.5	10.0	11.2	9.9	10.3	9.7	10.7	9.9	10.2

	RL1	RL2	RL6	RL4	RL3	RL7	RL5	H1A	H1B	H2A	H2B	H4	Mo Mean
					COAG Abnormal								
Oct	—	—	1.1	5.5	8.0	12.5	8.8	6.1	7.1	9.0	7.9	—	7.3
Nov	—	8.9	6.6	9.9	8.7	7.6	7.1	4.8	3.2	8.9	8.1	6.6	7.3
Dec	—	4.3	4.5	5.3	8.4	8.8	7.1	7.1	7.7	9.3	5.2	8.2	6.9
Jan	—	7.2	6.3	6.0	12.5	13.1	11.7	13.5	10.1	13.3	13.3	9.8	10.6
Feb	6.7	7.2	5.0	5.1	11.8	13.1	9.9	12.3	13.2	12.4	12.6	8.0	9.8
Mar	5.6	5.8	7.4	4.9	13.2	14	9.7	11.2	11.5	12.2	13.3	10.7	10.0
Apr	10.2	6.9	5.9	4.0	11.0	15	8.9	12.6	13.5	11.8	12.0	11.3	10.3
May	13.1	6.2	4.7	5.4	12.0	12.7	10.9	9.4	11.8	12.4	12.48	8.1	9.9
Jun	7.9	5.5	5.4	8.1	11.9	13.4	6.6	11.5	11.6	12.6	13.0	10.1	9.8
Site Average:	8.7	6.5	5.2	6.0	10.8	12.2	9.0	9.8	10.0	11.3	10.9	9.1	9.1

Clinic laboratories: RL1-7: Cold Springs, Lake Scranton, Moshannon Valley, Mount Pocono, Tunkhannock, Scenery Park, Lewistown.
Hospitals: H1: Geisinger Medical Center; H2: Geisinger Wyoming Valley; H4: Geisinger Shamokin Area Community Hospital.
Abbreviations: COAG-N, normal control material; COAG-ABN, abnormal control material.

and capacity needs of the site. Thus, the system includes XS-1000, XE-5000, XT-4000, and XN models. In 2015 the authors acquired Sysmex XN models for all of the hospital sites and began monitoring Sigma values for both XN and non-XN instruments. **Fig. 7** shows an example of the Sigma calculation trend plots and scatter plots for the Sysmex instrumentation using Sysmex level 3 QC material in the sequence XE-5000, XT-4000, and XS-1000 (left to right). The level 1 and level 2 and all 3 level XNs are on separate graphs. The analytes with calculated Sigma values are white blood cell count, platelet count, red cell count, hematocrit, and hemoglobin level. With the exception of hematocrit, all methods were consistently greater than the Sigma 4.0 threshold. These data are consistent and complementary with other recent reports on Sigma performance of Sysmex analyzers.[9]

A comprehensive discussion of actions taken for out-of-control events is beyond the scope of this report. However, it is important to note that reductions in false rejections occurred in the coagulation and hematology assays as frequently as with chemistry.

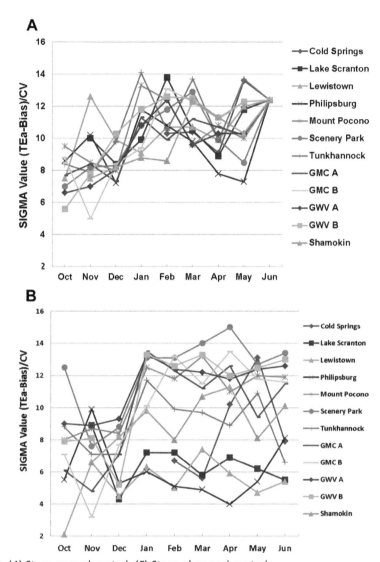

Fig. 5. (*A*) Stago normal control. (*B*) Stago abnormal control.

SUMMARY

Overall these results show the properties and value of serially measured Sigma values in specifying which methods may have ongoing QC limit adjustments made from high Sigma performance and those that require retention of the more traditional Westgard rules approach. Study of the month-to-month and year-to-year variation in Sigmas allows identification of continuously high-performing methods. It also demonstrates the value of monitoring ongoing Sigmas in managing an enterprise-wide analytical QC program that assures satisfactory performance among multiple sites in an integrated ACO (Accountable Care Organization) network. This monitoring assures providers and patients that they will receive comparable quality results independent of the site visited, an important consideration in a system that has distributive care and

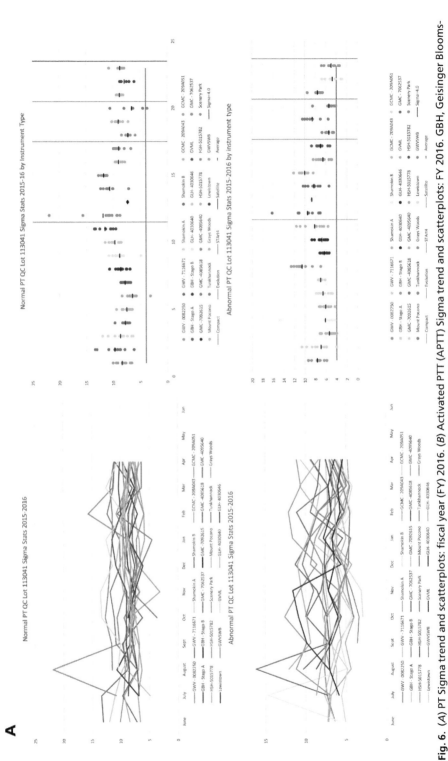

Fig. 6. (A) PT Sigma trend and scatterplots: fiscal year (FY) 2016. (B) Activated PTT (APTT) Sigma trend and scatterplots: FY 2016. GBH, Geisinger Bloomsburg Hospital; GCMC, Geisinger Community Medical Center; GHSH, Geisinger Holy Spirit Hospital; GLH, Geisinger Lewistown Hospital; GVML, Geisinger Viewmont Medical Laboratory; GWV, Geisinger Wyoming Valley; GWVSWB, Geisinger Wyoming Valley South Wilkes-Barre facility.

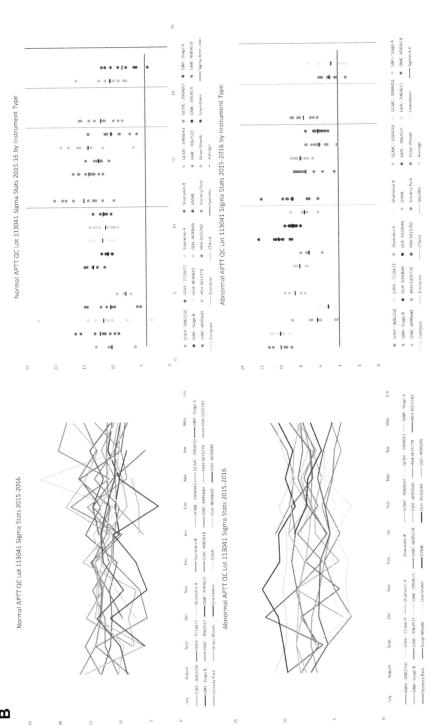

Fig. 6. (continued).

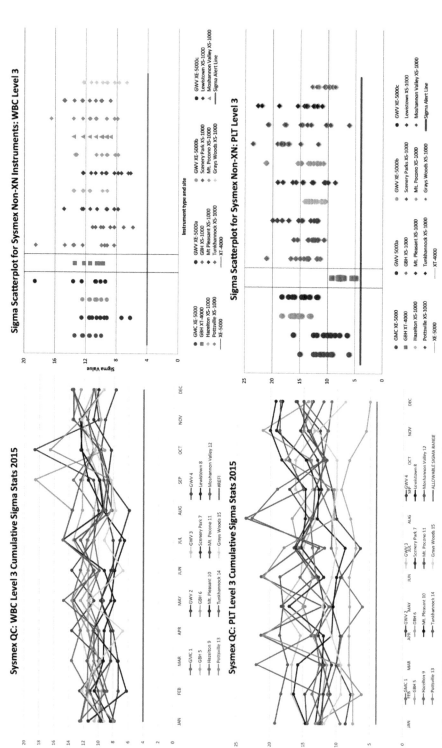

Fig. 7. Sysmex QC Sigma trend and scatterplots, non-XN: calendar year 2015. HCT, hematocrit; HGB, hemoglobin; PLT, platelet count; RBC, red blood cell; WBC, white blood cell.

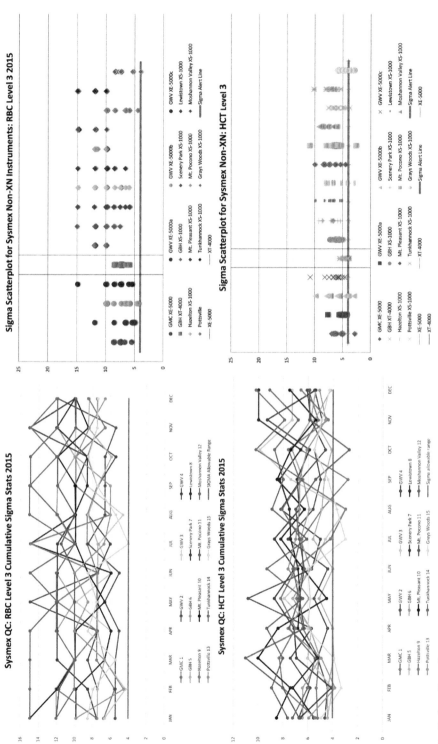

Fig. 7. (continued).

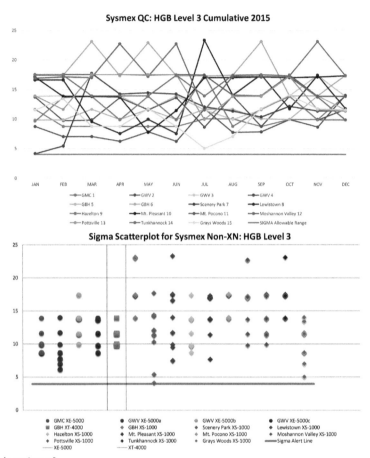

Fig. 7. (continued).

designated centers of excellence. Monitoring that demonstrates high Sigma maintenance also assures staff and regulators that the use of nontraditional QC rules is justified in an ongoing manner. Sustaining the program remains a challenge in situations of technical staff leadership turnover or acquisition of a new laboratory staff that is unfamiliar with the Sigma statistical approach to QC. The assimilation of these new sites requires a significant expenditure of effort in education and operational implementation of the program. However, once achieved, the benefits become readily apparent. The authors are currently in the process of applying the AAQC program to a new generation of laboratory instruments. Given the demonstrated stability of the Sigmas over time, they are also working to automate calculations and determine the optimal frequency of Sigma calculation and evaluation.

ACKNOWLEDGMENTS

The authors would like to thank Dr James Westgard, Sten Westgard, and Dr Conrad Schuerch for ongoing advice and encouragement. The authors would also like to thank the members of the AAQC Committee: Dr R. Patrick Dorion, Dr Elsie Yu, Dr Myra Wilkerson, Michele Adler, Janine Alexis, Ed Croall, Walter Fitt, Melissa Forsythe,

Karen Kile, Donna Kimmich, Margaret Knowles-Tuchman, Michael Lopatka, Robert Nowak, Larry Quinton, Duane Sargent, Marianna Sees, Melissa Whetstone, and Donna Young. Also, Kristie Walters, Andrea Popp, Christy Attinger and Henry Harrison provided graphics and spreadsheet assistance.

REFERENCES

1. Westgard JO. Internal quality control: planning and implementation strategies. Ann Clin Biochem 2003;40:593–611.
2. Westgard JO. Clinical quality vs. analytical performance: what are the right targets and target values? Accred Qual Assur 2004;10:10–4.
3. Westgard JO, Westgard SA. An assessment of sigma metrics for analytic quality using performance data from proficiency testing surveys and the CLIA criteria for acceptable performance. Am J Clin Pathol 2006;125:343–54.
4. Jones JB, Sargent D, Young D, et al. Integration of a multisite enterprise quality control program on a wide area network and use of sigma statistics to standardize Westgard QC rules. Clin Chem Suppl 2011;A107. Poster C40 for AACC Annual Meeting.
5. Jones JB, Young D, Smeal K, et al. Use of networked Westgard advisor quality control software and dashboards to reduce QC rejections in a regional laboratory system. Clin Chem Suppl 2012;A69. Poster B-29 for AACC Annual Meeting 2012.
6. Harrison HH, Young D, Sargent D, et al. Expansion of a multisite, advanced analytical qc program to include prothrombin time testing using sigma statistics and auto-generated peer values. Clin Chem 2013;59(Suppl 10):A147. Poster A-486 for AACC Annual Meeting 2013.
7. Plebani M, Sanzari MC, Zardo L. Quality control in coagulation testing. Semin Thromb Hemost 2008;34:642–6.
8. Geens T, Vertessen F, Malfait R, et al. Validation of the Sysmex CS5100 coagulation analyzer and comparison to the Stago STA-R analyzer for routine coagulation parameters. Int J Lab Hematol 2015;37:372–81.
9. Seo JY, Lee ST, Kim SH. Performance evaluation of the new hematology analyzer Sysmex XN series. Int J Lab Hematol 2015;37:155–64.

Moving?

Make sure your subscription moves with you!

To notify us of your new address, find your **Clinics Account Number** (located on your mailing label above your name), and contact customer service at:

Email: **journalscustomerservice-usa@elsevier.com**

800-654-2452 (subscribers in the U.S. & Canada)
314-447-8871 (subscribers outside of the U.S. & Canada)

Fax number: 314-447-8029

**Elsevier Health Sciences Division
Subscription Customer Service
3251 Riverport Lane
Maryland Heights, MO 63043**

*To ensure uninterrupted delivery of your subscription, please notify us at least 4 weeks in advance of move.

Printed and bound by CPI Group (UK) Ltd, Croydon, CR0 4YY

03/10/2024

01040391-0004